The Proceedings of the First International Food Data Base Conference held in Sydney, Australia, 22–24 September 1993.

Quality and Accessibility of Food-Related Data

Proceedings of the First International Food Data Base Conference

A satellite to the 15th International Congress of Nutrition

Edited by Heather Greenfield

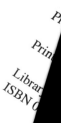

Pr
Prin
Librar
ISBN 0

Proceedings Sponsor

The publication of these Proceedings was generously assisted by the Nutrition Section, Department of Human Services and Health, Australia, in accordance with its educational role in the implementation of the national Food and Nutrition Policy.

Sponsors

The Conference was sponsored by:

Department of Industry, Trade and Commerce

AOAC INTERNATIONAL

Department of Food Science and Technology,
University of New South Wales

Food Industry Development Centre,
University of New South Wales

Eurofoods-Enfant

Australian International Development Assistance Bureau

National Food Authority

Australian Institute of Health and Welfare

McDonald's Australia Ltd

NSW Dairy Corporation

Goodman Fielder Ltd

Xyris Software (Australia) Pty Ltd

National Association of Testing Authorities

First International
Food Data Base Conference

Scientific Programme Committee

D.A.T. Southgate (UK) Chair

N-G. Asp (Sweden)

G.R. Beecher (USA)

R. Bressani (Guatemala)

R. English (Australia)

J.N. Thompson (Canada)

Aree Valyasevi (Thailand)

C.E. West (The Netherlands)

Organizing Committee

H. Greenfield

J. Barnes

B. Burlingame

K. Cashel

Contents

Preface

This Conference arose from the charge of IUNS Committee II/4 *Techniques for Measuring the Value of Foods for Man* (Chair: D.A.T. Southgate (UK)) "… to review techniques for the measurement of nutrients and other constituents in food … to improve and expand existing food composition data banks …"

The Conference was designed to recognize all aspects of food composition data production, management and use, and included papers, posters and computer demonstrations. All papers were invited in order to represent the diverse range of activities in the field. Sessions covered national and international food composition programmes, methods and conventions of nutrient analysis, quality control of food composition data and databases, a workshop on computer systems, food composition data and population studies, copyright considerations, and food industry and food safety considerations.

These Proceedings comprise the invited papers and selected posters. The authors of all but two of the invited presentations provided papers which were sent to two referees each and revised in accordance with the referees' comments prior to acceptance for publication. Posters were not refereed.

Thanks are due to the following who kindly reviewed manuscripts: K. Baghurst, P. Baghurst, D.H. Buss, K.M. Cashel, I. Coles-Rutishauser, J. Craske, J. Cunningham, J. DeVries, M. Filadelfi-Keszi, G. Greenleaf, W. Horwitz, J. Jin, M. Lawrence, S. Lee, J. Lewis, D. Mackerras, J. Klensin, R. Richards, G. Sevenhuysen, N. Slimani, D.A.T. Southgate, K.K. Stewart, A.S. Truswell, I. Unwin, J. Vanderslice, A. Walker, C.E. West and R.B.H. Wills.

Special thanks are due to Jane Barnes for assistance with editing, Sharon Debrezceni for word-processing and Michael Wyatt of Keyword Editorial Services for preparation of the camera-ready text. Krystyna McIver of AOAC INTERNATIONAL kindly provided editorial advice.

Heather Greenfield
Sydney
January 1995

National and International Food Composition Programs

The Conference was opened by Senator the Honorable Graham F. Richardson, Minister for Health. The Session was chaired by Professor A. Stewart Truswell, Boden Professor of Human Nutrition, University of Sydney, in his capacity as Vice-President of the International Union of Nutritional Sciences.

A keynote address was delivered by J. Lupien of the Food Policy and Nutrition Division, Food and Agriculture Organization, entitled *Developing Comprehensive Policies and Programs for Improved Food Supplies and Nutrition*, and this address was followed by papers by D. Slamet on *The Food Composition Program of Indonesia: Past, Present and Future* and L. Masson on *CHILEFOODS: Food Composition Activities in Chile and Latin America*, which are published on the following pages along with a print version of the poster entitled *Nutrient Composition of Wild-Gathered Foods from Mali* by M.B. Nordeide, A. Oshaug and H. Holm.

Posters displayed after Session I also were:

- *The Composition of Indian Restaurant Foods in Sydney*, Bishop, C.G., Pratap, S.W., & Arcot, J., Department of Food Science and Technology, University of New South Wales, Sydney NSW, Australia.
- *Tables of Composition of Australian Aboriginal Bush Foods*, Brand Miller, J.C., James, K.W., & Maggiore, P., Human Nutrition Unit, University of Sydney, Sydney NSW, DSTO, Scottsdale, TAS, and School of Public Health, Curtin University of Technology, Perth, WA, Australia.

- *The Food Composition Program of Nepal*, Karki, T., Central Food Research Laboratory, Kathmandu, Nepal.
- *The New Zealand Food Composition Database and Analytical Program*, Burlingame, B., Arthur, J., Cook, F., Duxfield, G., Gibson, J., Milligan, J., & Monro, J., Nutrition Programme, NZ Institute for Crop & Food Research, Palmerston North, New Zealand.
- *The UK Nutrient Databank,* Buss, D.H., Corkill, M.J., & Holland, B., MAFF, 17 Smith Square, London, and RSC, Thomas Graham House, Science Park, Milton Rd, Cambridge, UK.
- *Ingredient Composition of Australian Manufactured Foods*, Cassidy, S., Dietitians' Association of Australia, Canberra, ACT, Australia.
- *Determination of the "Pseudo-vitamins" in Dairy Products*, Indyk, H., & Woollard, D.C., Anchor Products, Waitoa, and Ministry of Agriculture and Fisheries, Auckland, New Zealand.
- *Nutrient Composition of Australian Ration Packs*, James, K.W., Hancock, A.T., Coad, R.A., Sheedy, C.J., Lichon M.J., & Walker, G.J., DSTO, Materials Research Laboratory, Scottsdale, TAS, Australia.
- *Cholecalciferol and 25-hydroxycholecalciferol Contents of Some Fish Species*, Mattila, P., & Piironen, V., Department of Applied Chemistry and Microbiology, University of Helsinki, Finland.
- *A Nutritional Survey of Sydney Bread*, Mugford, D., Griffiths, P., Walker, R., McGuirk, M., & Tomlinson, D., Bread Research Institute Inc., North Ryde, NSW, Australia.
- *Nutrient Composition of South African Beef*, Schönfeldt, H.C., Irene Animal Production Institute, Irene, South Africa.
- *The Cholesterol and Fatty Acid Composition of South African Beef Carcasses*, Schönfeldt, H.C., & Benadé, A.J.S., Irene Animal Production Institute, Irene, and Nutritional Intervention Programme, Medical Research Council, Tygerberg, South Africa.
- *Composition of South African Beef Carcasses*, Schönfeldt, H.C., Naudé, R.T., & De Bruyn, J.F., Irene Animal Production Institute, Irene, South Africa.

Developing Comprehensive Policies and Programs for Improved Food Supplies and Nutrition

John R. Lupien

Food Policy and Nutrition Division, Food and Agriculture Organization of the United Nations, Viale delle Terme di Caracalla, Rome 00100, Italy

In developing comprehensive policies and programs for improved food supplies and nutrition, governments need accurate information on food composition. The International Conference on Nutrition (ICN) 1992 emphasized food composition in its consideration of ways to improve household food security, prevent and control micronutrient deficiencies, assess, analyze and monitor nutrition situations and enhance food quality and safety. This paper summarizes the leading role FAO plays in international food and nutrient composition databases: developing global guidelines and standards; introducing food composition into countries' development activities; setting guidelines for laboratory facilities; disseminating standard techniques and references to improve analytical quality; supporting Codex Alimentarius, USDA and AOAC INTERNATIONAL; training in analytical techniques and data compilation; and documenting legal aspects of food composition. The potential role of FAO in collaboration with INFOODS and the Flair Eurofoods-Enfant Project in evaluating data quality and use; food nomenclature and foods to be included in nutrient databases; and criteria for setting food and nutrient data priorities is highlighted.

The International Conference on Nutrition (ICN) held in Rome from 5-11, 1992, encompassed nine themes, three of which are related to food composition work (1). These three themes were improving household food security, preventing and controlling specific micronutrient deficiencies and assessing, analyzing and monitoring nutrition situations. A government cannot make informed decisions regarding the food supply and meeting the food and nutritional needs of the population through an improved food supply without an understanding of the food that is eaten, particularly in the area of combating micronutrient deficiencies.

■ International Work in Food Composition

An initial step in planning food supplies is to assess the energy and nutrient situation by determining the composition of the diet. For this purpose the Food and Agriculture Organization (FAO) developed its expertise and reputation in international food composition with the development of the Food Balance Sheets. This work led to the production of regional food composition tables, the last being the Near East tables, published in by FAO in 1982 (2).

FAO is committed to maintaining its leadership role in the area of international food and nutrient composition databases. To this end a two-day meeting was held from 14-15 December 1992, hosted by FAO in Rome, with additional funding assistance from INFOODS, a UNU project, and the Flair EUROFOODS-Enfant Project (funded by the European Community). The participants at this meeting and subsequent forums welcomed FAO's renewed activity in international food composition and recognized its comparative advantage in developing worldwide guidelines and standards as well as the opportunity to introduce food composition into the overall development activities of the country.

Specifically FAO can be instrumental in setting guidelines for improving planning for laboratory facilities; improving analytical quality through the dissemination of standard techniques including inter-laboratory tests and reference materials; supporting the work of *Codex Alimentarius,* AOAC INTERNATIONAL and national laboratories involved in determining the composition of foods in identifying protocols for suitable, yet cheaper analytical techniques; supporting the education and training for composition work related to sampling, analytical techniques, and data compilation, through publications and programs at country level; providing documentation on the legal aspects of food composition data and their use in various jurisdictions which would assist the documentation required for food analysis and data quality.

A number of areas exist in international food composition work that require future input and attention. These include: evaluation of data quality and the need to relate the quality of the data to the use for which they are intended; food nomenclature and foods to be included in nutrient databases; criteria for setting food and nutrient data priorities.

As part of the follow-up activity to the ICN, FAO is initiating work at the developing country level in the areas mentioned above. In addition a joint FAO and UNU meeting in Tunis in March, 1994, has evaluated the progress in international food composition activities since the Bellagio meeting in 1983 (3) and formulated a long-term program of work suitable for attracting outside funding and participation.

Policies and Programs to Improve Nutrition

The title of this paper suggests that policies and programs in many countries are not comprehensive enough to improve nutrition. In fact better nutritional status depends on the kind of coordination across agricultural, health, educational, trade and development policies, that is rarely achieved. In part this situation occurs because the link between these policies and improved nutritional status is not clear. Of course all countries have policies that affect nutrition in some way, and the challenge is to find ways that enhance the piecemeal effects of separate initiatives into a larger sum.

There is agreement on a number of general policy orientations to improve nutritional status. For example, agricultural policies must be oriented towards rational and effective development of better food supplies, including the production, processing and effective marketing of all of the elements of an adequate and nutritionally balanced diet. Health policies must give specific attention to a wide range of preventive activities, such as immunization, vitamin and mineral supplementation of vulnerable groups such as infants and pregnant or nursing women, and effective treatment of diarrhoeal diseases. Agricultural and health policies must stress the assurance of adequate food quality and safety from the point of production, through harvesting, storage, processing/preservation and marketing. Educational policies must assure adequate basic education for all, and include appropriate elements of nutrition education for all, in elementary and secondary schools, and for use in the mass media.

International Conference on Nutrition

The extent to which these policies reinforce the separate impacts they have will determine the kind of improvement in nutritional status that may be expected. In this context it is important to discuss the International Conference on Nutrition (ICN) which was held in Rome during December 1992. Well before the Conference started, the two sponsoring agencies, the Food and Agriculture Organization (FAO) and World Health Organization (WHO), met together to decide which were the basic policy elements and activities necessary to improve nutrition for all and to define the objectives of the ICN in this regard. Needless to say, the issues were complex and expressed in many and varying views. However, after extended discussions it was clearly agreed that proper nutritional status depends on the effective preparation and implementation of a wide range of agricultural, health, educational, trade and development policies, carried out by a variety of government agencies, academia, industry and the public at large.

During the ICN, discussions were organized according to the following nine themes:

- incorporating nutritional objectives, considerations and components into development policies and programs
- improving household food security
- protecting consumers through improved food quality and safety
- promoting breast-feeding
- preventing and managing infectious diseases
- caring for the socio-economically deprived and nutritionally vulnerable
- preventing and controlling specific micronutrient deficiencies
- promoting appropriate diets and healthy lifestyles
- assessing, analyzing and monitoring nutrition situations.

These themes form the basis for vertical and potentially free-standing activities. They are in effect the essential elements of policy which must be considered, formulated and implemented in each country. A number of cross-cutting, or broad, issues discussed at the ICN provide important integration of policies and activities. These issues included education, environmentally sound and sustainable development, gender and population concerns, and resource allocation in the implementation of specific nutrition improvement activities.

In discussing these general and specific themes it became clear that implementing effective nutrition improvement activities needs to be inter-sectoral and inter-disciplinary, if sustained success is to be attained.

The Need for Food Composition Data

The fundamental importance of knowledge about the composition of food in the themes discussed at the ICN was recognized by FAO, and the Food Policy and Nutrition Division has reactivated work on food composition as one part of a number of activities initiated to follow-up on the ICN resolutions. FAO is currently committed to working with all of the agencies and professionals active in food composition in an effort to make more reliable data available worldwide.

Food composition work does not only depend on the global ICN objectives, but is in a real sense needed to support projects and interventions to improve nutrition. Information on the nutritional composition of food is essential for the provision of adequate and appropriate diets for individuals and populations. In this context food composition data are a major requirement for action in nutrition education, interventions on micro-nutrients, nutritional support for health care plans, food trade, food labeling and regulations, and the integration of nutrition concerns in agricultural policies.

Given that this variety of actions is implemented by a wide range of ministries and agencies, the uses and limitations of data on food composition need to be clear. A large number of users therefore require reliable and unambiguously labeled data and FAO can make a particular contribution in this area. In addition, the common use of data in different policy arenas will help in some ways to promote the kind of integration of action referred to earlier.

Collaboration in Food Composition

FAO published a number of international food composition tables in the 1960's and 1970's for use in regions such as Latin America, Asia, the Near East, and Africa (4, 5, 6). The work was carried out in collaboration with the US Department of Agriculture, the US Department of Health and Human Services, and the Institute of Nutrition of Central America and Panama (INCAP) in Guatemala. Following the production of these publications FAO and its Food Policy and Nutrition Division de-emphasized international activities on food composition for several years and other agencies increased their activities in this area.

Important progress in food composition has been made over the last ten years, in large part due to the International Food Data Systems Project, or INFOODS. Their publications contain the basis for world-wide standards in the development of food composition development (7, 8, 9, 10).

But perhaps an even more crucial contribution by INFOODS is the regional system of data generation and management for food composition data. Relying on a few key institutions around the world that are capable of coordinating a variety of food composition activities on a regional basis, INFOODS has greatly expanded the support for food composition work in developing countries. FAO intends to cooperate fully with INFOODS to participate in, and build on, such regional networks in future activities.

At the same time, the EUROFOODS group has achieved exemplary improvements in food composition data used in Europe as a result of improving the quality and compatability of the data from many sources, cultural environments and jurisdictions. The experience of EUROFOODS demonstrates the procedures which may be used in promoting the collaboration of countries in other regions of the world.

Particularly important are the advances of EUROFOODS in data quality related to food nomenclature and food coding systems that were developed to integrate the national food composition databases of European countries. For example, the names of foods in different European countries may be the same, but refer to products with a different formulation. Conversely, different food names may refer to the same food, but express differences in culturally determined food preparation. The achievement of the EUROFOODS group in maintaining data quality in the face of such diversity has provided those who are faced with integrating food composition databases in their own regions with important examples and lessons.

■ FAO's Strengthened Food Composition Program

The overall purpose of FAO's program in food composition is to promote the generation and dissemination of reliable food composition data that meets the needs of local users, or at least at national level. The work itself will be implemented in collaboration with other agencies, institutions and groups, according to the following program objectives:

■ to promote and expand existing activities at international, regional and national centres active in food composition work, such as data gen-

eration, data management, and the distribution of data to users

■ to publish standards on terminology required for the identification of food and nutrients, sampling procedures for food, requirements for handling food samples, analytical methodology, assessment criteria for data quality

■ to support training of staff involved with all aspects of food composition work, including the collection, preparation and analysis of samples, as well as the management of resulting data using electronic media, and utilization of reliable data in a wide range of nutrition improvement activities, projects and programs

■ to set standards for minimum laboratory environments required in developing countries to ensure acceptable data quality and comparability, and promote regional efforts for such standards

■ to provide a forum for exchange of information between professionals on new developments and solutions to common problems

■ to create a world-wide directory of sources, quality and availability of food composition data, where actual compositional data will be kept in a large number of national or regional centers

■ to monitor the regulatory and legal ownership aspects of food composition data and their use in food labeling and food standards, in order to assist the documentation required for food analysis and data quality.

In order to achieve these objectives, FAO has several ongoing activities and will start new ones. The most important of these include:

■ Support for new analytical work in developing countries in particular, where conditions for generating data are difficult. For example, assistance to the Ethiopian Nutrition Institute for laboratory upgrading, staff training and the preparation of a new food composition database is currently being organized. Such work is carried out in close collaboration with laboratories at Wageningen Agricultural University in The Netherlands.

- Formulation of criteria for the assessment of data quality and data sampling. The activity requires extensive communication with laboratories in many countries to find the optimum detail to be included. FAO is working closely with USDA where staff are producing expert systems for the evaluation of data quality.

- For a better view of the active institutions in the field, and the type of compositional data they generate and manage, FAO is collecting details for a "Directory of institutions" and a "Directory of databases". Again, the FAO effort in this area complements the work organized by others and close collaboration with INFOODS and EUROFOODS is maintained.

- FAO recognizes that a major revision is needed for the food composition data used to calculate the nutrient content of national food supplies for each of the countries for which FAO Food Balance Sheets are published. In cooperation with the FAO Statistics Division, which publishes the Food Balance Sheet databases, the Food Policy and Nutrition Division is helping with a major update of the system and data values. The work will give us new and more reliable estimates of the nutrient supply in the near future.

- The FAO Food Policy and Nutrition Division actively supports training for food composition related activities, such as learning new analytical techniques or modifications of techniques for different product groups, as well as learning computer based systems for the management and storage of compositional data. For example, FAO support for training workshops at the Wageningen, Agricultural University, where participants from developing countries have the opportunity to increase their skills in analysis. The Di-

vision expects that more training opportunities will become part of the program of work.

- Lastly, FAO and the UNU organized a meeting to discuss the progress of worldwide food composition activities over the last ten years and identify a program of work for the years to come. The meeting held in Tunis at the end of March 1994 is seen as the first major update on activities since the 1983 meeting on food composition in Bellagio (3). The Tunis meeting provided an opportunity to share issues related to food composition work in many countries and identify ways to support the activities. Participants considered criteria that are appropriate for selecting and managing food composition data (11). With the recent changes in analytical techniques, knowledge of the sources of error in nutrient values, and electronic means for sharing data, the meeting came at an appropriate time to take stock and plan innovations for the next decade.

■ Changes in Food Composition Data

It is interesting to note that over time food composition data have changed not only because of improved analytical techniques and better knowledge of representative sampling, but also because of real changes in the formulation of foods. For example, the plethora of low fat / low energy products with sensory characteristics of full fat formulations, have the potential to lower the fat intakes of people in many developed countries. Or, the dwindling choice in variety of potatoes in several developing countries since the last century to leave only a few commonly used ones, which reduces the variability in nutrient intake from potatoes and can reduce the food security for several population groups.

We know some of the factors that determined these changes, as well as others. These factors demonstrate the interrelationships between the agriculture, health, education and trade that can potentially affect nutritional status. The positive effects should be the objectives of interventions at any level of government or international cooperation. The detrimental effects of such changes need to be avoided or minimized, especially for disadvantaged groups.

■ Conclusion

The integrated nature of actions to improve nutrition shows the wide range of coordinated work which needs to be done and the importance of food composition activities to overall efforts. Nutrition problems cannot be resolved by nutritionists alone, or by the use of one policy strategy or one program approach. Each initiative intended to improve nutrition needs to be based on the theory and experience appropriate to it, and implemented with explicit expectations for nutritional improvement. The development of reliable, internationally comparable food composition data is one crucial element in achieving this integration and FAO is fully committed to that goal.

■ References

(1) FAO & WHO (1992) *Final Report of the International Conference on Nutrition*, Rome

(2) FAO (1982) *Food Composition Tables for the Near East*, Rome

(3) Rand, W., & Young, V. (1983) *Food Nutr. Bull.* **5**, 15-76

(4) INCAP-ICNND (1961) *Food Composition Table for Use in Latin America*, Interdepartmental Committee on Nutrition for National Defense, Washington, & Institute of Nutrition of Central America and Panama, Guatemala

(5) FAO (1970) *Food Composition Tables for Use in Africa*, Rome

(6) FAO (1972) *Food Composition Table for Use in East Asia*, Rome

(7) Klensin, J.C., Feskanich, D., Lin, V., Truswell, A.S., & Southgate, D.A.T. (1989) *Identification of Food Components for INFOODS Data Interchange*, UNU Press, Tokyo

(8) Rand, W.M., Pennington, J.A.T., Murphy, S.P., & Klensin, J.C. (1992) *Compiling Data for Food Composition Data Bases*, UNU Press, Tokyo

(9) Klensin, J.C. (1992) *INFOODS Food Composition Data Interchange Handbook*, UNU Press, Tokyo

(10) Greenfield, H., & Southgate, D.A.T. (1992) *Food Composition Data. Production, Management and Use*, Elsevier Applied Science, London

(11) FAO & UNU (1994) *Report of Discussions on Food Composition for Developing Countries* (in press)

The Food Composition Program of Indonesia: Past, Present and Future

Dewi S. Slamet

Nutrition Research and Development Center, Bogor, Indonesia

Indonesia is a country of diverse geography, culture and dietary patterns. The national food and nutrition policy aims to achieve food self-sufficiency, and diversification of food supplies and food consumption. For this reason the need for complete, accurate and up-to-date food composition tables has been recognized. This paper reports the progress towards this goal.

Indonesia is an archipelago of some 13,000 islands with an aggregate land area of 1,900,000 km² (Figure 1). The population of Indonesia is about 180 million, of which about 80 per cent live in rural areas. Thousands of kinds of foods are available in Indonesia. The staple foods are rice, maize, sago, cassava and sweet potato, and the diet can be classified according to three distinct consumption patterns, namely (a) rice pattern (West Java, Sumatra, Kalimantan); (b) rice and maize pattern (Central and East Java, Sulawesi, Bali, Nusa Tenggara Islands, with cassava being consumed especially by the low income groups in all these regions); (c) sago and sweet potato pattern in Maluku and Irian Jaya (1,2).

The Food and Nutrition Policy of the Fifth Five Year Nutritional Development Plan (1989–1994) is aimed towards achieving food self-sufficiency and the diversification of the food supply and consumption, i.e. away from total reliance on rice. A recommendation arising from the Fourth National Workshop on

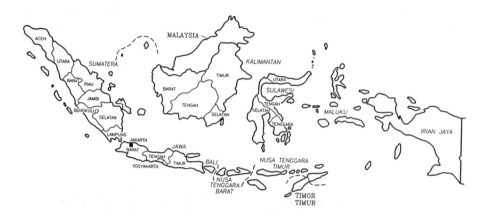

Figure 1. Map of Indonesia

Nutrition in Jakarta, June 1988, was made to assist this aim. This recommendation embraced the need to improve and develop information available to nutritionists including food composition tables, so that nutrition education directed towards broadening food choice could be carried out. Thus Indonesia fully recognized the need for complete, accurate and up-to-date food composition data as an important tool in developing the entire range of food and nutrition research and activities in the country.

■ Historical Background of Food Composition Tables in Indonesia

The first food composition tables (FCT), in Indonesia were produced by the Institute of Volksvoedings (1930-1940), during the Dutch occupation, from the data available at that time. In the period between the liberation of Indonesia in 1945 up to 1967, the name of FCT of Indonesia changed several times. Since 1967 the FCT of Indonesia were called *Daftar Komposisi Banan Makanan (DKBM)*, compiled by the Directorate of Nutrition Department of Health and published by Bhratara Jakarta (3rd printing, 1981). Most of the analytical data were generated by the Nutrition Institute since 1950 and some were taken from other international FCT. The tables contained 410 food items of which 283 were raw foods.

From 1970 till the present time the Nutrition Research and Development Centre (NRDC), Department of Health, Bogor, has been the only institution in Indonesia conducting the analyses of the nutrient composition of foods, with the specific objective of producing the national Indonesian FCT. Analytical data for 483 food items, raw, processed and prepared, obtained from various regions of Indonesia, have been produced for several nutrients: moisture, protein, total fat, carbohydrate (by difference), calcium, phosphorus, iron, vitamin A, carotenes, thiamin, ascorbic acid and total energy. The 483 food items included 10 per cent snacks, 5 per cent fermented foods, and 1 per cent dried, salted fish. Only 116 food items were analyzed for amino acids and niacin (3, 4).

∎ Recent Activities in Generation and Compilation of Indonesian Food Composition Data

Food analyses are also carried out at the following institutions such as the Indonesian Institute of Science, the National Institute for Chemistry, the Department of Agriculture, the Department of Trade, Department of Industry, the Atomic Energy Agency and private laboratories (e.g. food industry). The analyses carried out in these laboratories are limited by their functions and their facilities. In many cases the analytical data produced cannot be used for food composition tables since the data cannot easily be related to the food as consumed.

To generate and compile the food composition data to produce Indonesian FCT, a meeting between all interested parties was needed. Therefore in 1984, to tackle the problem of food composition data, a meeting was organized by the NRDC in Bogor, involving all the various government institutions which had a special interest in food composition data. The meeting was attended by about 19 representatives from 12 institutions. The meeting agreed that: the available DKBM should be revised to fulfil the increasing needs related to the Nutrition Program; the name of the DKBM should be changed to *Komposisi Zat Gizi Pangan Indonesia* (KZGPI); and the tables should

contain nutrients such as proximate constituents, minerals and vitamins, analyzed per 100 g edible portion. Priority should be given to those foods most commonly consumed by the people. These data would be most needed for the Food and Nutrition Program (5).

Similar meetings were organized also by the Research and Development Centre for Applied Chemistry (LIPI) in 1986 in Bandung, to review the existing problems which included updating the existing food composition data, development of food composition data systems, quality assurance programs for food analyses and a food composition network (6).

Also of importance was a workshop held under the auspices of the Association of South East Asian Nations (ASEAN) Sub-committee on Protein and Food Habits Research and Development in Jakarta, 20–23 October, 1986, and attended by representatives from Indonesia, Thailand, Malaysia and the Philippines. This technical workshop on food composition data was an initial activity towards the development of the ASEAN Food Data Network (7). The workshop was an important step towards a united effort to systematize, standardize and update the generation and compilation of food composition data in the ASEAN countries and to facilitate the interchange and use of the data throughout the region. Special objectives were adopted such as to exchange and share information on current trends in food composition data generation and compilation, and to develop a plan to standardize sampling, methods of analyses and compilation of food composition data in the ASEAN countries.

Further regional progress was made at the next ASEAN workshop on food data systems held in Bangkok, 25-27 October 1989, funded by Japan. The Indonesian representative reported the current activities of the food composition program in Indonesia (8). These activities continued under national guidance, the most recent being a small workshop on nutritive composition of foods conducted by the Nutrition Research and Development Centre at Bogor, March 22-24, 1990 (9).

■ Current Status

A collaborative food composition program has recently been carried out between the NRDC and the Directorate of Nutrition. The data obtained were compiled together with the food analytical work previously done by NRDC from 1970 to 1989 and published in journals (10-17). This new set of *KZGPI* was published in 1990 by the Directorate of Nutrition and NRDC (18). These tables contain nutrients for raw, processed, traditional and fast foods. The foods were analyzed for proximate composition, minerals and vitamins. The table is divided according to food groups: Table A, the nutritional composition of cereals, tubers, nuts, legumes, vegetables, fruits, eggs, fish and miscellaneous (total of 281 raw food items); Table B, the nutrient composition of processed and fast foods, (total of 153 food items); Table C, riboflavin and niacin content of foods (total of 142 food items); Tables D and E, essential and non-essential amino acids of 71 food items (18).

Advice on compiling FCT, preparing a manual of food composition analyses, and equipping the laboratory for future work was provided by Associate Professor Heather Greenfield, from Australia, who was invited by the National Institute for Health Research and Development as a consultant. The revised and expanded manual was published in 1990 by the Directorate of Nutrition and NRDC (19), and includes information on food sampling, sections on direct analysis of sugars, starch, total dietary fibre, fatty acids and cholesterol, as well as a chapter on quality assurance.

Presently, there are three FCTs available in Indonesia: *DKBM* (20); *KZGPI* (18); and *DABM*. The *DABM* (*Daftar Analisa Bahan Makanan*) has been published by the Medical Faculty of the University of Indonesia, Jakarta and is comprised of data compiled mainly from international FCT (21).

■ Future Program

Indonesia has recognized that the past and present available data of food composition are inadequate both in terms of food items and nutrients and other food constituents. Furthermore in the last decade, Indonesia has grown rapidly in the realm of research and technology, with particular emphasis in the field of food technology, resulting in a rapid development of the local food industry. These food manufacturers produce processed foods, fast foods, and new food formulas. The development of new techniques in the production and processing of foods and the availability of a demand for new food products have created dramatic changes in the food consumption pattern of the population, particularly in urban areas. These situations may have a negative or positive effect on the nutritional status of the Indonesian people.

Because of the need to provide family income, men and women work long hours and may not have enough time to prepare food at home. Most employed men and women have their meals outside of the home, and the quality of food consumed depends on the environment and the capacity to buy food. Nutritional information about pre-prepared and street foods is in great demand.

According to the Department of Health, Indonesia currently still has four main nutritional problems, i.e. vitamin A deficiency, protein energy malnutrition, iron deficiency and iodine deficiency. These are still prevalent in the poorer areas of eastern Indonesia which require more urgent attention. At the same time as changes in environmental and economic conditions occur, other nutritional problems are also arising in Indonesia such as degenerative disease (coronary heart disease, diabetes, hypertension and cancer), possibly related to the dietary changes caused by alterations in food habits. Processed foods might be higher in animal fats, cholesterol, sugars, salt, and food contaminants (including potentially carcinogenic substances) than traditional foods. Knowledge of the nutrient composition of foods forms the backbone of clinical therapeutic diets. These are important in the management of diseases such as hypertension, heart disease and diabetes. Without knowledge of nutrient composition data dietitians and nutritionists in government health agencies would be unable to assess the adequacy of patients' diets and the nutrient intake of the people. The FCT would be used to calculate the nutrients of a typical daily intake, and based on these calculations nutrient intakes could be compared to the Recommended Dietary Intakes (RDI). If there appears to be a tendency of low or excessively high intake of any nutrient, advice and diet plans could be supplied by the dietitian or the nutritionist.

A new project of the Nutrition Research and Development Centre will analyze the macro-nutrients, micro-nutrients and fatty acids of various food items (especially traditional foods, fast foods and foods from marine resources) in collaboration with other research institutions. This project will produce new information on Indonesian foods, e.g. sugars, dietary fiber and ω-3 and ω-6 fatty acids. The project will require additional equipment (such as LC and GLC) and more trained food analysts, as well as a high degree of collaboration between laboratories.

In the future, as recommended at the 5th National Nutrition Conference held in Jakarta, April 20-22, 1993, the government has decided that Indonesia should possess an up-to-date Indonesian national food composition table incorporating all the latest data. In the last decade there has been increasing interest in food composition data in relation to diets, food habits and degenerative diseases. The next FCT will be critical to the success of projects in these areas as well as other aspects of the Food and Nutrition Program.

∎ References

(1) Karyadi, D., & Hermana (1985) in *Proceedings of the First Asian Foods Conference*, Bangkok, pp.56-58

(2) Lie, G.H., Hermana, Suwardi, & Ismyati, S. (1978) *Proceedings of First ASEAN Seminar - Workshop on Food Habits*, Manila, pp.34-39

(3) Greenfield, H. (1991) *Study of Nutritive Composition of Foods in Indonesia*, World Health Organization SEARO, New Delhi

(4) Slamet, D.S., & Tarwotjo (1980) *Penelitian Gizi dan Makanan* **4**, 21-23

(5) *Workshop on Food Composition Data* (1984) Bogor

(6) Slamet, D.S. (1986) in *Workshop on Food Composition Data,* Bandung

(7) *Workshop for the ASEAN Food Composition Table,* (1986) Jakarta

(8) Sumardi (1989) in *Proceedings of the ASEAN Workshop on Food Data Systems*, Bangkok, pp.104-108

(9) Slamet, D.S. (1990) in *Workshop of Indonesian Food Composition Tables*, Bogor

(10) Slamet, D.S., & Purawisastra (1979) in *Proceedings of Food Technology Meeting*, Jakarta, pp.158-175

(11) Slamet, D.S., & Komari (1985) *Media Teknologi Pangan* **1**, 56-60

(12) Slamet, D.S., & Komari (1986) *Penelitian Gizi dan Makanan* **9**, 63-76

(13) Slamet, D.S., & Komari (1986) *Penelitian Gizi dan Makanan* **9**, 77-84

(14) Slamet, D.S., & Ubaidillah (1987) *Penelitian Gizi dan Makanan* **10**, 77-81

(15) Slamet, D.S., & Ubaidillah (1988) *Penelitian Gizi dan Makanan* **11**, 59-73

(16) Slamet, D.S., Komari, & Ubaidillah (1988) *Penelitian Gizi dan Makanan* **12**, 58-71

(17) *Study on Nutritive Composition of Foods* (1990) Directorate of Nutrition and Nutrition Research and Development Center, Bogor

(18) Mahmud, M.K., Slamet, D.S., Apryantono, R.R., & Hermana (1990) *The Indonesian Food Composition Table,* Directorate of Nutrition and Nutrition Research and Development Center, Bogor

(19 Slamet, D.S., Mahmud, M.K., Muhilal, Fardiaz, P., & Sumarmata, J.P. (1990) *Manual of Food Analysis,* Directorate of Nutrition and Nutrition Research and Development Center, Bogor

(20) Directorate of Nutrition, Department of Health (1987) *Food Composition Table,* Bhratara Karya Aksra, Jakarta

(21) Oei, K.N. (1992) *Nutrient Analysis Tables for Food,* University of Indonesia, Jakarta

CHILEFOODS: Food Composition Activities in Chile and Latin America

Lilia Masson

University of Chile, Department of Food Science and Chemical Technology, Casilla 233, Santiago 1, Chile

This paper describes the history and coverage of the food composition tables of Chile. The computerization of the most recent tables is discussed, together with the development of software packages to access and use the database. The links with food composition activities in other Latin American countries, via the LATINFOODS network, are also covered.

C hile is a modern country situated in the South West extreme of South America. It can be considered the longest country in the world with more than 4,000 km of Pacific Ocean coastline. It is narrow with a mean width of about 180 km. The total area is estimated as 1,992,000 km^2; 740,000 km^2 represents the continental area plus different islands including Easter Island while 1,250,000 km^2 corresponds to the Antarctic territory (Figure 1).

The total population is about 13 million, most of whom are concentrated in the central zone of the country. The Metropolitan Region, where the capital Santiago is located, has about 5 million residents, representing about 40 per cent of the total population.

Chile is mainly an urban country, with about 87 per cent of the total population living in cities and the remaining 13 per cent living in rural areas. Literacy levels are high at 92 per cent. The Chilean population is a mixture of people from Spain and other European countries to-

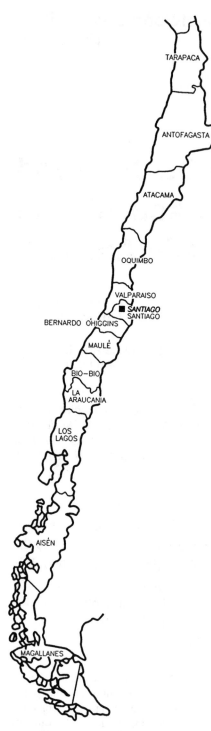

Figure 1. Chile regions

gether with people of indigenous ancestry. The latter are mainly in the Araucania Region (about 200,000 Araucanos or Mapuches) and the First Region close to the border with Bolivia and Perú (Aymará natives), while the inhabitants of Easter Island are mainly Polynesian.

In South America the countries of Chile, Argentina and Uruguay have a mainly European ethnic influence, while in the other Latin American countries, a high predominance of people of indigenous or other ethnic origins is found.

Latin America has supplied many of its different native foods to the rest of the world. The 18 native foods from Latin America which have found their way around the world are: maize, tomatoes, aji or chilli, palta or avocado, beans, potatoes which are from Perú and Chile, lupin, quinoa, tapioca, yuca, pineapple, cocoa, banana, coconut, lucuma, chirimoya, papaya (the last three from Ecuador, Perú and Chile) and strawberries from Chile. All of these foods are still very important in the Latin American diet and are an integral part of the Chilean diet, with the exception of yuca and tapioca which are confined to the Amazonian Region. In general the Chilean diet is homogeneous throughout the country, with typical meals being prepared from maize, beans, potatoes, tomatoes and chilli.

The main cereal in the Chilean diet is wheat, with a high consumption of different kinds of bread, pasta and noodles. Beef, poultry, pork, fish and shellfish, eggs, and milk and derivatives are the most important sources of dietary protein. Raw and boiled vegetables are always present in the Chilean diet as are fresh fruits, both groups being good sources of vitamins and minerals. For more than 30 years, wheat flour has been enriched by law with thiamin, riboflavin, niacin and iron. Long-standing government policies have been in force in Chile to promote good nutrition for infants, pre-schoolers and school children. Different programs to cover the main nutritional requirements of these groups have been established and thanks to these actions, which have been maintained for many years, it has been possible to reduce levels of infant malnutrition in the country to low levels of prevalence at about 5-6 per cent. The situation is not as favorable in other Latin America countries, which still seek adequate solutions for this problem.

In the Chilean food composition database system the description of the foods and meals has received considerable attention, including the main ingredients used, and the English language name. This helps the understanding of these local preparations for other users in Latin America or elsewhere. Of course, in other Latin countries there are many different meals based on their native foods that will be included in their own food databases.

■ Chilean Food Composition Activities

Activities in the field of food composition have been maintained in Chile for over 30 years, initiated by Dr Hermann Schmidt-Hebbel and continued by the group of food chemists belonging to the Department of Food Science and Chemical Technology at the University of Chile. This permanent work has permitted the publication of eight editions of the Chilean food composition tables (1). The most recent edition was published in 1990 (2), listing more than 400 different food items, including data for the proximate analysis, energy content, and major minerals and vitamins. Supplementary tables are included for the various fractions of dietary fiber in legumes and cereals; retinol and cholesterol in different foods; fluoride in some beverages, seafoods and fruits; some trace minerals in vegetables; and amino acids. Other complementary

tables are also included, e.g. energy conversion factors; essential amino acids in different foods compared with the provisional amino acid combination; servings weights and their equivalence in grams or millilitres; and the US Recommended Dietary Allowances (3)

These different published editions of the tables have permitted Chilean professionals not only in the health field, from government and private agencies, but also in the food technology and education areas, to obtain current comprehensive national information about the nutritive value of the main foods normally included in the Chilean diet.

The different food items were organized in 15 groups:

- milk and its derivatives
- avian and wild animals
- fish and shellfish (53 different fish and shellfish species, including low fat fish with less 1 per cent fat, e.g., golden congrio (*Genypterus blacodes*), hake or merluza (*Merluccius gayi*), corvina (*Micropogon furnieri*); semi-fat fish with about 3 per cent fat, e.g., albacora (*Xiphias gladius*), pejerrey (*Odeteshes regia*), reineta (*Lepidotus australis*); and fatty fish, e.g.., mero (*Dissosticuus eligenoides*) with 20 per cent fat, cojinoba (*Seriolella caerulea*) 13 per cent fat; Spanish sardine (*Sardinops sagax*) 10 per cent fat
- shell fish, mainly natives, e.g., piure, (*Pyura chilensis*), macha (*Mesodesma donacium*), loco (*Concholepa concholepas*), sea urchin gonads (*Lexoxhinus albus*)
- fats and oils
- cereals and derivatives (including quinoa (*Quenopodium quinoa*) a native with a higher protein content at 13 per cent than wheat, maize or rice; together with 17 different varieties of bread, some flours, pasta and spaghetti and ten varieties of cookies
- legumes, including beans, peas, lentils, and three varieties of lupin seeds (*Lupinus albus*)

- vegetables, including native seaweeds and mushrooms
- fruits, including close to 50 different species, produced for local consumption and export, comprising introduced species, e.g., kiwi fruit (*Actinia chinensis*); native or characteristic fruits, e.g., chirimoya (*Annona cherimolia*), lucuma (*Lucuma abovata*), sweet pepino (*Solanum muricatum*), and Chilean papaya (*Carica papaya*); and, wild fruits and seeds e.g., rosa mosqueta (*Rosa moschata mill*), arrayan (*Mireengenella apiculata*), maqui (*Aristotelia chilensis*), murtilla (*Ungi molina*), Chilean hazelnut (*Guevuina avellana*), and piñon (*Araucaria imbricata*)
- sugar and derivatives including fruit jams, honeys, instant desserts, juices, chocolates, cakes, baked specialities, jellies
- beverages comprising non-alcoholic, e.g., carbonated beverages and natural fruit juices, and alcoholic beverages, e.g., different varieties of white and red wine and beers
- miscellaneous, e.g., salad dressings and sauces, spices, different ready-to-eat meals, and snacks
- special dietary foods, e.g., infant formulas, breakfast cereals, baby foods
- others, e.g. yeast, seasoning tablets.

Another activity in the field of food composition has been the production of a publication in Spanish entitled *Fats and Oils Habitually and Potentially Consumed in Chile: Fatty Acid Composition* (7). This issue contains data obtained by the Food Chemistry Laboratory, University of Chile, for the main fatty acids present in the different fats and oils. General information about saturated, monounsaturated and polyunsaturated fatty acids is given. The publication also includes explanations about structure; physiological roles; families derived from essential linoleic and linolenic acids; and their requirements. The recommended dietary relationship between the three groups of fatty acids is also dis-

cussed as well as the potentially adverse effects that could be produced by excessive consumption of polyunsaturated fatty acids, and additional recommendations for vitamin E intake according to the amount of polyunsaturated fatty acids (PUFA) in the diet.

Five groups of different fats and oil are discussed in relation to the main fatty acids present in their structure. They are summarized in five tables, according to the following distribution: Table I, Vegetable fats and oil with less 40 per cent linoleic acid; Table II, Vegetable oils with more than 40 per cent linoleic acid; Table III, Fats of animal origin; Table IV, Fats and oils of marine origin; Table V, Hydrogenated fats and oils.

In total 62 different fats and oils with their respective fatty acid compositions are tabulated. The fatty acid composition of the fat extracted from different native seeds, is also included, e.g., Chilean hazelnut or avellana (*Guevuina avellana*), mayu (*Soffora macrocarpa*), Rosa mosqueta (*Rosa moschata mill*), quinoa (*Quenopodium quinoa*), pelu (*Sophora tetraptera sensu R*), tamarugo (*Prosopis tamarugo phil*), maracuya (*Passiflora edulis*), cardo (*Cynara cardunculus*), and the fruit of the Chilean avocado (*Persea gratissima*). In general, the linoleic acid content is high and special mention should be made of *Rosa mosqueta* seed oil which has about 43 per cent linoleic acid and 35 per cent linolenic acid.

Among the ω-3 fatty acids present in different seafoods of Chilean origin, eicosapentaenoic acid C20:5-ω-3 (EPA) and docosahexaenoic acid C22:6-ω-3 (DHA) are the most important. For example, in jurel (*Trachurus murphyi*) DHA is about 25 per cent of the total fatty acid methyl esters and EPA about 10 per cent, while piure (*Pyura chilensis*) has EPA present at a higher percentage compared with DHA.

This kind of work has continued and in recent years new items of vegetable, animal and marine origin have been studied, which will be incorporated in forthcoming editions of this publication and in the database system.

■ Food Composition Data Network in Latin America

Due to its strong national food composition program, Chile was invited to participate in the LATINFOODS organization (8,9), whose second meeting was held in Santiago in 1988 with the participation of many Latin countries.

The main recommendation from this meeting was that each country should start with the design of a local database system. In the meantime it was decided to organize CHILEFOODS as a branch of LATINFOODS and different groups of Chilean experts in food chemistry and nutrition, mainly from universities, government agencies and scientific societies were invited to participate. The group started to create a computer system able to support efficient handling of information about the composition of food produced in Chile.

In order to fulfil these objectives, suggestions from LATINFOODS were considered (10). Composition tables from other countries and the Eurocode 2 system from Eurofoods-Enfant for food classification were reviewed. In addition through a series of CHILEFOODS meetings, the different groups of Chilean experts in the field of food composition contributed their opinions and suggestions for improving the project. To design the system it was necessary to identify the output and input requirements, and then the archival and procedural specifications were identified.

First, the number of nutrients that should be included in the system was decided. A total of 171 nutrients was selected, then coded and classified into nine groups: proximate analysis, amino acids, vitamins, minerals, fatty acids, sterols, carbohydrates, dietary fiber and special constituents. A procedure for food classi-

fication and coding was also studied, and 14 groups were designated:

01	Milk and milk products
02	Eggs and derivatives
03	Meats and derivatives
04	Avian, wild animals and derivatives
05	Finfish and shellfish products
06	Fats, oils and derivatives
07	Cereals and derivatives
08	Legumes, seeds, oily fruits and derivatives
09	Vegetables, seaweeds and derivatives
10	Fruits and derivatives
11	Sugar products
12	Beverages
13	Miscellaneous, soups, sauces and derivatives
14	Special dietary foods.

A range of parameters to identify the different foods was also considered. Other variables were: identification of the samples, the analytical procedures employed and the source of information. A short code of eight digits was chosen, two digits to indicate the food group, two digits for the sub-group and the other four digits to identify the food.

In order to individualize a specific food, four parameters were considered: common name, synonyms, scientific name and English language name; weight and type of individual serving were also considered.

Printed forms were developed to facilitate one of the main tasks of LATINFOODS and CHILEFOODS, the compilation of data about food composition. These forms are being distributed among information generators and compilers. A total of 14 tables will gather all the necessary information. Along with the forms, a user handbook was produced with instructions for their correct use.

The program was created in CLIPPER (11), a language for handling databases and screens for program display. To run this program it is possible to use any computer compatible with PC DOS or MS DOS in 3.3 version or later. This program improves the information processing function that CHILEFOODS encourages. Additionally, it is able to develop input modifications, elimination operations, interactive consultations, nutrients for which information is compiled, information sources, analytical methods. Since the system has the facility to generate reports, it permits the distribution of information, another objective of LATINFOODS and CHILEFOODS.

The other project was to design a computing system to determine energy and nutritional requirements, and to assess nutrient contributions and quality of the diet of an individual.

We started with a comparative analysis of the different methods for dietary intake estimation, with the purpose of selecting the most adequate method for a computing system that could evaluate the diet quality of an individual; the dietary recall and the dietary record were the methods selected for the system.

For the estimation of dietary intake, the required energy and nutritional composition of the foods was supplied by the computerized Chilean food composition table (2), together with the Latin American and international dietary recommendations (12, 13).

The activities to design the system began with the identification of the required outputs, then the input requirements were studied, and finally the specifications for files and procedures were identified.

The program was created in dBASE III Plus, a package for handling databases that does not present learning difficulties. To run this program it is possible to use any computer compatible with PC-DOS or MS-DOS in 3.3 version or later.

The program was called PROARCAN, since the evaluation of dietary quality is based on a comparison between the individual's nutritional requirements and the actual nutrient intake. PROARCAN also adjusts the nutritional requirements for age, sex etc., and also computes

the nutritional contribution of a specific diet, or a particular food.

Once established both the CHILEFOODS and PROARCAN programs were tested to validate their performance.

The CHILEFOODS and PROARCAN programs (14,15) now constitute an important part of the Chemical Information Center (CIQ) at the Faculty of Chemical and Pharmaceutical Sciences at the University of Chile. This offers a fast and up-to-date information service to users in the food field and other areas of chemistry.

Other Latin American countries have carried out different actions in the field of food composition, many publishing their own national tables. When their tables are computerized, it should be possible in the future to establish an international data network around Latin America connected by the LATINFOODS organization.

■ References

(1) Schmidt-Hebbel, H., Pennacchiotti, I., Masson, L., et al. (1961-85) *Table of Composition of Chilean Foods,* 1st Ed. - 7th Ed., University of Chile, Santiago

(2) Schmidt-Hebbel, H., Pennacchiotti, I., Masson, L., et al. (1990) *Table of Composition of Chilean Foods,* 8th Ed., Cramer SACI, Santiago

(3) National Research Council (1989) *Recommended Dietary Allowances,* 10th Ed., National Academy of Sciences, Washington DC

(4) Pak, N., Ayala, C., Araya, H., Pennacchiotti, M., & Vera, G. (1989) *Arch. Lat. Nutr.* **60**, 116-125

(5) US Department of Agriculture (1976–) *Composition of Foods: Raw, Processed Prepared,* Agric. Handbook No.8 series, USDA, Washington, DC

(6) Masson, L., Mella, M.A., & Cagalj, A. (1990) *Rev. Chil. Nutr.* **18**, 257-265

(7) Masson, L., & Mella, M.A.(1985). *Fats and Oils Habitually and Po-*

tentially Consumed in Chile, Fatty Acid Composition, University of Chile, Santiago

(8)   Masson, L., Araya, H., & Mella, M.A. (1987) *Arch. Lat. Nutr.* **37**, 683-690

(9)   Bressani, R. (1987a) *Arch. Lat. Nutr.* **37**, 591-602

(10) Bressani, R. (1987b) *Arch. Lat. Nutr.* **37**, 793-802

(11) Straley, S.J. (1988) *Programming in Clipper: the Definitive Guide to the Clipper dBASE Compiler,* 2nd Ed., Addison-Wesley Publishing Co. Inc., Reading MA

(12) Latin American Society of Nutrition (1988) *Arch. Lat. Nutr.* **38**, 383

(13) FAO/WHO/UNU (1985) *Energy and Protein Needs,* Report of an Expert and Consultative Meeting, Technical Report No. 724, WHO, Geneva

(14) Masson, L., Elías, P., & Chavez, H. (1990) *Computing System for Chemical Food Composition Data Management,* Department of Food Science and Chemical Technology, University of Chile, Santiago

(15) Masson, L., Rousseau, I., Elías, P., & Chavez, H. (1992) *Computing System to Determine Caloric and Nutritional Requirements, Dietary Contribution and Diet Quality of an Individual,* Department of Food Science and Chemical Technology, University of Chile, Santiago

Nutrient Composition of Wild-Gathered Foods from Mali

Marit Beseth Nordeide, Arne Oshaug, Halvor Holm

Nordic School of Nutrition, University of Oslo, PO Box 1046, 0316 Oslo, Norway

The aim of this collaborative project between Mali and Norway is to initiate food analysis which will lead to a food composition table in Mali. The food composition table presently used is the FAO food composition table for Africa which does not have data from Mali. The first foods selected for analysis were important staples used by nomads. Laboratories in Norway and in Sweden have been involved in both chemical and biological analysis. The analytical results are used to discuss improvement of food quality/utilization by combined use of locally-produced and gathered foods in Gourma.

■ Methods

Foods. Wild-gathered *Cenchrus biflorus* (grains), *Panicum laetum* (grains) and *Maerua crassifolia* (leaves) were collected in the dry season, May 1992. The foods were studied as raw material and as processed. The grains of *Cenchrus biflorus* and *Panicum laetum* were boiled in water for 40 minutes. Leaves from *Maerua crassifolia* were washed and boiled with water for 6 hours, with water replaced every hour.

Chemical Analysis. Dry matter, crude protein (N 6.25), ash, gross energy, lipids, 12 minerals and amino acid patterns were determined.

Biological Analysis. The protein digestibility, biological value and net protein utilization of *Cenchrus biflorus*, *Panicum laetum* and *Maerua crassifolia*

Table I. Composition of wild-gathered foods from Gourma (per 100 g edible portion)

Food	Dry matter	Protein	Fat	Energy	Ash	K	Ca	Fe	Zn
Name	g	g	g	kJ	g	mg	mg	mg	mg
Cenchrus biflorus whole grains (n=7)	96.9	22.1	7.3	1880	6.4	382	43	234	6.5
Panicum laetum whole grains (n=4)	96.7	9.5	4.8	1580	11.5	340	51	211	3.8
Panicum laetum bran (n=2)	96.7	8.2	8.8	1430	23.3	603	78	310	4.7
Panicum laetum dehusked (n=1)	98.1	12.4	2.2	1630	1.4	178	13	24	3.0
Maerua crassifolia dried leaves (n=4)	97.5	26.0	4.1	1500	13.2	2262	1978	130	1.5

were determined in N-balance experiments in young growing rats.

∎ Results

Table I shows the composition of wild-gathered foods from Gourma; and Table II shows the protein quality. The data are provisional and require validation.

∎ Conclusion

Food quality can be substantially improved by processing and combined use of locally gathered wild foods.

Wild-gathered grains of *Cenchrus biflorus* and *Panicum laetum* were found to have high energy content and the minerals potassium, iron and zinc. These grains had a relatively high protein concentration, but low protein quality. The protein quality was increased by adding lysine to the grains during preparation (initial CS 28 increased to 100).

Leaves of *Maerua crassifolia* had high protein quantity, but low availability of protein in raw unprocessed material. Processing the green leaves of *Maerua crassifolia* yielded an acceptable food, which can be an important source of protein and energy in the dry seasons.

The use of unprocessed grains and leaves as foods is recommended. *Cenchrus biflorus* is used both as raw and as boiled grains. Using raw foods causes waste and reduced quality. Processing and combination are necessary to reach a high nutritive value of food resources in the area.

∎ Reference

(1) FAO/WHO/UNU (1985) *Energy and Protein Requirements,* WHO Tech. Rep. Ser. No. 724, WHO, Geneva.

Table II. Protein quality[a] of wild-gathered foods from Gourma (per 100 g edible portion)

Food	Protein	Chemical score[b]	Limiting amino acid	Biological value	True digestibility	Net protein utilization
Name	g	%		%	%	%
Cenchrus biflorus whole grains	22	28	Lys	41	89	36
Cenchrus biflorus whole grains, boiled	22	28	Lys	41	87	34
Cenchrus biflorus whole grains boiled + lysine	22	103	Thr	65	80	52
Panicum laetum whole grains	9.5	34	Lys	44	81	35
Panicum laetum bran	8.2	62	Lys	39	56	22
Panicum laetum dehusked grains	12.4	23	Lys	34	95	32
Panicum laetum dehusked grains, boiled	12.4	23	Lys	43	82	35
Maerua crassifolia dried leaves	26	116	Lys	–	ca 60	–
Maerua crassifolia dried, boiled	28	102	Lys	65	70	46

[a] N-balance experiments in rats; [b] reference pattern for preschool children 2 to 5 years (FAO/WHO/UNU 1985)

Methods and Conventions of Nutrient Analysis

Supported by AOAC INTERNATIONAL

This session was chaired by Dr Doreen Clark, Managing Director of Analchem Bioassay, Sydney. The keynote address *AOAC IN-TERNATIONAL-Validated Methods for Nutrient Analysis — Method Availability and Method Needs* was given by J. DeVries. This was followed by papers on *Analysis and Classification of Digestible and Undigestible Carbohydrates* by N-G. Asp, *Recent Developments in the Determination of Water-soluble Vitamins in Food — Impact on the Use of Food Composition Tables for the Calculation of Vitamin Intakes* by P.M. Finglas, *Update on the Analysis of Total Lipids, Fatty Acids and Sterols in Foods* by A.J. Sinclair and *Conventions for the Expression of Analytical Data* by D.A.T. Southgate. All of these papers are published on the following pages.

G.R. Beecher, F. Khachik and J.T. Vanderslice did not provide a print version of their presentation *Recent Advances in the Analysis of Fat-Soluble Vitamins in Foods*. They can be contacted at the Nutrient Composition Laboratory, Beltsville Human Nutrition Research Center, ARS/USDA, Beltsville MD 20705, USA for further information.

AOAC INTERNATIONAL-Validated Methods for Nutrient Analysis — Method Availability and Method Needs

Jonathan W. DeVries

Medallion Laboratories, General Mills Inc., 9000 Plymouth Ave No., Minneapolis, MN 55427, USA

Adequate analytical methods for nutrients in foods, food ingredients, and food products are the basic first step in determining the nutritional adequacy of a food supply. Whatever the ultimate use of nutrition data, i.e. consumer education via the food label, or databases for nutrient and deficiency disease studies, the assay used to provide the data must determine the analyte of interest adequately. AOAC INTERNATIONAL (formerly the Association of Official Agricultural Chemists then the Association of Official Analytical Chemists) has been systematically validating methods for nutrition analysis for over 100 years. This validation includes a complete peer review system, with study of the method in multiple laboratories and multilevel review of the study results to assure adequacy of a proposed method for its intended purpose. With the passage in the USA of the Nutrition Labeling and Education Act, concern arose regarding the availability and adequacy of validated analytical methods to meet the requirements of the labeling act. A special AOAC task force with members drawn from regulatory agencies, the food industry, academia, and analytical suppliers was formed to address the concerns. In this paper, results of the task force assessment of adequacy of current Official Methods for nutrition analysis are presented. Method matrix combinations where updated methods or method modifications are needed are covered. In addition, a number of special issues addressed by the task force relating to the analysis of fat, moisture, and carbohydrate, reference materials (certified and in-house), and the methods validation process are discussed.

Adequate analytical methods for nutrients in foods, food ingredients, and food products are the basic first step in determining the nutritional adequacy of a food supply. Whether the nutrition data are ultimately used to inform consumers with information on the food label, or to build databases to study correlations between nutrient(s) and deficiency diseases, the assay used to provide the data must determine the analyte of interest adequately. AOAC INTERNATIONAL (formerly the Association of Official Agricultural Chemists and then the Association of Official Analytical Chemists) has been systematically validating methods for nutrition analysis for over 100 years. These validated methods provide competent laboratories with a means of supplying dependable data for nutrition labels of databases regarding the nutrition content of foods and food products.

This paper covers three areas, first, the history of AOAC INTERNATIONAL, and its processes and criteria for validation and acceptance of a method as an AOAC Official Method; second, recent activities of AOAC carried out in response to the recently proposed *Nutrition Labeling and Education Act* (NLEA)(1) in the US; and third, ideas for a methods validation scheme that might be used to improve the method validation process for foods, providing better comparative data and more rugged methods for laboratory use.

■ History and Procedures of AOAC INTERNATIONAL

In 1884, a group of regulatory agricultural chemists formed the Association of Official Agricultural Chemists to adopt uniform methods for the analysis of fertilizers. The collaborative study was adopted as a means of validating methods and evaluating their performance. One of the active participants during the early years of the Association, Dr. Harvey W. Wiley carried out extensive studies on the adulteration of foods and drugs using AOAC methods. This ultimately led to the passage of the US Federal Pure Food and Drug Act of 1906. By 1912, the As-

sociation had begun publishing its validated methods as Official Methods in USDA bulletins. By 1920, the volume of validated methods had grown to the point where it warranted its own volume, and the *Official Methods of Analysis* was established. It has been revised and updated every five years since then (2).

In 1965, the name of the association was changed to Association of Official Analytical Chemists. As the Association's activities grew to include microbiologists and other scientists, the membership base became international in scope. As a result, the name was updated to AOAC INTERNATIONAL in 1991. Membership now includes scientists from many fields worldwide interested in improving analytical methodology and results.

Method validation under AOAC INTERNATIONAL auspices includes a complete peer review system, with study of the method in multiple laboratories and multilevel review of the study results to assure adequacy of a proposed method for its intended purpose. The key to rugged effective validated methods in AOAC INTERNATIONAL lies with the Associate Referee. The Associate Referee is appointed on a recommendation of a methods committee or a General Referee on the basis of the Associate Referee's expertise in an analytical area, i.e. active in methods development work, actively carrying out work assignments or projects relating to the analyte of interest, etc. Quite frequently the Associate Referee develops an analytical method to meet a need, or through knowledge of the literature selects an applicable method for study. After a requisite number of laboratories have been found to carry out a collaborative study, the Associate Referee distributes the methodology and samples. After the collaborative study is complete, the Associate Referee collects the data, develops a study report and submits a recommendation for method adoption to the Association. Assisting the Associate Referee is the General Referee, appointed on the basis of expertise and experience in broad analytical areas, who brings this broad knowledge base to bear on the study and its results.

When the General Referee and the Associate Referee agree that a method performs sufficiently well (see below for a discussion of criteria) to be considered as an Official Method, the method is submitted to an AOAC statistician and a safety advisor for review. Upon completion of these reviews, the method is sent to an appropriate Methods Committee for review and recommendation regarding Official Status. Methods committees are constituted of members chosen for their broad expertise in a given analytical area such as Food Nutrition, Food Toxins, or Drug Residues. Recommendation to the Official Methods Board to adopt a method as Official First Action requires agreement of two-thirds of the members of the Methods Committee. If members of the Methods Committee raise significant questions with regard to the method or its performance, the method cannot be recommended for Official Status until those questions have been addressed by the Associate Referee. Upon recommendation from the Methods Committee, the method is considered for Official Status by the Official Methods Board. The Board reviews the actions taken on the method, the review process, and assures consistency between methods and between methods committee reviews. If the method is given "First Action Official Status", it is published in the Official Methods of Analysis. After "First Action" status for two years, methods which have no unresolved negative comments or issues can be considered for "Final Action Status", a status achieved through ballot of the entire AOAC INTERNATIONAL membership. There is no difference in the Official Status of Methods, whether "First Action" or "Final Action". "Final Action" only indicates that a method has withstood some test of time with no substantive questions raised regarding its performance. Any method achieving Official Status through the AOAC process has had both substantial performance testing in multiple laboratories and peer review by scientists who are experts in the analytical area. In addition, it has had intense scrutiny by scientists in related endeavors.

Criteria for validation of a method for Official Status are well established (3). The method must be submitted to participating laboratories written exactly as it is intended to be run. Participating laboratories are expected to run the method exactly as written. For a given collaborative study, participation by no fewer than eight laboratories analyzing a minimum of five sample materials is required for quantitative methods. For qualitative methods, no fewer than 15 laboratories analyzing a minimum of two analyte levels per matrix, five samples per level, and five negative controls are required. Obviously in both cases participation by more laboratories and the inclusion of more samples is encouraged. In extenuating circumstances, for example a particular method being considered has significant regulatory or commercial importance, but can only be carried out in five laboratories anywhere because only they have key instrumentation special consideration is given. Obviously, such circumstances are rare.

After the collaborative study is complete, statistical outliers (laboratories and/or data points) are removed (3). Rejection of data from more than two-ninths of the laboratories (without a valid explanation such as failure to follow the method) is basis for the rejection of the method as being insufficiently rugged to be adequate for intended purpose. Method performance (in statistical terms) will vary depending on analyte, matrix, and/or analyte quantity. Ultimately, therefore, a method must be accepted based on its performance in collaborative study as judged by scientific peer review by experts from government, academia, industry and other organizations. These experts are cognizant of the ultimate use of the methods being validated and judge adequacy for intended purpose. Working together in concert through AOAC INTERNATIONAL, these experts have produced high quality methods for the analytical community to use.

■ Methods Needs for Nutrition Labeling

With the recent passage in the USA of the *Nutrition Labeling and Education Act,* concern arose amongst food consumers, producers, regulators, and laboratories providing nutrition analytical services, regarding the availability and adequacy of validated analytical methods to meet the requirements of the labeling act. The act was passed by the US Congress in November of 1990. The act required the US Food and Drug Administration to promulgate proposed regulations for nutrition labeling of nearly all foods sold in the US. The US Department of Agriculture, although not legally required to do so, initiated activities to adopt labeling regulations essentially equivalent to those of the USFDA. The proposed regulations of November 1991, were open for public comment for a number of months, with final regulations due in November of 1992. The final regulations were actually issued in January 1993, with an effective date for new label implementation of May 8, 1994 (July 8, 1994 for products under USDA jurisdiction).

The NLEA will have a significant impact on industry, consumers, and government agencies. It is estimated that it will cost industry upwards of $1.5 billion for the relabeling required, an estimated $1500 per product for small firms and $900 per product for large firms. Analytical costs will probably range from $750 for the 40 per cent of US foods that need label changes to $1800 for the 60 per cent of foods that had not been previously labeled. Research and development costs for products that will be modified somewhat for marketing advantage under the provisions of the act are hard to estimate, but run anywhere from $20,000 to $400,000 per product. Typically two to five months will be needed to redesign and print new packages. For consumers the cost of relabeling will be passed along in higher product prices. No money has been allocated for "Education", so it is expected that significant consumer confusion will exist after the label changes occur. Governmental agencies will incur extra costs for interpretation, analysis, and enforcement of the act.

The effective date for NLEA was May 8, 1994, however other aspects of labeling had different effective dates, i.e. juice labeling in May, 1993, health claims in May 1993, and metric weight declarations in February, 1994. The NLEA now mandates nutrition labeling of most products and allows specified uses of nutrient descriptors and health claims related to nutrition.

Label format(s) is(are) rigidly specified under the NLEA (e.g. Figure 1). Mandatory declarations include calories, calories from fat, total fat, saturated fat, cholesterol, sodium, total carbohydrate, dietary fiber, sugars, protein, vitamin A, vitamin C, calcium, and iron. Voluntary declaration is allowed for calories from saturated fat, polyunsaturated fat, monounsaturated fat, stearic acid (USDA products), potassium, soluble fiber, insoluble fiber, sugar alcohols, other carbohydrates, thiamin (vitamin B_1), riboflavin (vitamin B_2), niacin, vitamin D, vitamin E, folate, cyanocobalamin (vitamin B_{12}), phosphorus, iodine, magnesium, zinc, copper, biotin, and pantothenic acid.

Labels will list the quantity of a given nutrient, along with a percentage of a daily recommended dietary intake value guideline for the consumer to use for comparison. The percentage of daily value is determined against either a Reference Daily Intake (RDI) value (typically for micronutrients) or against a Daily Reference Value (typically for macronutrients). For example, the daily reference value (based on 2000 calories/day) for fat is 65 g, for saturated fat is 20 g, for cholesterol is 300 mg, and for dietary fiber is 25 g. To encourage consistency in reporting of daily values, reference amounts relating to serving sizes have been published for common food items, e.g. 30 g for ready to eat cereals and cookies, 55 g for cake. Label serving sizes are to be in common household units, e.g. cups, teaspoons etc.

Nutrient claims can be made regarding the food product. However, if fat, saturated fat, cholesterol, or sodium exceed certain levels, this must be disclosed on the package label along with the nutrient claim. Adequate analytical methods are obviously needed to assure compliance both with the spirit of the nutrient claim, as well as to monitor the disclosure level compliance.

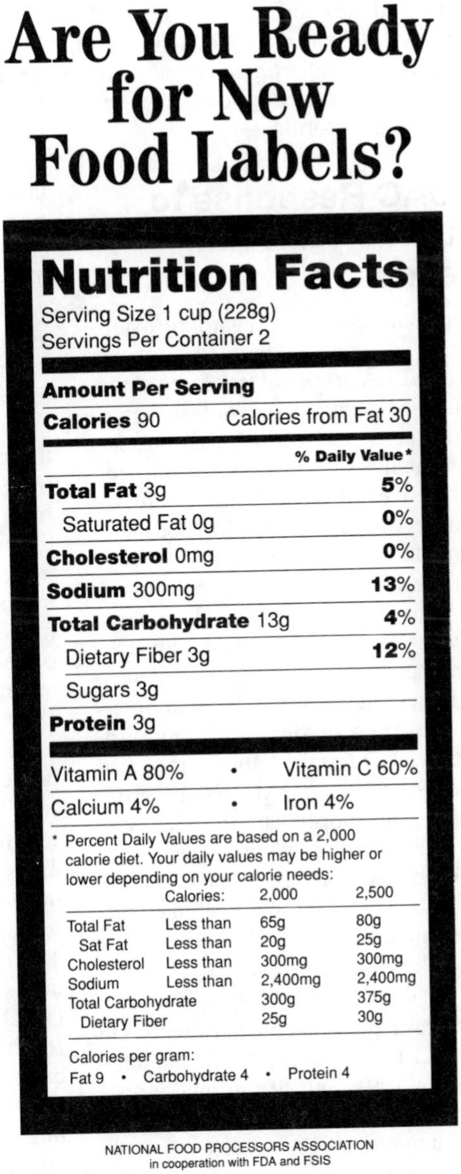

For added nutrients (referred to as Class I nutrients), the nutrient must be present at 100 per cent or greater than declared. For naturally occurring nutri-

Are You Ready for New Food Labels?

Nutrition Facts

Serving Size 1 cup (228g)
Servings Per Container 2

Amount Per Serving

Calories 90   Calories from Fat 30

	% Daily Value*
Total Fat 3g	**5%**
Saturated Fat 0g	**0%**
Cholesterol 0mg	**0%**
Sodium 300mg	**13%**
Total Carbohydrate 13g	**4%**
Dietary Fiber 3g	**12%**
Sugars 3g	
Protein 3g	

Vitamin A 80%	•	Vitamin C 60%
Calcium 4%	•	Iron 4%

* Percent Daily Values are based on a 2,000 calorie diet. Your daily values may be higher or lower depending on your calorie needs:

	Calories:	2,000	2,500
Total Fat	Less than	65g	80g
Sat Fat	Less than	20g	25g
Cholesterol	Less than	300mg	300mg
Sodium	Less than	2,400mg	2,400mg
Total Carbohydrate		300g	375g
Dietary Fiber		25g	30g

Calories per gram:
Fat 9 • Carbohydrate 4 • Protein 4

NATIONAL FOOD PROCESSORS ASSOCIATION
in cooperation with FDA and FSIS

Figure 1. Example of food label conforming with NLEA requirement.

ents, (Class II), the nutrient must be present at a level at least 80 per cent or greater than declared, but less than or equal to 120 per cent of declared. Examples of nutrients that must be greater than 80 per cent of declared are dietary fiber and potassium. Examples of nutrients that must be less than 120 per cent of declared are fat, saturated fat, and sugar. Analytical variability is taken into account for enforcement, so well-characterized validated methods are necessary for compliance monitoring.

■ AOAC Response to Nutrition Labeling Needs

To deal with concerns regarding availability of adequate methods to meet the needs of NLEA, a special task force of the AOAC with members drawn from regulatory agencies, the food industry, academia, and analytical suppliers was formed. The objectives of the task force were to: determine which Official Methods are adequate to meet current nutrition labeling analysis requirements; determine which Official Methods need revisions or modifications to meet current nutrition labeling analysis requirements; determine which nutrient-matrix combinations require the development and validation of Official Methods; propose means by which AOAC INTERNATIONAL can supply needed methods and/or modifications; identify means by which reference materials might be incorporated into AOAC Official Methods and into the validation process for AOAC Official Methods, further assuring the quality and performance of those methods.

The task force began informally at the AOAC INTERNATIONAL Annual Meeting in 1991, and was formally appointed by the board of directors in December of that year. Efforts were initiated immediately to obtain feedback regarding the status of Official Methods used for nutrition labeling. A survey was conducted of laboratories carrying out nutrition analysis and using AOAC methods. An information gathering session was also held in March of 1992. A number of task force meetings were held in the succeeding months to carry out the assigned objectives and fulfill the task force's mission.

Under the proposed nutrition labeling regulations, up to 54 nutrition-related items were either required or could be placed on the label, everything from A (ash) to Z (zinc). To organize the task of evaluating methods for these analytes, the task force divided foods into 20 different matrix groups that were felt at the time to cover the scope of foods and food products. This resulted in 1080 analyte-matrix combinations to be assessed regarding availability of adequate methods. Individual committee members took upon themselves assignments to review AOAC methods on an analyte-matrix basis. After this preliminary review was done, the entire task force, along with aid solicited from others, reviewed the assessments of the individual members. The analyte-matrix grid of adequate methods began to fill in. As the task force progressed, the information being generated was regularly reported in *The Referee* to keep the AOAC membership informed of progress and to allow feedback. For example the assessment of adequate methods under the proposed regulations was published in the July 1992 issue of *The Referee* (4).

Initial review of adequate methods under the proposed regulations, indicated that 947 of the 1080 possible matrix-analyte combinations had adequate methods. This meant that 88 per cent of the methods needs were addressed. In some cases, the Official Methods were deemed adequate for the need, but newer technologies can be brought to bear on the analyte-matrix combination to provide better methods at this point in time. An example might be vitamin A. The Carr-Price (5) method provides adequate results for labeling purposes, however most laboratories today would rather use liquid chromatography (e.g. (6)) and avoid handling the corrosive antimony trichloride. Therefore, although the task force accepted the adequacy of the Carr-Price method, it is recommending that validation of liquid chromatography methods be undertaken.

As the list of adequate methods was being generated, a complementary list of methods in need of validation or revision was also developed. This was published in October 1992 (7) to alert members of methods needs.

Special Nutrition Labeling Issues

As the task force evaluated methods for nutrition analysis, a number of issues were raised, in particular, methods for fat, dietary fiber, moisture, carbohydrates, standards and reference materials for Official Methods, and the need for a clear-cut means of determining if a particular Official Method is applicable to all foods. Subcommittees of the task force were formed to address each of these issues.

Fat has traditionally been analyzed by a variety of methods depending upon matrix, analyst carrying out the analysis, and intended use of the resulting data. Typically, the result was dependent upon determination of some solvent-soluble (solvents varied depending on the method) fraction of the food being analyzed. The task force realized that a single concise definition for fat was needed. AOAC INTERNATIONAL does not set definitions for nutrients, but provides validated analytical methods to quantify defined nutrients. Therefore, the subcommittee recommended, and the task force concurred, that the regulatory agencies, the USDA and FDA, adopt a single concise definition for fat. The agencies responded by adopting a definition of fat as the sum of the fatty acids (regardless of source) in the food, expressed as triglycerides (8). This concise definition provides a "gold standard" for evaluating fat analysis methods in the future.

The carbohydrates subcommittee determined that methods for total, soluble, and insoluble dietary fiber are adequate. Sugar methods, in particular the liquid chromatography methods with defatting steps, while adequate, should be further studied to assure validity across a broader matrix base. Complex carbohydrates as a nutrition label item had been included in the labeling proposal, but eliminated from the final regulations due to the lack of a clear definition of the nutrient, and

lack of analytical methods to measure it. The subcommittee (and the task force) recommends a concise definition for complex carbohydrates be adopted and has committed AOAC to validating appropriate methodology when a definition is adopted.

A complete listing of moisture methods, along with their characteristics has been published by the moisture subcommittee (9). As with complex carbohydrates, a clearer definition of moisture will be helpful in validating more concise methodology for this analyte.

The subcommittee on reference materials published a listing of commercially available reference materials for the nutrients requiring mandatory labeling in August, 1992 (10). The subcommittee further went on to publish *Guidelines for the Preparation of Inhouse Quality Assurance Materials* in the May, 1993 issue of *The Referee* (11). Recognizing that assuring an adequate supply of reference materials was an ongoing task, requiring significant follow-up long after the nutrition labeling task force would be disbanded, the task force supported the formation of the first technical division of AOAC INTERNATIONAL, namely the Technical Division on Reference Materials. This division will continue the efforts initiated through the task force and will expand to reference materials beyond food nutrition. This division already has over 125 members and held its first annual meeting in conjunction with the AOAC INTERNATIONAL Annual Meeting in July, 1993.

■ Method Validation Needs

After the final regulations for Nutrition Labeling in the US were issued by the USDA (12) and the USFDA (13), the task force reassessed methods adequacy and needs. The updated listings were published in the March (14) and April (15), 1993 issues of *The Referee*, respectively. In particular, methods and/or collaborative studies are needed for β-carotene, biotin, sugar alcohols, sugars (verification for certain matrices), cholesterol, copper, cyanocobalamin, defatting of samples for dietary fiber, fat (total, saturated, monounsaturated, and stearic acid), folate, iodine, niacin (microbiological method), pantothenate, protein (eliminating mercury use), pyridoxine, tryptophan (microbiological method), vitamin A, vitamin C (where erythorbate is present), and vitamin E. Some of these nutrients do have adequate methods, however, the methods are in need of modernization and therefore are recommended for further study.

■ The Food Triangle as a Systematic Approach to Method Validation

A question that arose during the task force deliberations was: How does one ascertain with reasonable confidence that a method is applicable to all foods without a substantial history of trouble-free application to a wide variety of food samples? Clearly, a defined systematic approach might be helpful to assure method ruggedness across all food types while minimizing the analyst's efforts in assessing the method. The task force Subcommittee on Definition of Foods for Analytical Purposes has proposed an approach that is currently being considered by the Foods committees and the Official Methods Board (16).

The idea of requiring a collaborative study of 40 or more samples can be very discouraging, both for the associate referee organizing the study and for potential participants. There are five macronutrient components of any given food that have a significant impact on the performance of a method, no matter what the analyte being measured. The macronutrients impact analysis of various analytes by causing extraction difficulties or analyte interferences. The five macronutrients are moisture, ash, protein, fat, and carbo-

hydrate. Moisture of nearly all samples can be adjusted if the level affects an assay. Water can be added, or the sample dried. Ash content of a sample usually has little effect on assays, particularly for organic nutrients. Therefore, the remaining three macronutrients, fat, protein, and carbohydrate have the major impact on the effectiveness of an analytical method. In a picture of a triangle with fat, protein, and moisture at the apices, all food samples will fit somewhere on that triangle, assuming the sum of fat, protein, and carbohydrate is normalized to 100 per cent, and these components are expressed as a percentage thereof. For example, a sample with 10 per cent fat, 30 per cent carbohydrate, and 10 per cent protein will have normalized values of 20 per cent fat, 60 per cent carbohydrate, and 20 per cent protein.

The triangle can be split equally in nine subtriangles, with any particular nutrient lying between 0–33 per cent, 33–67 per cent, and 67–100 per cent, respectively. By choosing 18 samples (two from each subtriangle), the analyst would be reasonably certain of covering foods characteristic of most foods. To develop further confidence in a method, samples taken from a subtriangle can be purposefully chosen to represent particular characteristics, i.e. for the 67–100 per cent carbohydrate subsection, a high fiber and a high starch sample might be used. For the 67–100 per cent fat section, a milk or animal fat and a vegetable fat might be chosen. The system could be applied to any nutrient being analyzed by using a Youden pairing technique [closely matched sample pairs as opposed to blind duplicates] (3) for determination of within laboratory variability for the analyte of interest. If difficulty is experienced with getting acceptable results for the method in question for samples from certain subtriangles, this information could be quite helpful for understanding and delineating the cause of the ineffectiveness. A similar approach had earlier been suggested for reference materials for nutrition analysis (17). The concept is extended by Tanner et al. (18).

■ Conclusion

The task force has completed its objectives and reported the results of its deliberations on an ongoing basis in *The Referee,* the official house organ of AOAC. The final report has been published (19). The task force disbanded at the July 1993 Annual Meeting of AOAC INTERNATIONAL.

■ References

(1)   Anon. (Nov 27, 1991) *Federal Register* **56**, no 229, 60301-60891

(2)   *Official Methods of Analysis,* (1920, 1925, 1930, 1935, 1940, 1945, 1950, 1955, 1960, 1965, 1970, 1975, 1980, 1985, 1990) Association of Official Analytical Chemists, Arlington, VA

(3)   *Manual for the Development, Study, Review, and Approval Process for AOAC Official Methods* (1993) AOAC INTERNATIONAL, Arlington, VA

(4)   Nutrient Labeling Task Force (1992) *The Referee* **16**, 1, 7-12

(5)   *Official Methods of Analysis* (1990) 15th Ed., secs **1045-1047,** AOAC, Arlington, VA

(6)   DeVries, J.W. (1985) in *Methods of Vitamin Assay*, J. Augustin, B.P. Klein, D. Becker, & P.B. Venugopal, (Eds.), John Wiley and Sons, New York, NY

(7)   Nutrient Labeling Task Force (1992) *The Referee* **16**, 5-10

(8)   Anon. (1993) *Federal Register* **58**, 2086-2093

(9)   Anon. (1993) *The Referee* **17**, 6-9

(10)   Anon. (1992) *The Referee* **16**, 4-5

(11)   Anon. (1993) *The Referee* **17**, 6-8

(12)   Anon. (1993) *Federal Register* **58**, 631-2063

(13)   Anon. (1993) *Federal Register* **58**, 2065-2964

(14)   Nutrient Labeling Task Force (1993) *The Referee* **17**, 6-10

(15)   Nutrient Labeling Task Force (1993) *The Referee* **17**, 6-8

(16)   Anon. (1993) *The Referee* **17**, 1, 6-7

(17)   Southgate, D.A.T. (1987) *Fres. J. Anal. Chem.* 326, 660-664

(18)   Tanner, J.T., Wolf, W.R., & Horwitz, W. (1995) in *Quality and Accessibility Food-Related Data*, H. Greenfield (Ed.), AOAC INTERNATIONAL, Arlington, VA, pp. 99-104

(19)   *Methods of Analysis for Nutrition Labeling* (1993), D.M. Sullivan, & D.E. Carpenter, (Eds.), AOAC INTERNATIONAL, Arlington, VA, pp. 33-83

Analysis and Classification of Digestible and Undigestible Carbohydrates

Nils-Georg Asp

Department of Applied Nutrition and Food Chemistry, Lund University, Chemical Center, PO Box 124, S-221 00 Lund, Sweden

The current interest in the nutritional properties of various food carbohydrates has increased the demand for compositional data. The small-intestinal digestibility is the most important nutritional property. The digestible carbohydrates provide glucose to body tissues, whereas the undigestible carbohydrates are partially fermented and provide fermentation substrate and bulk in the colon. Mono-, di- and oligosaccharides, as well as polyols, can be determined with specific enzymatic methods, but gas-liquid chromatography (GLC) and especially liquid chromatography (LC) methods are preferable when a range of sugars is to be analyzed. Dietary fiber determination should aim to differentiate between digestible ("available") and undigestible ("unavailable") carbohydrates. Gravimetric and component analysis methods are complementary for different purposes. Resistant starch, i.e. undigestible starch, as well as lignin should be included in the dietary fiber. Starch is preferably analyzed with specific enzymatic methods, that should have the same cut-off as for starch removal in dietary fiber analysis.

Dietary guidelines in Western countries recommend that the carbohydrate intake be increased to at least 55–60 per cent of the energy (1). In diets consumed in other parts of the world carbohydrates may contribute more than 70 per cent of energy. Originally, the carbohydrate recommendations came as a consequence of the fat and protein recommendations. In recent years, however, the nutritional importance of the carbohydrates as such has been more and more emphasized, and new developments call for a more nutritional classification of the different food carbohydrates as a basis for more specific recommendations about intake.

Labeling of foods regarding carbohydrate content is a separate, but closely related issue. Most carbohydrate content figures on food labels are still being calculated "by difference", i.e. the material remaining after moisture, ash, fat and protein determinations. In view of the quite variable nutritional effects of different carbohydrates, this is unsatisfactory.

A thorough characterization of the various digestible and undigestible carbohydrate fractions is required whenever investigating the physiological properties of a carbohydrate-containing food or diet. Compositional data on the food carbohydrates are also essential in epidemiological research.

Table I shows the food carbohydrates that are quantitatively most important. Starch generally occurs in the largest amount in diets, followed by sucrose and — when milk products are consumed — lactose. Glucose, fructose and sucrose are present naturally in fruits, berries and vegetables, and also may be added as refined sugars. Polyols and fructans such as inulin are increasingly used as low-calorie bulking agents, as is polydextrose. Since many dietary guidelines recommend a limited use of refined sugars (sucrose, fructose, corn syrups, high fructose corn syrup etc.), the contribution of such "extrinsic" sugars is of special interest. However, it is not possible analytically to distinguish between "extrinsic" sugars and the "intrinsic" sugars present naturally.

Table I. Main food carbohydrates

Monosaccharides	**Polysaccharides**
Glucose	Starch
Fructose	– amylopectin
Galactose	– amylose
Polyols	– modified food starches
Disaccharides	Non-starch polysaccharides (NSP)
Sucrose	– cellulose
Lactose	– hemicelluloses
Polyols	– pectins
	– fructans
Oligosaccharides	– gums
α-Galactactosides	– mucilages
– raffinose, stachyose	– algal polysaccharides
	other
Fructans	
– fructo-oligosaccharides	
Polyols	
Polydextrose	

■ Nutritional Properties of Food Carbohydrates

Small Intestinal Digestibility

Carbohydrates that are digested and absorbed in the small intestine provide glucose, fructose and galactose to body tissues. Undigestible carbohydrates, on the other hand, are delivered to the large intestine and fermented to various extents. The main products of this anaerobic fermentation are acetate, propionate and butyrate. Acetate and propionate are absorbed and metabolized in peripheral tissues and the liver, respectively, and their possible effects on carbohydrate and lipid metabolism are currently investigated. Butyrate is an important source of energy for the epithelial cells of the large intestine itself, and may be important in protecting against colonic cancer (for review, see e.g. 2). Various fermentable carbohydrates give different proportions of these fermentation products (3).

As early as 1929, McCance and Lawrence emphasized small-intestinal digestibility by introducing the term "available" carbohydrates, based on determination of starch and digestible sugars (4). Correspondingly the term "unavailable carbohydrates"was used for cellulose, non-cellulose polysaccharides and lignin (5). Within the European Community legislators have defined "carbohydrates" as digestible ("metabolizable") carbohydrates and including polyols (6).

Dietary fiber was first defined as the remnants of plant cell-walls not digested in the small intestine (7). With this definition it constitutes the non-starch polysaccharides of the plant cell-walls, but also undigestible protein, inorganic material, tannins, cutin etc. The redefinition by Trowell et al. (8) restricted the definition to polysaccharides and lignin, but enlarged it to include all undigestible polysaccharides. There were two reasons for this: First, purified polysaccharides such as pectins and gums were frequently used to study the physiological effects of dietary fiber constituents, and second, cell-wall polysaccharides could not easily be differentiated analytically from undigestible polysaccharides from other sources (9).

Dietary fiber includes a large number of polysaccharides with quite different properties, both from the chemical and physiological points of view. Insoluble, lignified types of dietary fiber have the most prominent fecal bulking effect due to their resistance to fermentation, whereas soluble, gel-forming polysaccharides are most efficient in lowering blood cholesterol and blood glucose after a meal (for review, see e.g. 10).

In the large intestine, the dietary fiber polysaccharides, oligosaccharides and resistant starches are fermented to various extent with production of acetate, propionate and butyrate in various proportions.

Rate of Carbohydrate Digestion and Absorption

In diabetes, patients have long been advised to choose carbohydrates that are slowly digested and absorbed, giving a limited and sustained blood glucose elevation with minimum insulin requirement. This has been demonstrated to improve the metabolic control in maturity onset diabetes (NIDDM) (11). Generally it has been believed that starch is slowly digested and absorbed due to its high molecular weight ("complex carbohydrate"). Sucrose and other low-molecular weight carbohydrates ("simple sugars"), on the other hand, have been regarded as rapidly absorbed. It is remarkable that this view has been so prevalent in spite of the lack of scientific evidence. On the contrary, data accumulated in the 70s and 80s showing that the height and shape of the blood glucose curve could be quite different after the intake of different foods, and that these differences were unrelated to the molecular size of the carbohydrates. Among the low molecular weight carbohydrates, fructose gives a very low glycemic response, and sucrose is intermediate between glucose and fructose (12). Starchy foods are found across the whole range of "slow" to "rapid" (for review see e.g. 13).

A number of other carbohydrate and food properties determining the glycemic response have now been identified and include gel-forming types of dietary fiber, degree of gelatinization and other properties of the starch, cellular structure and gross structure (14). There is increasing evidence that "slow" properties of food carbohydrates may also be beneficial in relation to blood lipid levels, satiety, physical performance and dental caries (12). The cariogenic properties of foods have mainly been related to added sucrose, but there is evidence that other fermentable carbohydrates are important as well. Even starch can lower dental plaque pH, and this property is related to the availability of starch for enzymatic degradation in the mouth (15).

The term "complex carbohydrates" was used in 1977 by the U.S. Senate Committee on Nutrition and Human Needs (McGovern Report) without any exact definition, but meaning in practice digestible polymeric carbohydrate, i.e. starch. From what has been said above, it is obvious that starch has no nutritional advantage per se, and therefore, the term "complex carbohydrates" is questionable. In Britain, it was reintroduced to mean starch and non-starch polysaccharides (16). Although the grouping together of starch and non-starch polysaccharides may be relevant from the chemistry point of view, its usefulness for nutritional classification is questionable. Recommendations regarding complex carbohydrate intake (1) are very complicated to interpret in terms of foods even for experts.

■ Overview of Analytical Methods

Mono-, Di- and Oligosaccharides including Polyols

Depending on the food matrix to be analyzed, an extraction of the free sugars may be necessary. Aqueous ethanol is preferable due to the toxicity of methanol, that was frequently used earlier. A final ethanol concentration of at least 80 per cent (v/v) should be used to avoid extraction of polysaccharides. However, some polysaccharides such as inulin and pectic substances may have considerable solubility also at this alcohol concentration. Some sugars, especially lactose, have a slow rate of dissolution and limited solubility, and may need lower alcohol concentration (e.g. 50 per cent v/v) at extraction with a final increase to precipitate polysaccharides (17).

The International Union of Pure and Applied Chemistry (IUPAC) defines oligosaccharides as having less than ten monomeric residues. In practice, however, oligosaccharides are defined as carbohydrates soluble or extractable in aqueous ethanol. Precipitation in 78-80 per cent ethanol (or dialysis/ultrafiltration) is generally used to separate oligosaccharides and starch degradation products from polysaccharides in dietary fiber analysis (9).

The α-galactosides in leguminous seeds and fructans in onions, artichokes etc. are the quantitatively most important groups of naturally occurring undigestible oligosaccharides. Inulin is a non-starch polysaccharide, but it is also not determined as dietary fiber with any of the current methods in spite of a degree of polymerization (DP) of 30 or more. Arabans in sugar beet fiber are another example of a dietary fiber polysaccharide that is extremely soluble in alcohol due to its extensive branching (18). Polydextrose also falls into this category.

Physical methods, such as polarimetry, refractive index, or density are

Table II. Resistant starch definition and determination

1. Difference in "NSP" glucan without and with KOH or DMSO solubilization (21).
2. Starch remaining in enzymatic, gravimetric dietary fiber residue (24).
3. Starch remaining after extensive α-amylase hydrolysis (27).
4. Difference of total starch and starch hydrolyzed after standardized milling during pancreatin/amyloglucosidase incubation for 120 min. Separate procedures for three forms of resistant starch available (38).

still useful in pure systems, e.g. in sugar production control. Methods based on the reduction of copper salts, and colorimetric methods based on condensation reactions with anthrone, orcinol and carbazol, can also be used in well known systems (17).

The enzymatic procedures based on specific, highly purified enzymes have been instrumental in providing means of specific and precise analysis of carbohydrates in mixtures without high capital investments. GLC and LC procedures, on the other hand, are preferable when a number of different carbohydrates are to be determined simultaneously. LC analysis has for long been hampered by the relative insensitivity of refractory index detectors. However, this has been overcome by systems using amperometric detection (17).

Polysaccharides

Starch. Starch is the predominant dietary carbohydrate, and the only polysaccharide that is digestible in the human small intestine. Enzymatic hydrolysis and specific glucose assay is the method of choice today because of glucose liberation also from for instance α-glucans at acid hydrolysis. However, the enzymes used have to be checked for contaminating activities (19).

A heat stable amylase (Termamyl) in a combined gelatinization and hydrolysis step, has turned out to be particularly useful (e.g. 20).

Resistant Starch. Resistant starch was first defined as a starch fraction resisting amylase hydrolysis unless it was first solubilized in KOH or DMSO (21).

It is now generally defined as the sum of starch and products of starch degradation not absorbed in the small intestine (22). It is then an undigestible polysaccharide, that should be included in the dietary fiber. There are different forms of resistant starch: Physically enclosed starch, raw α-type starch granules, retrograded amylose and chemically or physically modified food starches (23).

Originally, resistant starch was measured as the starch remaining associated with the dietary fiber if solubilizing agents were not used (21,24). This type of resistant starch has been identified as mainly retrograded amylose (25,26). Methods capable of measuring also other forms of resistant starch (27,28) are currently evaluated against in vivo measurements of starch absorption within the European FLAIR Concerted Action program (EURESTA).

Chemically modified food starches (29) and dry heated starches (30) are degraded by amylases to fragments that are soluble in alcohol. These fragments are neither determined as starch with enzymatic methods, nor as dietary fiber (30). Methods for resistant starch analysis are summarized in Table II.

Dietary Fiber. Dietary fiber is analyzed according to two different principles (for review, see 9). In the gravimetric methods the non-fiber components are removed and a residue weighed. The residue can be analyzed for e.g. protein and ash, and corrections used accordingly. The crude fiber and detergent fiber methods belong to this category. Enzymatic gravimetric methods such as those approved by the AOAC (31,32) use alcohol precipitation to recover soluble fiber

Table III. Advantages and disadvantages of various method for dietary fiber analysis (9).

	Enzymatic gravimetric	Component analysis	
		GLC/LC	Colorimetry
Equipment	Simple	Advanced	Simple
Information on composition	No	Yes	No/Yes
Risk of overestimation	Yes[a]	No	(Yes)
Risk of underestimation	No	Yes[b]	Yes[b]

[a] but residue can be analyzed
[b] if hydrolysis is complete

components and can be used to measure total dietary fiber (TDF) or soluble and insoluble components separately. Correction for protein and ash in the fiber residue is needed.

The component analysis methods use more or less specific determination of monomeric constituents, that are then summed to yield a total fiber value. As in gravimetric methods, soluble and insoluble components can be determined separately. It should be noted that the solubility of polysaccharides is method dependent and determined by the temperature, time and pH conditions used.

The Southgate procedure (33) employs colorimetric methods to determine hexoses, pentoses and uronic acids. The methods of Theander et al. (34) and Englyst et al. (35) use GLC for neutral sugar components and a colorimetric assay for uronic acids. LC determination is gaining in popularity. A colorimetric measurement of reducing sugars has been introduced as an alternative to the GLC determination by Englyst et al. (35).

Advantages and disadvantages of the two different ways of analyzing dietary fiber are summarized in Table III. Enzymatic gravimetric methods are simple and robust with no requirement of advanced equipment. There is a risk of overestimating the fiber content if other components remain in the residue. However, this can be analyzed for any such contaminating components. Colorimetric methods can

also be inflated by unspecific reactions. Specific, GLC or LC measurements on the other hand, require complete hydrolysis and quantitative recovery of monomers after hydrolysis of the polysaccharides. Incomplete hydrolysis or losses due to decomposition of monomers will lead to underestimation (for review, see 9).

The current component analysis methods employ acid hydrolysis and corrections for hydrolysis losses of the different components. As in amino acid analysis, conditions for the hydrolysis have to be chosen to obtain an optimal compromise between hydrolysis yield and monomer degradation. Quantitative hydrolysis yield is particularly difficult to obtain with acidic polysaccharides due to the high stability of glycosyl uronic acid linkages towards acid hydrolysis. This fact and the more rapid degradation of monomeric uronic acids at acidic condition are reasons why colorimetric methods are preferred for uronic acid determination (9).

Collaborative Studies of Dietary Fiber Analysis. A number of collaborative studies of enzymatic, gravimetric dietary fiber determination has been carried out within the AOAC. The component analysis method of Englyst and co-workers has been tested in studies carried out by the Ministry of Agriculture, Food and Fisheries in the UK (MAFF). The studies reported prior to 1990 were reviewed and compared (9). They show gradually improved performance with typical mean reproducibility (R95) values of 2-3 for both the gravimetric methods approved by the AOAC and for the Englyst method. An AOAC study with the method of Theander et al. is about to be finished. The best performance reported so far is a Swiss study with the enzymatic gravimetric AOAC method (R95=1.0-1.1) (36). An R95 value of 2.0 at a dietary fiber content of 10 g/100 g means that 19 out of 20 single determinations coming from various laboratories would fall in the range 9-11 g/100 g.

There are few formal collaborative studies covering more than one method. Usually, studies have included just one or a few laboratories running a different methods, which makes strict inter-method comparison difficult. In a recent study coordinated by the European Community Bureau of Reference (BCR) dietary fiber values with the AOAC method could be certified for three different materials. Indicative values only could be given for the Englyst GLC and colorimetric methods, but means with these methods were similar to those obtained with the AOAC method (37).

For most foods, estimates of total dietary fiber with the enzymatic gravimetric method of the AOAC or according to Theander et al. (both including the retrograded amylose type of resistant starch and lignin) would not be significantly different from estimates of non-starch polysaccharides with the Englyst methods. This means that the confidence intervals for the different methods overlap (9). It should be noted also that two collaborative studies have shown consistently higher values with the colorimetric Englyst method than with the original GLC variety (9). Only in foods with particularly high levels of resistant starch of the retrograded amylose type, or lignin, would Englyst values be expected to be significantly lower than estimates with methods including these components.

Delimitation problems in definition and analysis of dietary fiber have been much focused on the inclusion or not of resistant starch and lignin. Equally important, however, is the delimitation towards components that are not precipitated in the 70–80 per cent (v/v) ethanol used in all the methods to separate water-soluble fiber components. Inulin is an undigestible polysaccharide that is not precipitated and therefore not recovered in any of the methods. Polydextrose is another undigestible oligo-polysaccharide also not determined as dietary fiber. As discussed above, these components should be grouped together with the dietary fiber rather than with digestible carbohydrates. The same is true for the undigestible oligosaccharides. Specific enzymatic or HPLC methods then have to be employed for these components.

Difference methods are unspecific and accumulate analytical errors from the fat, protein, ash and moisture determinations. When keeping these limitations in mind, however, these methods are capable of giving a reasonable estimate of "total available carbohydrates" in many foods if the dietary fiber is measured, e.g. with the enzymatic gravimetric AOAC method. Difference calculations are also useful in the laboratory to check the standardization of methods for proximate analysis.

∎ References

(1) World Health Organization (1990) *Diet, Nutrition, and the Prevention of Chronic Disease. Technical Report Series*, 797, WHO, Copenhagen

(2) Rémésy, C., Demigné C., & Morand, C. (1992) in *Dietary Fibre — A Component of Food*, T.F. Schweizer & C.A. Edwards (Eds.), Springer-Verlag, London, pp. 137-150

(3) Edwards, C.A., & Rowland, I. (1992) in *Dietary Fibre — A Component of Food*, T.F. Schweizer & C.A. Edwards (Eds.), Springer-Verlag, London, pp. 119-136

(4) McCance, R.A., & Lawrence, R.D. (1929) Medical Research Council Special Report Series No. 135, London, HMSO

(5) McCance, R.A., & Widdowson, E.M. (1940) Medical Research Council Special Report Series No. 235, London, HMSO

(6) *Official Journal of the European Community* (1990) Directive NOL 276/40

(7) Trowell, H.C. (1972) *Am. J. Clin. Nutr.* **25**, 926-932

(8) Trowell, H.C., Southgate, D.A.T., Wolever, T.M.S., Leeds, A.R., Gassull, M.A., & Jenkins, D.J.A. (1976) *Lancet*, **i**, 967

(9) Asp, N.-G., Schweizer, T.F., Southgate, D.A.T., & Theander, O. (1992) in *Dietary Fibre - A Component of Food*, T.F. Schweizer & C.A. Edwards (Eds.), Springer-Verlag, London, pp. 57-101

(10) Asp, N.-G., Björck, I., & Nyman, M. (1993) *Carbohydrate Polymers* **21**, 183-187

(11) Brand Miller, J.C. (1994) *Am. J. Clin. Nutr.* **59** (Suppl), 747S-752S

(12) Truswell, A.S. (1992) *Eur. J. Clin. Nutr.* **46** (Suppl 2), S91-S101

(13) Würsch, P. (1989) *World Rev. Nutr. Diet.* **60**, 199-256

(14) Björck, I., Granfeldt, Y., Liljeberg, H., Tovar, J., & Asp, N.-G. (1994) *Am. J. Clin. Nutr.* **59** (Suppl), 699S-705S

(15) Lingström, P., Holm, J., Birkhed, D., & Björck, I. (1989) *Scand. J. Dent. Res.* **97**, 392-400

(16) The British Nutrition Foundation. (1990) *Complex Carbohydrates in Foods*, Chapman and Hall, London, pp. 1-164

(17) Greenfield, H., & Southgate, D.A.T. (1992) *Food Composition Data Production, Management and Use*, Elsevier Applied Science, London, pp. 94-104

(18) Asp, N.-G. (1990) in *New Developments in Dietary Fiber*, I. Furda & C.J. Brine (Eds.), Plenum Press, New York, pp. 227-236

(19) Åman, P., & Graham, H. (1987) *J. Agric. Food Chem.* **35**, 704-709

(20) Holm, J., Björck, I., Drews, A., & Asp, N.-G. (1986) *Starch/Stärke*, **38**, 224-226

(21) Englyst, H.N., Wiggins, H.S., & Cummings, J.H. (1982) *Analyst*, **107**, 307-318

(22) Asp, N.-G. (1992) *Eur. J. Clin. Nutr.* **46** (Suppl), S1

(23) Asp, N.-G., & Björck, I. (1992) *Trends Food Sci. Technol.* **3**, 111-114

(24) Johansson, C.-G., Siljeström, M., & Asp, N.-G. (1984) *Lebensm. Unters Forsch.* **179**, 24-28

(25) Siljeström, M., Eliasson, A.-C., & Björck, I. (1989) *Starch/Stärke*, **41**, 147-151

(26) Russel, P.L., Berry, C.S., & Greenwell, P. (1989) *J. Cereal. Sci.* **9**, 1-15

(27) Berry, C.S. (1986) *J. Cereal Sci.* **4**, 301-314

(28) Englyst, H.N., & Cummings, J.H. (1990) in *New Development in Dietary Fiber*, Furda, I., Brine, J. (Eds.), Plenum Press, New York, NY, pp. 205-225

(29) Björck, I., Gunnarsson, A., & Östergård, K. (1989) *Starch/Stärke* **41**, 128-134

(30) Siljeström, M., Björck, I., & Westerlund, E. (1989) *Starch/Stärke* **41**, 95-100

(31) Prosky, L., Asp, N.-G., Schweizer, T.F., DeVries, J.W., & Furda, I. (1988) *J. Assoc. Off. Anal. Chem.* **71**, 1017-1023

(32) Lee, S., Prosky, L., & DeVries, J. (1992) *J. Assoc. Off. Anal. Chem.* **75**, 395-416

(33) Southgate, D.A.T. (1969) *J. Sci. Food Agric.* **20**, 331-335

(34) Theander, O., Åman, P., Westerlund, E., & Graham, H. (1990) in New *Developments in Dietary Fiber*. I. Furda & J. Brine (Eds.), Plenum Press, New York, NY, pp. 273-281

(35) Englyst, H.N., Cummings, J.H., & Wood, R. (1987) *J. Assoc. Publ. Analysts* **25**, 73-110

(36) Schweizer, T.F., Walter, E., & Venetz, P. (1988) *Mitteilungen aus dem Gebeit der Lebensmitteluntersuchung und Hygiene* **79**, 57-68

(37) Hollman, P.C.H., Boenke, A., & Wagstaffe, P.J. (1993) *Fres J. Anal. Chem.* **345**, 174-179

(38) Englyst, H.N., Kingman, S.M., & Cummings, J.H. (1992) *Eur. J. Clin. Nutr.* **46**, S33-S50

Recent Developments in the Determination of Water-Soluble Vitamins in Food — Impact on the Use of Food Composition Tables for the Calculation of Vitamin Intakes

Paul M. Finglas

Nutrition, Diet & Health Department, Institute of Food Research, Norwich Research Park, Colney, Norwich, NR4 7UA, UK

There is a need for improvements in the determination of vitamins in food, in particular, the establishment of properly validated and robust techniques that are applicable to a wide range of food matrices. This paper addresses three main topics: first, recent developments in methods including LC techniques and biospecific methods utilizing antibodies and naturally occurring vitamin binding proteins which are both based on the microtitration plate format; second, results from a European Union project under the Measurement and Testing Programme concerned with the improvement in vitamin analysis in food by intercomparisons of methods, optimization of extraction conditions and the preparation of food reference materials (RMs); and third, the impact of the improvements in methods on the quality of vitamin data currently presented in UK food tables by comparing calculated vitamin intakes obtained using both the 4th and 5th editions of McCance & Widdowson's The Composition of Foods and direct analysis of duplicate diets.

It is important that the method of analysis chosen for any vitamin should be that which most closely reflects the vitamin activity of the food in question since the primary objective for use of the data is for nutritional purposes. The term "vitamin" reflects a certain physiological activity which is related to the chemical substances or "vitamers" responsible for this activity (1). Ideally methods would be chosen that could determine each vitamer separately and then by calculating the sum of the individual activities, a total activity of the food could be obtained (2). However, in practice this is rarely possible as procedures are not specific for the compounds of interest.

Methodology

Liquid Chromatography

The major advantage of this technique is that individual forms of the vitamin can be measured, and together with estimates of the biological activity of the various forms, can be used to provide better estimates of the vitamin activities of foods than are currently available in food tables.

Although LC techniques have been widely used for the determination fat-soluble vitamins in food, their application to water-soluble vitamin analysis has mainly been limited to vitamins B_1, B_2, B_6 and C. This has largely been due the availability of sufficiently sensitive and specific detection systems that are capable of quantifying several vitamers from a complex mixture of compounds. The use of LC with UV detection has been used for the determination of these vitamins in food but this form of detection is generally not sufficiently sensitive nor specific due to the low levels found, especially in unfortified foods (3). LC with fluorescence detection has been preferred using either the natural fluorescence of the vitamin (e.g. riboflavin), or with derivatization to form a suitable fluorescent complex (e.g. thiamin and vitamin C). This form of detection gives better sensitivity and specificity compared to UV detection (3). Examples of LC procedures available for selected water-soluble vitamins are given in Table I.

Thiamin and Riboflavin. These vitamins are usually extracted from foods using dilute mineral acids and autoclaving at 121°C, followed by enzymatic hydrolysis to release the bound forms of the vitamins. Riboflavin can be measured directly with fluorescence but thiamin requires conversion to thiochrome with alkaline potassium ferricyanide solution. The latter can be performed either manually prior to injection onto the analytical column, or by post-column derivatization. Reverse phase LC analysis of thiochrome invariably involves the injection of high salt concentrations on to the analytical column necessitating frequent washing and much reduced column life (4). This can be overcome to some extent by the use of guard columns but this may be uneconomic. Alternatively, thiochrome can be selectively extracted into an organic solvent, normally isobutanol, allowing fluorometric determination after a normal phase LC separation of thiochrome from any remaining fluorescing interferences (5). This approach can give increased sensitivity and rapid automated analysis without the need for post-column derivatization.

Thiamin methods based on the thiochrome reaction after acid hydrolysis and treatment with enzyme to release the phosphorylated forms give total thiamin concentrations. The separation of thiamin and its phosphorylated forms [thiamin monophosphate (TMP), thiamin di- or pyro-phosphate (TPP) and thiamin tri-

Table I. Selected LC procedures available for some water-soluble vitamins

Vitamin	Principle	Column	Mobile phase	Detection[a] (nm)	Reference
Thiamin	1 Post-column oxidation to thiochrome	Silica (rad-pak)	0.05M Phosphate buffer:EtOH	F (265/418)	37
	2 Pre-column oxidation to thiochrome	μ-Bondapak C-18	MeOH:H_2O	F (365/435)	38
	3 Free thiamin + phosphorylated forms	Micropak Ax5	Ammonium phosphate	UV (245)	6
Riboflavin	Native fluorescence (B_2, FMN)	Apex ODS 2	MeOH:H_2O	F (450/510)	37
Vitamin B_6	1 Acid digestion with autoclaving (PM, PL, PN)	Spherisorb ODS 2	0.04M H_2SO_4:MeOH	F (290/395)	2
	2 $HClO_4$ extraction + post-column reaction with bisulphate (PM, PL, PN, PMP, PLP)	Lichrosphere RP 18	0.03M Phosphate buffer: MeOH:ion pair	F (340/400)	9
	3 TCA extraction + post-column reaction with KH_2PO_4	Lichrosphere RP18	0.1M KH_2PO_4:EtOH acetonitrile: ion pair	F (325/385)	7
	4 Acid phosphatase hydrolysis. PM→PL using glyoxylic acid/Fe2+; PL→PN using $NaBH_4$/NaOH	Octysilyl	0.05 KH_2PO_4: acetonitrile:ion pair	F (290/395)	10
Vitamin C	1 Acid extraction + oxidation with ascorbate oxidase) (AA + DHAA)	Hypersil ODS	0.8 M Phosphate buffer:MeOH	F (367/418)	39
	2 Acid extraction (AA only)	Partisil P5	H_2O:MeOH: acetic acid	UV (248)	Leatherhead Food RA
	3 Acid extraction, homocysteine reduction (Total AA, AA)	Apex ODS 2	Acetate buffer:NaOH	EC	11
Folates	Hog kidney deconjugation, anion exchange cleanup, post-column reaction with $Ca(OCl)_2$	μ-Bondapak phenyl	Phosphate buffer: acetonitrile	F(9295/365)	14

[a] Fluorescence (excitation and emission wavelengths); EC, electrochemical; UV, ultraviolet

phosphate (TTP)] has also been reported (6).

Results from the manual thiochrome procedure agree well with the LC fluorometric procedures but are generally lower when compared to the microbiological results (7). The main cause of variability between laboratories for the determination of thiamin was found to be the extraction/enzyme hydrolysis step (7).

Similarly, for riboflavin, LC methods generally give lower results compared to the microbiological assay (MA). Most test organisms used in the MA give an equivalent growth response to riboflavin and flavin mononucleotide (FMN), which are both vitamin active. In LC procedures, riboflavin is separated from

FMN and the latter is not measured. In the same study as above several laboratories reported incomplete conversion of FMN to riboflavin and thus lower LC results compared to the MA. The enzyme conversion of FMN to riboflavin needs to be improved if LC is used for quantification (7).

Vitamin B6. LC provides a technique that is capable of measuring in a single chromatographic run all vitamin B_6 forms [pyridoxamine (PM), pyridoxal (PL), pyridoxine (PN), pyridoxamine phosphate (PMP) and pyridoxal phosphate (PLP)] and is now more widely used than the microbiological assay in food composition work. All these five forms have equal biological activity (1).

A major limitation of the MA is the lower growth response to PM compared to PL and PN obtained using some organisms. This can obviously result in a substantial underestimation in the total vitamin B_6 activity of foods that are high in the PM form (8). Two approaches have been used in the development of LC methods for vitamin B_6 depending on whether the separation and quantification of the phosphorylated forms are required in addition to PM, PL and PN. The normal acid digestion with autoclaving and enzymatic digestion is used for the extraction of total amounts of PM, PL and PN and these forms can be quantified using a reverse phase LC system with fluorometric detection (2). This type of extraction gives an array of potential interfering compounds that can make accurate quantification difficult. In addition, the conversion of PMP to PM can be incomplete unless autoclaving for 2 hours is performed. However, such conditions may lead to thermal degradation of vitamin B_6 vitamers (9).

The second type of extraction system developed for vitamin B_6 employs less vigorous conditions in order to keep the phosphorylated forms (PMP and PLP) intact. Typical acids used include sulfosalicylic acid, SSA (8), trichloroacetic acid, TCA (7) and perchloric acid, PER (9).

The SSA procedure uses anion exchange sample clean-up to remove SSA and interfering compounds prior to separation and quantification on a similar column with fluorometric detection. All five B_6 forms and the internal standard, 3-hydroxypyridine, are measured by means of detector wavelength switching. The inclusion of an internal standard before sample extraction is useful as corrections for any dilution errors and instrument variation can be made. This method has been compared to a microbiological assay and satisfactory agreement obtained for meat samples (8). Differences were found, however, between the two methods for fruits and vegetables. This was attributed to incomplete extraction of vitamers for the LC procedure (8).

The other two systems with TCA and PER use reverse-phase LC with ion-pair regents and a post-column reaction with potassium dihydrogen phosphate (7) and sodium bisulfite (9), respectively, to enhance the flurometric response of the various forms. The internal standard used was 4-deoxypyridine. Chromatograms for these procedures tend to give fewer interfering peaks and better resolution compared to those LC methods measuring total amounts of PM, PL and PN forms. For the determination of vitamin B_6 in fortified foods where PN is predominantly present, LC systems can be greatly simplified.

A recent LC procedure using ion-pair reagent and fluorometric detection has been reported (10). After dephosphorylation using acid phosphatase, PM is transformed to PL with glyoxylic acid/Fe^{2+} as catalyst, followed by conversion of PL to PN using alkaline sodium borohydride. The conversion of PM to PL was reported to be 95 per cent but it was found the conversion of PL to PN was always less than 100 per cent and variable from food to food. The procedure was only tested on four foods [yeast, wheat germ and two types of breakfast cereals (with bran and muesli)] and no comparison with the MA was made. However, the method has the advantage of much simplified chromatograms with only the separation and quantification of PN required.

Vitamin C. Vitamin C activity is exhibited by L-ascorbic acid (AA) and L-dehydroascorbic acid (DHAA) but not by D-isoascorbic acid (erythorbic acid, IAA) (1). The latter is also used as an antioxidant in foods and it is therefore important to have methods that can measure both AA and DHAA either separately or together, and differentiating them from IAA (1).

A variety of LC methods have been reported for the determination of vitamin C in food and biological materials have been reported either as a total value (AA+DHAA), or with separate determinations of each form. The latter can increase the complexity and length of the procedure and introduce additional errors and thus LC methods which give total vitamin C values are preferred (1). Three types of detection systems have been used. Fluorescence detection requires the oxidation of AA to DHAA with ascorbate oxidase or charcoal followed by a reaction with o-phenylenediamine to form a fluorescent quinoxaline derivative (1). These methods measure total vitamin C, i.e. ascorbic and dehydroascorbic acids.

Those LC methods that employ UV detection are less specific and can only measure AA since DHAA is non-UV absorbing (2). In addition, they may not separate AA from IAA (2).

The most recent form of detection used for vitamin C is electrochemical which is extremely sensitive. DHAA is reduced to AA by homocysteine and the total AA measured electrochemically-chemically using an Ag/AgCl electrode (11). Concentrations of DHAA have been found to be fairly low in individual foods and mixed diets compared to AA (12). Good agreement between the vitamin C results obtained using various types of LC methods and the manual fluorometric procedure has been found (7).

Folates. Various LC methods have been developed for the determination of folates but most of these procedures have only been applied to standard mixtures and fortified foods such as infant foods and breakfast cereals where pteroylmonoglutamic acid (PGA) is the predominant form. When these methods have been applied to natural levels found in most foods, extensive sample clean-up and purification is required (13).

Most of the LC methods developed have concentrated on the analysis of folate monoglutamates which requires conjugase treatment of samples prior to analysis. The selection of a deconjugase enzyme and of reaction conditions that provide complete hydrolysis of folate polyglutamates to the monoglutamate level is essential for accurate LC quantification (14). Three types of deconjugase enzymes are available: hog kidney (HK), human plasma (HP) and chicken pancreas (CP). The first two enzymes produce mainly monoglutamate products whereas CP gives essentially diglutamates. Although CP may be less susceptible to inhibition by certain food components compared to HP and HK enzymes (15), it is not advisable to use this enzyme in chromatographic studies as identification and quantification of diglutamate products is difficult due the lack of availability of commercial standards for these forms.

Although HK enzyme gives essentially monoglutamate products, deconjugase activity can be low compared to CP necessitating extensive enzyme clean-up and purification before use (16).

There has been renewed interest in the use of HP as the deconjugase enzyme because it is readily available, it can be used without any purification, it contains low levels of folate and it gives a monoglutamate end-point (17). However, a recent collaborative study has found it may not be as effective as CP or HK in three foods (wheat flour, milk flour and yeast powder) (Lumley & Finglas, unpublished data). A triple enzyme combination consisting of CP (acetone preparation; Difco), α-amylase (*Aspergillus oryzae*; Sigma) and Pronase (Calbiochem-Be-

Table II. Folate content (nmol/g) and distribution in selected foods using LC and microbiological assay (MA)[a]

Food	LC				MA
	THF	5-CH3-THF	5-CHO-THF	Total	
Whole cow's milk	nd[b]	0.07	nd	0.07	0.03
Fresh cabbage	0.07	0.11	nd	0.18	0.29
Orange juice	nd	0.37	nd	0.37	1.90
Wholewheat flour	nd	nd	nd	0	1.59

[a] Adapted from (14)
[b] nd, not detected

hring Corp.) has been reported to give higher folate values in some starchy foods compared to CP alone (18). Similar results have also been found in cereal products using CP, a heat resistant α-amylase (Termamyl; Novo) and amyloglucosidase (Sigma) (19). It is clear that whatever conjugase enzyme is used for folate deconjugation, it should be fully optimized for each food analyzed.

There has also been recent interest in being able to use LC in quantifying not only any type of folate in respect to its carbon substitution but polyglutamate forms as well (20). This would obviously eliminate the need for the lengthy deconjugation step and facilitate the use of simplified extraction systems.

The most promising LC procedures are those based on methods incorporating anion-exchange clean-up followed by hog kidney deconjugation and quantification using the native fluorescence of the reduced folates in an acidic mobile phase (14). Extraction conditions were chosen so that 10-formyl-tetrahydrofolic acid (10-CHO-THF) was quantitatively converted to 5-formyl-tetrahydrofolic acid (5-CHO-THF). While tetrahydrofolic acid (THF) and 5-methyl-tetrahydrofolic acid (5-CH3THF) can be readily quantified using their natural fluorescence, the relatively weak fluorescence of 5-CHO-THF is a limiting factor and requires careful control of the slit widths of the fluorometer during the chromatographic run to give greater sensitivity. For PGA,

THF and dihydro-folic acid, a oxidative post-column derivatiation system using calcium hypochlorite converts these compounds to highly fluorescent pterin compounds. The agreement between this LC procedure and the MA for six foods was found to be poor (Table II) and further work is needed to explain the reasons for this.

Microbiological Procedures

Despite many of the drawbacks concerning the use of microbiological assays for the analysis of water-soluble vitamins, they are still widely used for folate, vitamin B12, pantothenic acid, niacin and biotin. Over the years MAs have received a great deal of attention especially for folates (17). Although the MA has been modified and improved, the basic concept of the assay has not changed.

In our laboratory, the response of folate monoglutamates to *L. rhamnosus* (formerly *L. casei*) has been extensively studied (21-23) and a pH of 6-6.2 found to give equivalent response of the major forms over the 0-1 ng calibration range.

The most recent development in the MA for folates has been the introduction of the 96-well microtitration plate based assay (24, 25). In our experience this has improved assay reliability and increased sample through-put dramatically. Bacterial growth in each well is measured using a microplate reader at 600–670 nm, the entire plate taking 2–3 minutes to read

Table III. Biospecific methods currently developed for the determination of water-soluble vitamins in food[a]

Vitamin	Type	Immunochemicals	Foods analysed	Reference
Biotin	EBPA	1. Avidin-HRP[b], Biotin-KLH	1. Liver	1. 27
		2. Avidin/Streptavidin[b] Biotin-HRP	2. Breakfast cereal	2. 39
Biotin	ELISA	1. Anti-biotin antisera[c] Biotin-KLH	1. Liver	1. –
		2. Anti-biotin antisera[b] Biotin-HRP		
Pantothenic acid (PA)	ELISA	Anti-pantothenic acid[c] antisera, PA-KLH	Milk, eggs, bread, potatoes, liver, lettuce	26
			Bread, milk, rice, vegetables, chicken, beef	30
Pyridoxamine Cyanocobalamin (B_{12})	ELISA EPBA	Anti-pyridoxamine antisera[c], PL-KLH R-protein-HRP, B_{12}-KLH	Breakfast cereals	29
Folates, total	EPBA	1. FBP-HRP, PGA-KLH	1. Vegetables, animal feeds	1. 27
		2. FBP-HRP, BSA-KLH	2. Breakfast cereals, fruit juices	2. 39
PGA	ELISA	3. Anti-folate antisera[b] PGA-KLH	3. Standard mixtures	3. –
5-CHO-THF 5-CH₃-THF		4. Anti-folic antisera[b] PGA-HRP	4. Multivitamin preparations	4. 39

[a] Adapted from (44)
[b] Commercially available
[c] In-house antisera

completely. Seven levels of standard and 16 samples (all in quadruple) are included on each plate, with ten plates in an assay run. Considerable time is saved using the microtitration plate assay over conventional procedures using test tubes.

Biospecific Procedures

During the last five years biospecific methods of analysis using either antibodies [enzyme-linked immunosorbent assay (ELISA) format], or naturally occurring vitamin binding proteins [enzyme protein-binding assay (EPBA) format], have been shown to be capable of producing sensitive and specific assays for a number of B-group vitamins (Table III). Both types of assay are based on the microtitration plate format which is ideally suited to high sample through-put. ELISAs have the greater potential for the measurement of specific vitamers, whereas EPBAs is more useful for broad specificity assays where the analysis of a group of vitamers is required (e.g. folates).

Most of the ELISAs developed at Norwich have used in-house antisera which can take several months to produce. Antisera have been raised against the major, naturally occurring forms of each vitamin. There is, however, a range of commercial antisera (polyclonal and monoclonal) currently available to several vitamins including PGA, 5-MTHF, 5-CHO-THF, vitamin B_{12} and biotin. This should facilitate the development of suitable ELISAs for food use.

There are limited comparative data available comparing results from biospe-

Table IV. Food reference materials (RMs) currently under stability testing for fat- and water-soluble vitamins[a]

RM	Fat-soluble	Water-soluble
Margarine[b]	A, E, D, β-carotene	–
Wholemeal flour	–	B_1, B_2, B_6, folate, niacin, biotin
Milk powder[c]	A, E, D, β-carotene	C, folate, B_{12}, B_1, B_2, B_6
Brussels sprouts[d]	–	C, B_1, B_2, folate, B_{12}, niacin
Pig liver[d]	A, E, D, β-carotene	Folate, B_{12}, C, B_1, B_6, biotin
Mixed vegetables[d]	Carotenoids	C, B_1, B_2, folate, B_{12}

[a] Adapted from (45)
[b] Canned product
[c] Vtamin enriched
[d] Lyophilised

cific methods to MA and HPLC procedures. We have compared the determination of pantothenic acid by ELISA and MA (26); biotin , folate and vitamin B_{12} by EPBA and MA (27-29) and PM by ELISA and LC in a range of foods (30). In general, the agreement between the results obtained using the biospecific methods and the more conventional techniques has been good for those foods analyzed. These techniques also offer the potential of developing simplified extraction systems as it should be possible to measure bound vitamin forms.

■ Community Bureau of Reference (BCR)

In 1988, BCR undertook a research project to improve the quality of vitamin analysis carried out by its Member States for nutritional labeling purposes and the production of food composition data. The project involves about 50 European laboratories specialized in vitamin determinations and includes method intercomparison studies to identify and eliminate sources of error, and the preparation of suitably stable and homogeneous food reference materials (RMs).

Reference Materials (RMs)

The use of certified RMs is an essential part of quality assurance and provides a means by which results can be traced back to a certified value. RMs are especially useful in the development of new techniques. The range of RMs currently under stability testing are given in Table IV. The approach used in the preparation of RMs has been to produce dry foods but taking care to control the lyophilization conditions (time, temperature etc.) in order to minimize vitamin losses. The final materials have been packaged into food grade, aluminum sachets under an inert atmosphere. The homogeneity and stability of a wide range of vitamins are being vigorously tested for each RM.

Method Intercomparison Studies

The first intercomparison of methods for vitamins was organized to study the state of the art in a group of European laboratories experienced in vitamin determinations. A summary of the main results is given in Table V. The agreement between the participants for vitamins B_1 and C, and niacin was good and indicative values were given for three candidate RMs.

For vitamin B_6, two problem areas were identified. Firstly, the identification of the various vitamers proved difficult

Table V. Summary of the results of the First BCR Intercomparison of Vitamins in the candidate food reference materials

Vitamin	Methods used[b]	Number of laboratories	Within- and between- laboratory variation (%CV)		Comments
			%Cv$_W$	%CV$_B$	
Thiamin	LC, fluorometric, MA	10	3–5	11–18	Indicative values given for three RMs
Riboflavin	LC, MA	12	4–7	28–74	Problems in extraction/dephosphorylation step
Vitamin B$_6$	LC, MA	6	4–7	18–51	Problems in peak identification of extraction/hydrolysis
Niacin	MA	7	3–5	9–15	Indicative values given for three RMs
Vitamin C	LC, fluorometric	10	5	15	Indicative value given for one RM

[a] adapted from (7)
[b] LC, liquid chromotography; MA, microbiological assay

and consequently there were large variations in both individual vitamers and total B$_6$ values obtained by the participants (Table VI). Secondly, it was found that glucoside derivatives of pyridoxine were not hydrolyzed by phosphatase and takadiastase enzymes used and required an additional β-glucosidase enzyme to release these forms for LC analysis. However, these forms are unlikely to be absorbed by man and should therefore not be included in the total B$_6$ activity. The microbiological results for B$_6$ were higher due to inclusion of the glucoside forms. There was also large variation in the results for vitamin B$_2$ (Table V) and it

Table VI. Results for B$_6$ content and individual vitamers in three food reference materials (RM)[a]. Results for individual vitamers are means (with ranges in parentheses) from five laboratories using LC procedures.

RM	Individual vitamers (% of total B$_6$)			Total B$_6$ (mg/100 g dry mass)	
	PM[b]	PL[b]	PN[b]	Mean	%CV
Milk powder	25 (21–31)	70 (60–78)	6 (0–16)	0.33	18
Pork muscle	22 (0–47)	67 (53–76)	11 (0–31)	1.32	35
Haricot vert beans	50 (26–100)	31 (0–54)	19 (0–36)	0.17	22

[a] Adapted from (7)
[b] PM, pyridoxamine; PL, pyridoxal; PN, pyridoxine.

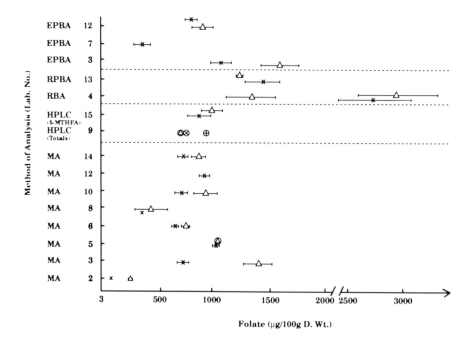

Figure 1. BCR-intercomparison on the determination of folates in food
Determination of folate in a brussels sprouts RM using microbiological assay (MA), enzyme protein-binding assay (EPBA), radioassay kit (RIA) and liquid chromatography (LC). (Δ), chicken pancreas, (x) human plasma and (+) hog kidney deconjugase enzymes. **Results are means +/- 1SD** (Reprinted with permission from *Food Chemistry*, Copyright 1992, Elsevier Applied Science Publishers Ltd).

was concluded that this was due to the hydrolysis/de-phosphorylation step of the procedure.

Few laboratories were able to perform analyses for folate and vitamin B_{12} and thus a second intercomparison was organized for folate analysis in a lyophilized brussels sprouts material using MA, LC, EPBA and radio-protein binding kit (RIA) (13). Three types of deconjugation were investigated: HP, CP and HK. Good agreement was obtained with laboratories using MAs (Figure 1). CP deconjugation gave about 20 per cent higher folate levels in this foodstuff compared to HP. The use of autoclaving followed by CP or HP deconjugation gave lower (10-20 per cent) levels determined by MA when compared to refluxing and deconjugation

with the same enzymes. Problems in the identification of peaks and poor calibration were found in the LC procedures used. In general, EPBA and RIA results were higher than MA and LC values but much more variable. It was concluded that the response of the individual folate forms to the binding protein used in the assay is crucial and careful control of assay pH and type of calibrant is required if an equivalent response to the main folate forms is to be obtained. Further work is needed before LC and other techniques can be used for routine folate analysis in food.

The extraction conditions for the LC determination of vitamins B_1, B_2 and B_6 in three food materials (pork muscle, milk powder and wholemeal flour) have also been investigated. The aim of this study was to optimize conditions for enzyme hydrolysis (pH, time, temperature and sample-enzyme ratio). Four commercially available enzymes which are most commonly used were selected: takadiastase (Pfaltz & Bauer, Serva), phosphatase (Sigma) and a mixture of takadiastase (Fluka) and phosphatase (Sigma). Optimum levels of B_6 in pork and milk powder were found using either takadiastase (Pfaltz & Bauer) or phosphatase (Sigma) with a pH of 4.8-5.5, an overnight incubation and a temperature of 37-45C. The minimum amounts of enzyme needed were 500 mg takadiastase or 50 mg phosphatase per gram of sample. For B_1 in pork and flour, optimum levels were only found using takadiastase (Pfaltz & Bauer) with a pH of 4 and incubation time of four hours. The minimum amount of enzyme needed was 100 mg/g pork and 20 mg/g flour. The conversion of thiamin monophosphate to free thiamin was only about 30 per cent using the takadiastase/phosphatase mixture and these enzymes should be avoided for LC work. Similar results were obtained for B_2 in pork and flour except an overnight incubation and higher enzyme levels (100 mg takadiastase/g pork, 20 mg takadiastase/g flour) were required. The conversion of flavin mononucleotide (FMN) to free vitamin was not complete using both enzyme preparations. The takadiastase/phosphatase mixture gave about 60 per cent conversion whereas takadiastase (Pfaltz & Bauer) gave nearly 80 per cent conversion. This is not a problem in the MA as FMN gives an equivalent growth response compared to riboflavin.

■ Impact of Improvements in the Determination of Water-Soluble Vitamins on the Quality of Food Composition Data in UK Food Tables

Many nutritional studies have relied upon the 4th edition of McCance and Widdowson's *The Composition of Foods* (MW4) for the calculation of nutrient intakes (31). This has been superseded by a revised 5th edition (MW5) (32) containing a much wider range of foods and new analytical data using improved methods of analysis.

One way of assessing the impact of improved vitamin methods is to compare vitamin intake values computed from food composition tables with values obtained by direct analysis of diets consumed. This is also important as many nutritional studies in the literature have relied on MW4 for the calculation of vitamin intakes and it is therefore essential to assess the likely impact on the interpretation of such studies if MW4 is now replaced with revised data given in MW5.

In a study in Norwich, nutrient intake data, collected from 54 adolescents using a 7-day weighed inventory (recorded every 6th day for 7 weeks), calculated using MW4 with the same data calculated using MW5. In addition, intake values obtained using MW4 and MW5 are compared with values obtained by direct analysis of duplicate diets collected on the same day of dietary recording (33, 34). In particular, MW5 versus analyzed values are examined for those nutrients where the agreement was found to be poor when calculated intake values were computed using MW4, for example folate and vitamin B_6 (33). A summary of methods used to analyze duplicate diets for selected water-soluble vitamins are given in Table VII. Typical methods used for

Table VII. Summary of methods used to analyse duplicate diets of schoolchildren in Norwich study for energy and selected water-soluble vitamins and typical methods used for UK food composition tables (MW4 & MW5)[a]

Nutrient	Methods[b] used for duplicate diet analysis (reference)	Methods[e] used for UK food composition folates (reference)	
		MW4	MW5
Energy	Bomb calorimetry corrected to metabolizable energy (40)	Calculation from protein, fat, carbohydrate and alcohol	Calculation from protein, fat, carbohydrate and alcohol
Thiamin (B$_1$)	LC/F (41, 42)	F (43), MA (35)	MA (34), F (43), LC/F (37)
Riboflavin (B$_2$)	LC/F (41, 42)	MA (34), F (43)	MA (34), LC/F (35, 37)
Vitamin B$_6$[c]	LC/F (2, 42)	MA (34)	MA (34), LC/F (2)
Vitamin C[d]	LC/EC (11,42)	T (AA only; 43), F (Total; 43)	T (AA only; 43) F (total; 43)
Folate (total)	MA (21, 42)	MA (34)	MA (34), MA (21)

[a] (31); (32)

[b] LC/F, liquid chromatography with fluorometric detection; LC/EC, liquid chromatography with electrochemical detection and MA, microbiological assay using *Lactobacillus rhamnosus* at pH 6.2

[c] Total vitamin B$_6$ = pyridoxamine (PM) + pyridoxal (PL) + pyridoxine (PN)

[d] Total vitamin C = ascorbic acid (AA) + dehydroascorbic acid (DHAA)

[e] F, fluorometric & T, titrimetric. For MW4, MA (riboflavin): *Streptococcus zymogenes*; MA (thiamin): *Lactobacillus viridescens* or *L. fermienti*; MA (B$_6$): *Saccharomyeces carlsbergensis* and MA (folate): *Lactobacillus casei*. For MW5, MA (thiamin): *L. viridescens*; MA (B$_6$): *Kloeckera apiculata*; MA (folate): *Lactobacillus rhamnosus* & MA (B$_2$): *Streptococcus zymogenes*

food composition data for these vitamins in MW4 and MW5 are also included.

The possible extent of under-recording of total food intake in this study was assessed using mean daily analyzed energy intake values and estimates of daily energy expenditure for similar subjects. It was concluded that there was no gross under-estimation of habitual energy intake and the calculated nutrient intake values represented a good reflection of their habitual intake (12). The results for energy and water-soluble vitamins are given in Table VIII for girls only. Similar trends were found for boys (34).

The major differences in vitamin intake values calculated from MW4 and MW5, and compared to analyzed intake values, were found for folate and vitamin B$_6$.

Folates

In the UK, the microbiological assay conditions of Bell (35) were used to obtain values for the folate content of foods given in MW4. Under these conditions, i.e. initial pH of 6.8 for organism growth and 0-1 ng calibration range, the growth response of *Lactobacillus rhamnosus* (*casei*) to 5-MTHF was poor in comparison to PGA, the normal folate used to calibrate the assay. If the pH is lowered to 6.2, the response of 5-MTHF and PGA is the same (21). Although PGA is used for food fortification because of its greater stability and lower cost, it does not occur naturally. The implication of this is that in foods that contain appreciable amounts of natural folates, the folate values given in MW4 are likely to be grossly under-estimated. This has subsequently led to an apparent underestimate in the true folate intake in the UK (22, 23). Analysis of 128 vegetables for folate using an improved

Table VIII. Average daily intakes of energy and water-soluble vitamins calculated from MW4, MW5 and direct analysis of duplicate diets

Values are means with standard errors for 35 girls (13–14 year olds) with ranges in parentheses.[a]

Nutrient	Calculated MW4[d]	Analyzed[b]	Correlation coefficient, r[c]	Calculated MW5[d]	Analyzed[b]	Correlation coefficient, r[c]
Energy (MJ)	7.23±0.26 (4.3–11.1)	7.36±0.24 (4.5–11.00)	0.94	7.18±0.24 (4.2–10.9)	7.36±0.24 (4.5–11.0)	0.95
Thiamin (mg)	1.1±0.05** (0.6–1.8)	1.5±0.1 (0.6–2.7)	0.43	1.3±0.07* (0.8–2.6)	1.5±0.1 (0.6–2.7)	0.19
Riboflavin (mg)	1.3±0.08* (0.4–2.6)	1.2±0.07 (0.4–2.3)	0.77	1.3±0.07 (0.4–2.4)	1.2±0.07 (0.4–2.3)	0.78
Vitamin B6 (mg)	1.1±0.04* (0.7–1.6)	0.7±0.04 (0.4–1.4)	NS[e]	1.7±0.08 (0.9–3.2)	0.7±0.4 (0.4–1.4)	0.35
Vitamin C (mg)	75±7 (19–182)	84±5 (43–153)	0.66	71±6 (26–144)	84±5 (43–153)	0.56
Folate (mg)	145±8** (61–278)	252±17 (96–510)	0.42	212±9* (103–340)	252±17 (96–510)	0.66

[a] Adapted from (42)
[b] For details of methods see Table VII
[c] Correlation coefficient (r) between calculated MW5 & MW4 and analyzed data for girls [statistical significance of r=P< 0.05]
[d] Calculated MW4/MW5 intake was significantly different from analyzed data: * P < 0.05, ** P < 0.001
[e] NS, not significant

MA found that the revised folate values were about two-fold higher compared to MW4 data (36).

In this study, calculated folate intake values using MW5 are considerably higher (50 per cent) than MW4 intake values and much nearer the values obtained by duplicate diet analysis. The revised folate content of several breakfast cereals, especially cornflakes and muesli, using the improved MA were much higher and made a significant contribution to the total daily intake for this vitamin. Although a weak correlation was found for between MW4 calculated and analyzed intake values for girls, no association was found for boys (33). However, the correlation between MW5 and analyzed intake values is improved, and significant for both sexes.

Vitamin B6

Some doubt has been expressed over the vitamin B6 data appearing in MW4, which has largely been obtained by MA using a variety of test organisms, some of which may not respond equally to all forms and thus total vitamin B6 activity may be underestimated (34). This possible underestimation will vary from food to food depending on the relative amounts of each vitamer present. Much of the newer data for vitamin B6 appearing in MW5 has been obtained using the MA with *Kloeckera apiculata* which should give better estimates for the total vitamin activity than other organisms used. This is likely to have contributed to the large increase in calculated intake values found when using MW5 compared to MW4. The vitamin B6 MW5 values of muesli and cornflakes, which are two of the major contributors to total daily intake of this vitamin, are considerably higher than values appearing in MW4 for these foods.

Some of the vitamin B6 values appearing in MW5, for example raw and cooked vegetables, have been obtained by an LC procedure which permits the separation and quantification of PM, PL and PN forms and the sum of which gives the total vitamin B_6 activity (36). Although the analyzed intake values are about 50 per cent lower than the revised MW5 calculated intake values for total vitamin B_6, there is now a significant correlation between the data for both sexes, which was not found for the MW4 calculated intake versus analyzed values. Clearly further improvements in LC methodology is needed for this vitamin, especially extraction and peak identification, before more reliable food composition data can be obtained.

■ Conclusions

There has been a steady improvement in methods for the determination of water-soluble vitamins in food over recent years notably with the development of LC and biospecifc procedures. These techniques allow the quantification of individual vitamers and thus give better estimates of the vitamin activities of foods than is currently available in food composition tables. Further work is needed on the optimization of extraction/dephosphorylation conditions and comparative data between methods. The availability of a range of certified RMs will greatly assist in method validation and improving the quality of data generated for food composition tables. Care should also be exercised when interpreting dietary intake data from nutritional studies particularly the source, limitations and reliability of the analytical techniques used to acquire them.

■ Acknowledgments

Various parts of this work were supported by the Office of Science and Technology and the European Communities' Community Bureau of Reference.

■ References

(1) Greenfield, H., & Southgate, D.A.T. (1992) in *Food Composition Data*, Elsevier Science Publishers, London

(2) Brubacher, G., Müller-Mulot, W., & Southgate, D.A.T. (1985) *Methods for the Determination of Vitamins in Food,* Elsevier Applied Science, London, pp. 129-140

(3) Finglas, P.M., & Faulks, R.M. (1987) *J. Micronutr. Anal.* **3,** 251-283

(4) Ang, C.Y.W., & Moseley, F.A. (1980) *J. Agric. Food Chem.* **28,** 483-486

(5) Bailey, A.L., & Finglas, P.M. (1990) *J. Micronutr. Anal.* **7,** 147-157

(6) Hilker, D.M., & Clifford, A. J. (1982) *J. Chromatogr.* **231,** 433-438

(7) Hollman, P. C. H., Slangen, J.H., Wagstaffe, P.J., Faure, U., Southgate, D.A.T., & Finglas, P.M. (1993) *Analyst.* **118,** 481-488

(8) Polansky, M.M., Reynolds, R.D., & Vanderslice, J.T. (1985) in *Methods of Vitamin Assay,* J.A. Augustin, B.P. Klein, D. Becker & P.B. Venugopal (Eds.), John Wiley & Sons, New York, pp.427-428

(9) Bitsch, R., & Moller, J. (1989) *J. Chromatogr.* **463,** 207-211

(10) Reitzer-Bergaentzle, M., Marchioni, E., & Hasselmann, C. (1993) *Food Chem.* **48,** 321-324

(11) Behrens, W.A., & Madere, R. (1987) *Anal. Biochem.* **165,** 102-107

(12) Finglas, P.M., Bailey, A.L., Walker, A., Loughridge, J.M., Wright, A.J.A., & Southon, S. (1993) *Br. J. Nutr.* **69,** 563-576

(13) Finglas, P.M., Faure, U., & Southgate, D.A.T. (1993) *Food Chem.* **46,** 199-213

(14) Gregory, J.F., Sartain, D.B., & Day, B.P.F. (1984) *J. Nutr.* **114,** 341-353

(15) Eigen, E., & Shockman, G.D. (1963) *Fed. Proc.* **42,** 2105

(16) Keagy, P.M. (1985) in *Methods of Vitamin Assay,* J. Augustin, B.P. Klein, D.A. Becker & P.B. Venu-

gopal (Eds.), John Wiley & Sons, New York, pp. 450-452

(17) Tamura, T. (1990) in *Folic Acid Metabolism in Health & Disease*, M.P. Picciano, E.L.R. Stokstad & J.F. Gregory (Eds.), Wiley-Liss, New York, pp.121-137

(18) De Souza, S., & Eitenmiller, R. (1990) *J. Micronutr. Anal.* **7,** 37-57

(19) Goli, D.M., & Vanderslice, J.T. (1992) *Food Chem.* **43,** 57-64

(20) Gregory, J.F. (1985) in *Methods of Vitamin Assay*, J.Augustin, B.P. Klein, D.A. Becker & P.B. Venugopal (Eds.), John Wiley & Sons, New York, pp. 473-496

(21) Phillips, D.R., & Wright, A.J.A (1982) *Br. J. Nutr.* **47,** 183-189

(22) Wright, A.J., & Phillips, D.R. (1985) *Br. J. Nutr.* **53,** 569-573

(23) Finglas, P.M., Wright, A.J.A., Faulks, R.M., & Southgate, D.A.T. (1990) in *Recent Knowledge on Iron and Folate Deficiencies in the World,* Vol. 197, S. Hercberg, P. Calan & H. Dupin, (Eds.), Inserm, Paris, pp.385-392

(24) Newman, E.M., & Tsai, J.F. (1986) *Anal. Biochem.* **154,** 509-515

(25) Horne, D.W., & Patterson, D. (1988), *Clin. Chem.* **34,** 2357-2359

(26) Finglas, P.M., Faulks, R.M., Morris, H.C., Scott, K.J., & Morgan, M.R.A. (1988) *J. Micronutr. Anal.* **4,** 47-59

(27) Finglas, P.M., Faulks, R.M., & Morgan, M.R.A. (1986) *J. Micronutr. Anal.* **2,** 247-257

(28) Finglas, P.M., Kwiatkowska, C., Faulks, R.M., & Morgan, M.R.A. (1988) *J. Micronutr. Anal.* **4,** 309-322

(29) Alcock, S.A., Finglas, P.M., & Morgan, M.R.A. (1992) *Food Chem.* **45,** 199-203

(30) Alcock, S.A., Finglas, P.M., & Morgan, M.R.A. (1990) *Food Agric. Immunol.* **2,** 197-204

(31) Paul, A.A., & Southgate, D.A.T. (1978) in *McCance & Widdowson's The Composition of Foods*, 4th Ed., HMSO, London

(32) Holland, B., Welch, A.A., Unwin, I.D., Buss, D.H., Paul, A.A., & Southgate, D.A.T. (1991) in *McCance & Widdowson's The Composition of Foods*, 5th Ed., Royal Society of Chemistry, Cambridge

(33) Southon, S., Wright, A.J.A., Finglas, P.M., Bailey, A.L., & Belsten, J. (1992) *Proc. Nutr. Soc.* **51,** 315-324

(34) Bell, J.G. (1974) *Lab. Pract.* **23,** 235-242, 252

(35) Kwiatkowska, C.A., Finglas, P.M., & Faulks, R.M. (1989) *J. Hum. Nutr. Diet.* **2,** 159-172

(36) Schrijver, J., Speek, A.J., Klosse, J.A., van Rijn, H.J.M., & Schreurs, W.H.P. (1982) *Ann. Clin. Biochem.* **19,** 52-56

(37) Finglas, P.M., & Faulks, R.M. (1984) *Food Chem.* **18,** 37-44

(38) Speek, A.J., Schrijver, J., & Schreurs, W.H.P. (1984) *J. Agric. Food Chem.* **32,** 352-355

(39) Rubach, K., & Reichert, N. (1991) *Deutsche Lebensmittel-Rundschau* **88,** 341-347

(40) Miller, D.S., & Payne, P.R. (1959) *Br. J. Nutr.* **13,** 501-508

(41) Bailey, A.L., & Finglas, P.M. (1990) *J. Micronutr. Anal.* **7,** 147-157

(42) Southon, S., Wright, A.J.A., Finglas, P.M., Bailey, A.L., & Loughridge, J.M. (1994) *Br. J. Nutr.* (in press)

(43) *Official Methods of Analysis* (1975) 12th Ed., AOAC, Arlington, VA

(44) Finglas, P.M., Alcock, S.A., & Morgan, M.R.A. (1992) in *Food Safety and Quality Assurance: Applications of Immunoassay Systems*, M.R.A. Morgan, C.J. Smith, & P.A. Williams (Eds.), Elsevier Applied Science, London, 401-409

(45) Finglas, P.M., Faure, V., & Wagstaffe, P.J. (1993) *Fres. J. Anal. Chem.* **345,** 180-184

Update on the Analysis of Total Lipids, Fatty Acids and Sterols in Foods

Andrew J. Sinclair

Department of Medical Laboratory Science, Royal Melbourne Institute of Technology, GPO Box 2476 V, Melbourne, Vic 3001, Australia

In the last 20 years, there has been an increasing awareness of the nutritional importance of lipids in foods. This has led to a requirement to improve the quality and quantity of data on food lipids in food databases. This paper discusses the extraction of lipids from different food matrices, the use of manual versus automated procedures and problems which occur during the extraction process. Methodological approaches are discussed for the analysis of fatty acid composition and concentration, and the analysis of the sterols by gas chromatography and high pressure liquid chromatography. This paper raises the future requirement for a wider range of food lipid data including quantitative information on tocopherols and tocotrienols, molecular species of triacylglycerols, distribution of fatty acids on the 2-position of the triacylglycerols, cholesterol oxides and other lipid oxidation products.

L ipids are an important group of substances found in food where they make major contributions to taste, flavor and the energy content of the food. Lipids are a heterogeneous class of compounds which makes it difficult to provide a precise definition, however they are classified as those substances insoluble in water and soluble in a range of organic solvents. The information required on lipids for a food database include the total lipid content for the calculation of energy content as well as comparison between foods, the fatty acid types which include the saturates, *cis*- and *trans*-monounsaturates and ω-6 and ω-3 polyunsaturates, and the sterol content and composition, including the proportion of cholesterol in the food. While greater than 95 per cent of most food lipids in westernized countries consist of triacylglycerols (TAG), there are other lipids which need to be considered because of their presence in high concentration in certain foods. These include wax esters (found in high concentration in certain species of fish (1) and phospholipids (found in high concentration in eggs). Fatty acids, although rarely present in foods as such, are major components of all food lipids apart from sterols. Interested readers are referred to specialized books on lipids and lipid analysis (2-5).

▪ Extraction of Samples

The choice of technique to be adopted for the analysis of total lipids can depend on a number of factors including the type of food being analyzed and therefore the lipid classes present, the number of samples to be analyzed and the laboratory facilities. The general approach to the extraction of lipids from biological materials is to denature lipoproteins and enzymes in alcohol and to extract the lipids into an organic solvent. Simple soxhlet extraction in ether has been used in the case of foods with very high concentrations of TAG, such as meat fat and milk fat however this can lead to poor extraction of the more polar lipids (6). There have been many different procedures published for the extraction of lipids (2, 5) including refluxing liver tissue in ethanol (7), use of n-butanol saturated with water for cereals (8), the use of iso-propanol as a preliminary extractant for plant tissue to inhibit phospholipase D activity (2), and a 5-stage extraction process using chloroform and methanol as well as acidic and basic solvents systems (9). A dry column method for the extraction of meat ground up with anhydrous sodium sulfate using columns containing celite followed by elution of the lipids from the column with a variety of solvents has been described (10). Extraction of lipids from lyophilized samples is known to result in difficulty of complete lipid extraction, as illustrated recently by poor recovery of TAG from oysters (11).

The most common process for animal and fish tissues, however, is to blend samples in ten volumes of methanol followed by the addition of 20 volumes of chloroform, with additional re-extraction of the sample (2, 5). This approach was developed by Folch et al. (12) and Bligh and Dyer (13). The addition of antioxidants to the solvents is recommended, at a level of 50-100 mg/L in the case of butylated hydroxytoluene. Use of glass containers with glass stoppers or Teflon-lined caps is mandatory for the extraction and subsequent processing steps and use of re-distilled solvents has been recommended, although highly purified solvents are available from suppliers.

Supercritical CO_2 can also be used to extract lipids from foods followed by weighing of the residue (5, 14). This technique has a number of advantages including extraction of the samples at relatively low temperatures, and use of a non-toxic and inert gas which may satisfy regulatory authorities who are concerned with the use and disposal of hazardous solvents in laboratories.

▪ Removal of Non-Lipid Contaminants

Most polar solvents also extract non-lipids such as sugars, urea, amino acids and salts. It has been claimed that pre-extraction with 0.25 per cent acetic acid will remove contaminants and destroy lipolytic enzymes (15), however this procedure has not been widely adopted. Most contaminants can be removed by washing the organic solvent extract with water or dilute salt solution, with the proportions of solvents to aqueous phase being important to prevent losses of polar lipids (2, 12, 13). These contaminants can also be removed by passing the solvent through Sephadex G25, a procedure which is strongly recommended by Nelson (16). He showed that the extraction of 20 mL of plasma yielded 83.2 mg of organic solvent soluble material before passing through Sephadex where the yield was only 50.1 mg of lipid. Since the total lipid content of foods is usually estimated gravimetrically, this example highlights the importance of removal of non-lipid material. This is particularly important when the individual fatty acid content of foods is based on total lipid value rather than using an internal standard to quantitate the fatty acids (17). Following this clean-up step, the solvent is removed in a rotary evaporator with the water bath set at or near room temperature to protect the lipids which are then transferred in chloroform to a storage tube/flask. The total lipid content is estimated by weighing an aliquot from which the solvent has been evaporated using a stream of nitrogen gas. The remaining lipids should then be stored at −20°C, prior to future analysis of lipid classes, fatty acids, and sterols. The procedures described above are very time consuming, labor intensive and require the use of large volumes of solvents.

■ Automated Lipid Extraction Procedures

There are a number of different automated techniques which can be used to analyze large numbers of food samples which would be ideally suited for the analysis of similar materials for quality control purposes. These include the soxhlet process either with or without acid digestion using solvents such as diethyl ether or chloroform:methanol (6). This technique can allow samples to be analyzed in a batch process, and following

extraction and evaporation of the solvent, the weight of the total fatty acids (after acid treatment) or total lipids is determined gravimetrically.

Another technique is to use a rapid automated procedure to remove water, extraction of the dry residue with dichloromethane and re-weighing the defatted residue which gives a figure for total lipids and percent water. This technique, using an instrument known as the CEM automated analyzer (CEM Corp., Indiana Trail, NC), allows the analysis of one laboratory sample at a time and is rapid (about 5 min/sample), however this process is not suited for further processing of the extracts due to loss of the lipid in the process. We have shown that this procedure does not extract all the phospholipids from meat and this can influence the total lipid value significantly in the case of the analysis of lean meats, such as lean pork, chicken breast and certain cuts of beef (18).

Supercritical CO_2 can be used to extract lipids from foods in a continuous process. The extraction apparatus can be connected to a gas chromatograph (GC) or super-critical fluid chromatography unit for the analysis of the component lipids or for pesticide analysis (5, 14).

Foods or feeds can also be analyzed using infrared analysis, which is a nondestructive technique, using a single sample at a time and which provides data on total lipids, water and protein.

The advantages of these automated techniques are speed of analysis and the use of less solvent or no solvent at all. Disadvantages include the small sample size, the necessity to standardize the infrared analyzer and the CEM analyzer for each food type and the fact that it would be necessary to use a separate conventional extraction technique for the analysis of fatty acids and sterols.

■ Sampling

A major problem exists in relation to determining a representative sample of food to be analyzed when the foods are not homogeneous, as is the case with fresh meat and fish. This problem is exacerbated if the technique adopted requires the use of only a small analytical portion. For example, we have experienced difficulty in taking representative samples for the analysis of meat using the CEM analyzer which uses only 3-5 g meat/analysis. The fat content of these retail meat samples can range from 4 to 50 per cent lipid (19) and the problem occurs at the stage where the lean meat and visible fat are mixed and blended together, and is most evident in meat with a high lipid content. It may be necessary to use a larger food sample to analyze foods which are not homogeneous.

■ Analysis of Lipid Classes

Prior to the analysis of unfamiliar tissues for fatty acid composition and sterols, it is considered essential to examine the lipid extract by thin layer chromatography using a solvent system to separate the non-polar lipids from the phospholipids which remain at the origin. The lipids can be visualized using cupric acetate-orthophosphoric spray (20), followed by heating in an oven at 100°C which leads to sterols showing a characteristic purplish color initially and finally all the lipids char. This procedure can assist in determining the likely identity of the lipid classes (e.g. presence of wax esters in fish flesh) as well as the approximate proportions of each class which is useful to estimate amounts of internal standards to be used in the fatty acid and sterol determinations. More sophisticated options include use of liquid chromatography (LC) (3, 5) or the Chromarod-Iatroscan technique to separate and quantitate lipid classes (5).

■ Determination of Fatty Acid Composition and Content of Foods

For a food database, information is required on chain length of saturates, *cis/trans* isomers of the monounsaturates, and ω-6 and ω-3 polyunsaturated fatty acids (PUFA) (21). There is also a developing interest in the positional distribution of fatty acids on TAG molecule (22) and the molecular species of TAG present in the sample (23). The general procedure for the analysis of the fatty acids is to hydrolyze the fatty acids, form derivatives and then analyze these by GC or LC with quantitation by use of internal standards. At the present time, GC is the method of choice for analysis of fatty acids as methyl esters. There are many different methods for forming the fatty acid methyl esters (FAME), including the use of BF_3 in methanol, 5 per cent anhydrous HCl in methanol, and 1–2 per cent H_2SO_4 in methanol (2). It is usually essential to purify the esters on a small column of fluorisil which removes sterols and oxidized material (2). The most common internal standard is heptadecanoic acid (C17:0), although other odd-chain fatty acids have been used including C13:0, C15:0, C19:0, C21:0 and C23:0. The choice depends on the fatty acids found in the food and the separation of the internal standard from the sample fatty acids. It is preferable to add the internal standard as the TAG if this is the main lipid class, rather than as a free fatty acid. There has been some discussion on the choice of internal standards when the food is rich in long-chain PUFA with Ackman (24) arguing for the use of a standard with a similar retention time (e.g. C23:0) as the fatty acids of interest.

The separation of the FAME is best achieved using polar capillary columns, with a wide range of columns of different lengths, internal diameters and phase thicknesses being commercially available. Columns designed for optimal separation of FAME are available (e.g.. BPX70[a], CPSil 88[a], SP-2560[a] and Omegawax[a]) and the choice depends on the specific separations required. The separation of *cis-* and *trans-*monounsaturated FAME as found in margarines can be achieved successfully on 50-100m columns of BPX70 (25) (Figure 1) and SP-2560[a] (26). Standards for determination of retention times are available commercially with a wide range of mixtures of known composition being available from Nu Chek Prep. Inc. (Elysian, MN). Craske and Bannon (27), amplifying the work of Ackman and Sipos (28) demonstrated that, for a number of common saturated and unsaturated fatty acids, the flame ionization detector theoretical response factors can be calculated from the content of carbon bonded to hydrogen in the molecule. However, primary standards are still essential to determine that both the gas chromatographic parameters and the analyst's manipulative skills are efficiently optimized. Assistance in the confirmation of the identity of unknown FAME can be gained by using non-polar capillary columns (e.g.. methyl silicone) since the unsaturated FAME elute before the saturated FAME using these phases (4). The use of GC mass spectrometry (MS) to confirm the identity of FAME is becoming more common with the wider access to modestly priced instruments. The use of picolinyl esters (13-OH methyl pyridine) of fatty acids for the GC-MS has been recommended for FAME with unusual structures (29).

∎ Determination of Sterol Composition and Content in Foods

The main sterol of interest from a nutritional viewpoint in foods is cholesterol and it is now widely acknowledged that the earlier spectrophotometric methods employed for the estimation of the cholesterol content of foods led to an overestimate of the true amount present (30). The general approach to the analysis of food sterols is to saponify the lipids, isolate the non-saponifiable fraction and analyze the sterols by GC or LC using appropriate internal standards. Cholesterol can also be determined enzymatically (31) using kit methods which are widely available.

In a review of the analysis of sterols by GC or LC (30), details of the direct saponification methods for the analysis of food sterols are discussed. The advantages include reduced solvent volumes and sample preparation times, excellent recoveries compared with the standard AOAC method (32), and application of this method to the analysis of eggs, meats and milk products. A disadvantage could be the very small analytical portion weight which is likely to be problematic with heterogeneous foods (e.g. in the case of eggs, the sample weight amounts to only 200 mg). The compounds present in the non-saponifiable fraction of foods, apart from cholesterol, include plant sterols, tocopherols and tocotrienols, cholesterol oxides and other hydrocarbons such as squalene (30).

A common approach to the separation of sterols in foods is the use of capillary GC with non-polar columns and using a GC with a flame ionization detector. Internal standards of 5 α-cholestane or 5 α-cholestanol have been used, however it is more difficult to separate cholesterol and 5 α-cholestanol, compared with 5 α-cholestane and cholesterol. Separation of the sterols as trimethyl silyl (TMS) ether derivatives has been the preferred method since it is regarded that this improves peak shape, decreases retention times and improves sensitivity, however problems associated with the use of TMS derivatives include hydrolysis and the fact that the reagents are toxic, flammable and corrosive (30). With the development of inert fused silica capillary GC columns, many workers no longer derivatize sterol samples prior to GC analysis (30). LC has been used to separate food sterols, however, while cholesterol does not have a strong absorption in the UV region, absorption at 205 nm can be used (30).

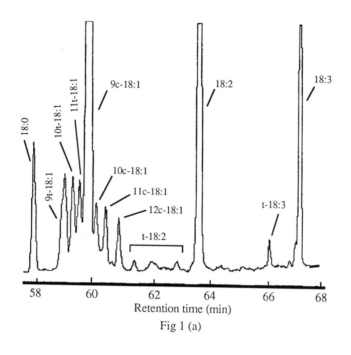

Fig 1 (a)

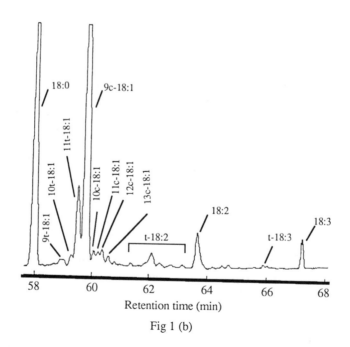

Fig 1 (b)

Figure 1. Gas chromatograms on 50 metre x 0.22mm BPX70 column of (a) margarine and (b) butter showing separation of the main *trans* 18:1 and *cis* 18:1 positional isomers (adapted from Mansour & Sinclair, 25)

■ The future

Cardiovascular disease is still the leading cause of death in most industrialized societies. Recent research into dietary aspects of cardiovascular disease have indicated that it will no longer be sufficient for food databases to have information on the total fat, cholesterol and major fatty acids types of different foods. Because of the increasing interest in oxidation of low density lipoproteins (33), oxidation of cholesterol in food (34, 35), the role of *trans* fatty acids in lipoprotein metabolism (36) and the beneficial effects of the ω-3 PUFA on various aspects of cell metabolism (37), in the future food databases will require detailed information on the tocopherol and tocotrienol isomers, *cis* and *trans* fatty acid isomers, cholesterol oxides and other oxidation products of food lipids, and molecular species and positional distribution of fatty acids in TAG (21-23). Another issue which is likely to emerge as a challenge for analysts in the near future will be the development of standard methods for the wide range of different fat substitutes which have been developed in recent years (38).

■ References

(1)   Vlieg, P., Body, D.R., & Burlingame, B. (1991) *J. N.Z. Diet. Assoc.* **45**, 29-30

(2)   Christie, W.W. (1982) *Lipid Analysis*, 2nd Ed., Pergamon Press, New York, NY

(3)   Christie, W.W. (1987) *High Performance Liquid Chromatography and Lipids*, Pergamon Press, New York, NY

(4)   Christie, W.W. (1989) *Gas Chromatography and Lipids*, The Oily Press, Ayr, Scotland

(5)   *Analysis of Fats, Oils & Derivatives* (1993) E.G. Perkins (Ed.), AOCS Press, Champaign, IL

(6)   Sahasrabudhe, M.R., & Smallbone, B.W. (1983) *J. Am. Oil Chem. Soc.* **60**, 801-805

(7)   Lucas, C.C., & Ridout, J.H. (1970) *Prog. Chem. Fats* **10**, 1-150

(8)   Morrison, W.R., Tan, S.L., & Hargin, K.D. (1980) *J. Sci. Food Agric.* **31**, 329-340

(9)   Rouser, G., Kritchevsky, G., & Yamamoto, A. (1967) in *Lipid Chromatographic Analysis*, Vol 1, G.V. Marinetti (Ed.), Edward Arnold Ltd., London, pp.99-162

(10) Marmer, W.N., & Maxwell, R.J. (1981) *Lipids* **16**, 365-371

(11) Dunstan, G.A., Volkman, J.K., & Barrett, S.M. (1993) *Lipids* **28**, 937-944

(12) Folch, J., Lees, M., & Sloane-Stanley, G.H.S. (1957) *J. Biol. Chem.* **226**, 497-509

(13) Bligh, E.G., & Dyer, W. (1959) *Can. J. Biochem. Physiol.* **37**, 911-917

(14) King, J.W. (1993) *INFORM (J. Am. Oil Chem. Soc.)* **4**, 1089-1098

(15) Phillips, F.C., & Privett, O.S. (1979) *Lipids* **14**, 949-952

(16) Nelson, G.J. (1993) in *Analysis of Fats, Oils & Derivatives*, E.G. Perkins (Ed.), AOCS Press, Champaign, IL, pp.20-59

(17) Weirauch, J.L., Posati, L.P., Anderson, B.A., & Exler, J. (1977) *J. Am. Oil Chem. Soc.* **54**, 36-40

(18) Mann, N.J., Sinclair, A.J., Watson, M.J., & O'Dea, K. (1991) *Food Aust.* **43**, 67-69

(19) Watson, M.J., Mann, N.J., Sinclair, A.J., & O'Dea, K. (1992) *Food Aust.* **44**, 511-514

(20) Fewster, M.E., Burns, B.J., & Mead, J.F. (1969) *J. Chromat.* **43**, 120-126

(21) Sinclair, A.J. (1993) *Food Aust.* **45**, 226-231

(22) Kritchevsky, D. (1988) *Nutr. Rev.* **46**, 177-181

(23) Currie, G.J., & Kallio, H. (1993) *Lipids* **28**, 217-222

(24) Ackman, R.G. (1991) *Lipids* **27**, 858-862

(25) Mansour, M.P., & Sinclair, A.J. (1993) *Asia Pacific J. Clin. Nutr.* **3**, 155-163

(26) Firestone, F., & Sheppard, A. (1992) in *Advances in Lipid Methodology*, Vol. 1, W.W. Christie (Ed.), The Oily Press, Ayr, Scotland, pp. 273-322

(27) Craske, J.D., & Bannon, C.D. (1987) *J. Am. Oil Chem. Soc.* **64**, 1413-1417

(28) Ackman, R.G., & Sipos, J.C. (1964) *J. Am. Oil Chem. Soc.* **41**, 377-383

(29) Harvey, D.J. (1992) in *Advances in Lipid Methodology*, Vol. 1, W.W. Christie (Ed.), The Oily Press, Ayr, Scotland, pp. 19-80

(30) Fenton, M. (1992) *J. Chromat.* **624**, 369-388

(31) Shen, C.J., Chen, I.S., & Sheppard, A.J. (1982) *J. Assoc. Off. Anal. Chem.* **65**, 1222-1224

(32) *Official Methods of Analysis* (1980) 13th Ed., AOAC, Washington, DC, sec. **43.235**

(33) Steinberg, D., Parthasararthy, S., Carew, T.E., Khoo, J.C., & Witztum, J.L. (1989) *New Eng. J. Med.* **320**, 915-924

(34) Chisolm, G.M. (1991) *Current Opinion in Lipidology.* **2**, 311-316

(35) Sarantinos, J., O'Dea, K., & Sinclair, A.J. (1993) *Food Aust.* **45**, 485-490

(36) Mensink, R.P., Zock, P.L., Katan, M.B. & Hornstra, G. (1992) *J. Lipid Res.* **33**, 1493-1501

(37) Sinclair, A.J. (1993) *Asean Food J.* **8**, 3-13

(38) Haumann, B.F. (1993) *INFORM (J. Am. Oil Chem. Soc.)* **4**, 1227-1235

Conventions for the Expression of Analytical Data

David A. T. Southgate

formerly of AFRC Institute of Food Research, Norwich Laboratory,
Colney, Norwich, NR4 7LY, UK

The modes of expression and the conventions used in citing analytical data in nutritional databases are critical for the accurate use of the database. This is especially true for the nutritionist who wishes to use data from a number of different databases or who wishes to merge data from databases in different countries for a specific study. While international agreement on the modes of expressions and conventions is the preferred approach, at the very least it is essential that the documentation of all databases describes in detail the modes of expression and conventions explicitly so that users will know where data are compatible. The major conventions in use are discussed and proposals made for establishing some common positions in the preparation of nutritional databases.

The nomenclature, conventions and modes of expression used to describe the nutrient values have a profound influence on the accurate use of nutritional databases. They are especially important when one is working using a series of different databases. Many nutritional epidemiological studies are being made internationally. For such studies it is often necessary to construct a special database from a number of different sources, and it becomes critically important to ensure that compatible data are being combined. This involves consideration of, first, the compatibility of the analytical methods used to generate the data (1) and, second, that the modes of expression, and for many nutrient values, the conventions used in deriving the values, are also compatible.

Where the analytical methods for a nutrient are specific and the range of methods in use is known to produce comparable values then expression on an appropriate weight basis is straight-forward (2).

There are three major categories of nutrients where the conventions and modes of expression are a major cause of incompatibility. First, where the nutrient values are calculated from some other analytical measurement. Second, where the nutrient is a complex mixture and some analytical compromises have been adopted in the measurement of the mixture. The third category includes those vitamins for which there are a number of active forms (vitamers) which differ in biological activity.

■ Nutrient Values Calculated from Other Analytical Measurements

These cover two of the most important conventions used in the expression of nutrient values in databases; the expression of values for energy and protein.

Energy Values of Foods

In nutritional databases (and in general nutritional usage) the energy values of foods are, strictly, the "metabolizable energy values" in other words, the energy that is available for use by the body. In formal terms metabolizable energy of the dietary intake is equal to the gross (the heat of combustion) energy intake minus the energy lost in feces and urine (other losses should also be included, for example, energy lost in other secretions or gases but in human nutrition these are customarily discounted). Metabolizable energy values thus are, in strict terms, an attribute of the dietary intake and the calculation of values for foods is a pragmatic approximation.

Metabolizable values for foods are calculated using energy conversion factors applied to the amounts of protein, fat, carbohydrates and alcohol in the food.

The energy conversion factors in use in most databases are based on the studies made by Atwater and his colleagues in the early years of this century and it is a tribute to their experimental skills that the system, despite the assumptions which had to be made at that time, remains a practical approximation (3). The Atwater factors adjust the protein, fat and carbohydrate heats of combustion to allow for the fecal losses of these constituents by multiplying the average heats of combustion for mixed proteins, fats and carbohydrates, by the respective apparent digestibilities of the three components. The energy loss in urine was allowed for by correcting the protein value for the energy per unit nitrogen lost in urine.

These calculations give the familiar, 4, 9, 4 factors (kcal per g of protein, fat, and carbohydrate, respectively), which are still widely used.

There are two other conventions used in nutritional databases.

Specific Energy Conversion Factors. This was originally developed by Atwater but not used by him. It was later advocated by Merrill and Watt (4). This convention is based on the premise that it would be better to use heats of combustion values specific for the different foods (or food groups) and to use specific apparent digestibility values for the constituents of each food (or group), rather than to use average values derived for mixed diets. This system depends on having experimental data for the heats of combustion for all components of foods and extensive data from human metabolic studies, and at the present time relies heavily on early data, some from Atwater himself. It is important that databases using this system document, precisely, which factors have been used for specific foods as the published account can be interpreted in different ways

Modified Atwater System Used in the UK Nutritional Database. In the United Kingdom a different system was developed by McCance and Widdowson (5). The need for this arose because these authors measured carbohydrates directly (as opposed to Atwater's use of the "by difference" method) and furthermore, they divided the food carbohydrates into two categories; "available" the digestible sugars and starches, which were glucogenic in man and "unavailable", those carbohydrates not digested in the small intestine and not providing the body with absorbable carbohydrates. For the available carbohydrates they assigned the energy conversion factor 3.75 kcal per g (this is the heat of combustion of monosaccharides) because available carbohydrates were expressed in this way. Unavailable carbohydrates were assigned a zero energy value, not because they did not provide energy but because these components were known to reduce the apparent digestibility of proteins and fats and therefore any energy from the short chain fatty acids produced by fermentation in the large bowel was discounted.

Detailed evaluation of this approach in experimental studies on a large number of subjects showed that it gave a good prediction of metabolizable energy intakes (6). The UK system gives lower energy values for plant foods that are rich in plant cell wall material (and incidentally organic acids).

Comparisons of the Three Conventions. In practical terms the three conventions give similar values. The Atwater system tends to give over-estimates of metabolizable energy and the UK system under-estimates energy intakes at very high unavailable carbohydrate intakes because of the increasing importance of the energy from the fermentation products of the unavailable carbohydrates. It has been suggested (7) that a radically different system based on measured heats of combustion of foods would be intellectually more satisfying but in practical terms the differences produced by the three systems are much smaller than the errors inherent in ignoring individual differences in digestibility and the errors in measuring food intakes. Provided that it is recog-

nized that these conventions are approximations and energy values are not cited to four significant figures the practical incompatibilities are not significant (2).

Protein

Virtually all nutritional databases give values for protein that are derived by calculation from measured total nitrogen values. These have been customarily measured by the Kjeldahl method. These calculated values should be called "crude protein" and recognized as a approximations and not as estimates of protein in a biochemical sense. The factors used for calculating protein are based on the percentage of nitrogen in a typical proteins. Thus 6.25 is appropriate for proteins with 16 g N per 100 g protein.

The FAO expert report on protein requirements in 1973 (8) recommended that different factors should be used for calculating "crude" protein values for different food groups to take account of the N-content of different food proteins and this approach has been followed in the UK nutritional database (5, 13). When the protein and energy requirements were reviewed again in 1985 (9), it was clear that the use of these factors produced anomalies when making recommendations for protein intakes. This arises because all the experimental studies on protein requirements have been based on the measurement of nitrogen metabolism and it has been argued that it would be better to avoid confusion by using only 6.25 as a conversion factor.

In nutritional terms it would be preferable to move to more biochemically coherent measures where protein values were based on estimates of amino acid nitrogen content using amino acid composition data. The practice of correcting for non-protein, non-amino acid nitrogen is desirable for some foods especially cartilaginous fishes and some fungi in order to avoid over-estimating the protein in these foods.

As a general principle it is desirable that all databases include total nitrogen values so that when merging data a consistent approach to calculating crude protein values can be adopted. It is important to ensure that users do not equate (N x a factor) with a biochemical concept of protein as functional polymers of amino acids and to recognize the conventional approximation.

■ Complex Nutrients Involving Analytical Compromises

The nutrients which fall into this category include fat, the carbohydrates and the folates. The essential difficulties arise because these nutrients are very complex mixtures the determination of which requires time-consuming separations which are not widely used in routine food analysis. This means that most of the data available to database compilers is based on simple methods and the values obtained tend to be method-dependent.

Fat

The values for fat in most databases are for "total lipid-solvent soluble material", which includes the triacylglycerol compounds, sterols and depending on the method used, phospholipds. Several of the methods in common use do not extract the lipids efficiently from some food matrices and the values cited in databases may be incompatible because of this method-dependence. In the compilation of databases preference should be given to values obtained using methods that give complete extraction such as those used to prepare extracts for fatty acid analysis (2) with all values documented by method.

Carbohydrates

The main difficulties arise from the incompatibility between carbohydrates values obtained "by difference" and by direct analysis. Direct analysis provides values for the different classes of sugars, mono-, di- and oligo-saccharides starch and non-starch polysaccharides (the major components of dietary fiber) (10). The sum of the individual components approximates to the total carbohydrate "by difference" if the food does not contain substantial amounts of non-carbohydrate components. It is important to recognize that "by difference" values also include errors in the measurement of water content, ash, protein and total lipid.

In the UK database the available carbohydrates are expressed as monosaccharides, which means that the summation of the values will exceed the total carbohydrate "by difference" by a significant amount especially in starch-rich foods because of the addition of water on hydrolysis of disaccharides and polysaccharides.

The ideal from the analytical point of view is to move away from the technically obsolete "by difference" method; but at the present time it is essential to identify the method used when giving carbohydrate values. This is especially true for dietary fiber where the methods in use measure conceptually different fractions. Thus dietary fiber values should be cited (measured as total dietary fiber, AOAC, or as non-starch polysaccharides etc.).

Folates

A large number of folate vitamers exist in foods. The biological availability of them is an active topic of research and there are chromatographic methods for the separation of the different forms, although these are technically exacting and not suitable for routine use at the present time. Most values in nutritional databases are based on microbiological determinations using either *Streptococcus faecalis* or *Lactobacillus caseii* (*rhamnosus*). Deconjugation of the polyglutamyl chain has to be used to measure total folates. At one time it was assumed that a value measured before deconjugation represented free monoglutamyl folates but is now clear that this value includes contributions from the polyglutamyl forms and has no value for the nutritional classification of the folates. *S. faecalis* does not respond to some folates and the values obtained are significantly lower than when using *L. rhamnosus*. It is thus critically important to identify the organism used in the assay when citing folate values (11).

■ Assigning Biological Activity to Different Vitamers

This concerns those vitamins where there are a range of vitamers in foods which have differing biological activities and where it is customary in nutritional databases to give some kind of aggregated value for the vitamin activity of the food. The major vitamin which falls into this category is vitamin A, where it has become accepted to give a vitamin A value expressed as micrograms retinol equivalents, based on summation of the amounts of retinol and the activity of different carotenoids. An analogous convention has been proposed for vitamin E where the aggregated α-tocopherol equivalents are being estimated by summing the weighted values of the different tocopherols and tocotrienols.

Vitamin A Activity

The accepted convention is to take the values for the provitamin carotenoids and divide by factors which reflect the efficiency of conversion to retinol. These conversion factors are based on studies with mixed diets and there is growing evidence that the efficiency of conversion is profoundly affected by the amount of fat in the diet and on the structure of the food matrix, so that under some conditions the carotenoids may not contribute to vitamin A status. The convention is to divide β-carotene values by 6 and other carotenoids by 12 to convert them to retinol equivalents. Some authors argue that the conversion efficiency of the β-caro-

tene in dairy foods is under-estimated by the use of 6 and suggest 3 but the evidence for this is not totally convincing (12).

At the present time there is growing evidence that the carotenoids are important nutrients in addition to their role as provitamin A compounds and this suggests that databases should firstly, give values for retinol and the different carotenoids separately. If a total vitamin A activity is deemed useful in addition, the convention used must be described. Such an approach permits users to assign their own convention and to use different conventions as understanding of the factors determining the efficiency of conversion improves.

Vitamin E Activity

The biological activity of the tocopherols and tocotrienols vitamers is related in this convention to the activity of α-tocopherol. The biological evidence for calculating the biological activity factors is limited but the approach is being used in the UK database (13).

Once again it is desirable that the databases contain the values for the different forms so that users can apply their own consistent conversion conventions. Should the compilers wish, in addition, to give a total vitamin E activity value in the database then the convention must be documented.

■ Development of Agreed Conventions and Modes of Expression

The interchange systems developed by INFOODS (14) allow for the documentation of data values within the exchange tags which incorporate units and details of method where values are method-dependent. In the context of this paper "method-dependence" is restricted to those instances where different methods give different values, not to differences arising because of differences in the performance of the method. Values that have been calculated by conventions, such as energy and protein are similarly assigned different tags where this is appropriate. One has therefore within the INFOODS interchange scheme a system that should prevent the aggregation of incompatible data. The primary need at present for those involved in merging data from databases where different conventions have been used is to resolve the differences so that they can bring the values into a consistent compatible form. This depends on having access to complete documentation of all databases, and at the primary data source level, avoiding any tendency to aggregate original analytical data.

Thus if a database has values for protein, fat and carbohydrate (however expressed) it is possible to recalculate energy values de novo to avoid incompatibilities. Similarly total nitrogen values give the possibility of calculating protein values using either one or several factors.

At the present time some carbohydrate values are incompatible without more detailed analytical information than is currently available. This is especially true for dietary fiber values because the crude fiber values still given in some databases are incompatible with dietary fiber values. In principle TDF values should be higher than NSP values but taken across the whole range of plant foods resistant starch may be of the order of 3–6 g per day and lignin intakes rarely exceed 1 g per day so in practical terms great errors will not flow from combining these two types of values .

In the case of the vitamins the biological equivalents will undoubtedly change as more evidence emerges and it is essential to accumulate and give the actual analytical values for the different vitamers in databases to permit reappraisal in the future.

Finally documentation as part of the database should be seen as the ideal. We really should be aiming for imbedded information (15) so that the user can easily establish what a nutrient name implies and where analytical methods may make the values method-dependent.

Conventions should be recognized as such and the values they provide recognized as approximations of biological phenomena and treated as one would treat all derived values, with caution.

■ References

(1)   Southgate, D.A.T. (1985) *Ann. Nutr. Metab.* **29**, Suppl., 49-53

(2)   Greenfield, H., & Southgate, D.A.T. (1992) *Food Composition Data: Production, Management and Use,* Elsevier Applied Science, London

(3)   Allison, R.G., & Senti, F.R.(1983) *A Perspective on the Application of the Atwater System of Food Energy Assessment,* Federation of American Societies for Experimental Biology, Bethesda, MD

(4)   Merrill, A.L., & Watt, B.K. (1955) *Energy Value of Foods,* US Dept of Agriculture, Handbook 74, USDA, Washington, DC

(5)   Paul, A.A., & Southgate, D.A.T (1978) *McCance and Widdowson's The Composition of Foods,* 4th Ed., HMSO, London

(6)   Southgate, D.A.T., & Durnin, J.V.G.A.(1970) *Br. J. Nutr.* **24**, 517-535.

(7)   Livesey, G. (1991) *Proc. Nutr. Soc. Aust.* **16**, 79-87

(8)   FAO/WHO Expert Group (1973) *FAO Nutrition Series,* No.52, FAO, Rome

(9)   FAO/WHO/UNU (1985). *WHO Technical Report Series 724,* WHO, Geneva

(10) Southgate, D.A.T (1991) *Determination of Food Carbohydrates,* 2nd Ed., Elsevier Applied Science, London

(11) Finglas, P.M., Faure, U., & Southgate, D.A.T. (1993) *Food Chem.* **46**, 199-213

(12) WHO (1967) *WHO Technical Report Series* 362, WHO, Geneva

(13) Holland, B., Welch, A.A., Unwin, I.D., Buss, D.H., Paul, A.A., & Southgate, D.A.T. (1991) *McCance and Widdowson's The Composition of Food,* 5th Ed., Royal Society of Chemistry, Cambridge

(14) Klensin, J.C., Feskanich, D., Lin, V., Truswell, A.S., & Southgate, D.A.T. (1989) *Identification of Food Components for INFOODS Data Interchange,* UNU Press, Tokyo

(15) Southgate, D.A.T. (1992) in *The Contribution of Nutrition to Human and Animal Health,* E.M. Widdowson & J.C.Mathers, (Eds.), Cambridge University Press, Cambridge, pp.369-378

Quality Control of Food Composition Data and Databases

This Session was chaired by Dr Dorothy Mackerras of the Department of Public Health, Sydney University. The keynote address entitled *Food Classification and Terminology Systems* was given by J.A.T. Pennington. This was followed by papers on *Nutritional Metrology: the Role of Reference Materials in Improving Quality of Analytical Measurement and Data on Food Components* by J.T. Tanner, W.R. Wolf and W. Horwitz, *Strategies for Sampling: the Assurance of Representative Values* by J. Holden and C.S. Davis, and *Assuring Regional Data Quality in the Food Composition Program in China* by G. Wang and X. Li, and *Quality Control for Food Composition Data in Journals — a Primer* jointly presented by K.K. Stewart and M. R. Stewart. These papers are published on the following pages.

The paper by B. Perloff and S. Gebhardt, *Building Data Quality in the Data Base Management Process*, is not included. The authors can be contacted at the US Department of Agriculture, 4700 River Road, Riverdale, MD 20737, USA.

Posters presented after Session III were:

- *Criteria Used for Analytical Data Evaluation*, Buick, D., Mottershead, R., & Scheelings, P., Australian Government Analytical Laboratory, Seaton, SA, Australia.

- *Evaluation of Foods as Analytical Control Samples,* Buick, D., Pant, I, Trenerry, C., & Scheelings, P., Australian Government Analytical Laboratory, Seaton, SA, Australia

- *Development of an In-house Nutrition and Food Science Bibliographic Database Using Micro CDS/ISIS,* Chia, W.Y., & Greenfield, H., Department of Food Science and Technology, University of New South Wales, Sydney NSW, Australia.

- *APINMAP - an Integrated Database of Medicinal and Aromatic Plants,* Henninger, M., School of Information, Library and Archive Studies, University of New South Wales, Sydney, NSW, Australia.

- *Food Analysis Reference Materials for the Asia-Pacific,* James, K.W., DSTO, Materials Research Laboratory, Scottsdale, TAS, Australia.

- *International Survey on Dietary Fiber Definition, Analysis and Reference Materials,* Lee, S.C., & Prosky, L., Kellogg Company, Battle Creek, MI 49016, and US FDA, Washington, DC 20204, USA.

- *Desktop Publishing of Food Tables,* Mikkelsen, B.E., Danish Catering Centre, Institute of Food Chemistry and Nutrition, National Food Agency, Søborg, Denmark.

- *Information Sources in Nutrition and Food Science and Technology,* Mobbs, S.L., & Siu, C.S., Biomedical Library, University of New South, Sydney NSW, Australia.

- *Interface Standard for Food Databases,* Pennington, J.A.T., Hendricks, T.C., Douglass, J., Peterson, B., & Kidwell, J., Center for Food Safety and Applied Nutrition, US FDA, Washington, DC 20204, USA.

- *Development of ASEANFOODS Reference Materials,* Pustawien, P., & Sungpuag, P., Institute of Nutrition, Mahidol University, PO Box 31, Talingchan, Bangkok 10170, Thailand.

Food Classification and Terminology Systems

Jean A.T. Pennington

Food and Drug Administration, 200 C Street, S.W.,
Washington, DC 20204, USA

Food classification systems organize foods in databases among groups and subgroups based on food type (e.g., grain products, fruits) and/or food use (e.g., beverages, main dishes). The food groups and subgroups vary among databases according to the number and types of foods in the database, the cultural uses of the foods, and specific decisions made by the database compiler. Terminology systems are structured methods of applying descriptive terms (e.g., terms relating to packaging, processing, color, maturity) to foods. Faceted terminology systems assign descriptive terms for specific characteristics of foods, allowing these characteristics to be considered independently. Eurocode is a food classification, coding, and terminology system. Langual/Interface Standard is a faceted food description system with standardized vocabulary, and the INFOODS system is a free-text faceted food description system.

The words used to classify, name, and describe foods are a mixture of traditional, fanciful, technical, and sensory terms. Sometimes these terms convey a clear picture of what a food is, especially if one is already familiar with it. For a food that is not familiar, the mental image conveyed by the terms is important to understanding the food and the data associated with it. Food names and the terms associated with them are key to the use of information in food-related databases. There should be sufficient descriptive information about the food to clearly understand what the data represent.

Table I. Food classification systems (number of groups in each database)

References	(1)	(2)	(3)	(4)	(5)	(6)	(7)	(8)	(9)
Food Type Classifications									
Milk and eggs						1			
Milk and milk products	1	1	1	1	1		1	1	1
Eggs	1	1	1	1	1		1	1	1
Meat, poultry, fish							1	1	
Meat and poultry	1	1	1	1	1				1
Meat						3			
Poultry						1			
Luncheon meat &sausages						1			
Fish and shellfish	1	1	1	1	1	1			1
Fats and oils	1	1	1	1	1	1	1		1
Grain products	1	1	1	1	1	3	1	1	1
Fruits and vegetables								1	
Fruits	1		1	1	1	1	1		1
Fruits and nuts		1							
Fruit juices/nectars		1							
Legumes, nuts, seeds	1						1		
Nuts and seeds				1	1	1		1	1
Vegetables	1	1	1	1	1	1	1		1
Legumes						1			1
Potatoes and roots			1						1
Food Use Classifications									
Beverages	1	3		1	1	1	1	1	1
Alcoholic beverages		1			1				
Sugars/syrups/sweets	1	2		1	1		1	1	1
Special nutritional use	1								
Herbs/spices/ flavourings		1			1	1		1	
Snacks						1		1	
Soups/sauces/gravies/dressing					1	1		1	
Fast foods						1			
Baby food						1			
Prepared products								1	
Miscellaneous/other	1	3	1	1				7	1
Number of major groups	13	19	10	12	14	21	10	29	14

References

(1)	Eurocode 2	(6)	USDA Agriculture Handbooks
(2)	Germany	(7)	USDA Nationwide Food Consumption
(3)	Sweden		Survey
(4)	Australia	(8)	Langual
(5)	Britain	(9)	Near East

∎ Classification Systems

Classification systems refer to the groupings and subgroupings of foods in databases, based on food type (e.g., vegetables, dairy products) and/or food use (e.g., beverages, fast foods, snacks) (Table I). Most food composition databases, except those arranged alphabetically, are organized by such groupings. These groupings assist database users in locating foods and comparing the nutrient content of similar products. They also reduce the repetition of group and subgroup headings. The number of major food groups found in nine selected databases (1-9) ranges from 10 to 21 (Table I).

Foods in the major groups are usually subgrouped by more precise food names or by descriptive terms, creating hierarchies within each major group. For example, meats may be subgrouped by beef, lamb, and pork, and desserts may be subgrouped by cakes, cookies, and pies. Beef may be further subgrouped by specific cuts (brisket, loin, steak), grade (choice, good, prime), and/or fat trim (0", ¼", ½"). Cookies may be further subgrouped by flavor ingredients (chocolate chip, oatmeal, peanut butter, sugar) or source (commercial, homemade).

As Table I shows, food type classifications vary somewhat among countries. For example, some databases group all vegetables together. Others have separate groupings for legumes and root vegetables; some group legumes and nuts together. However, there is probably better international agreement for food type than for food use groupings because the use of foods in daily diets varies among ethnic and cultural groups. Food use categories are particularly useful to group together products with common dietary use that could be "lost" among food type classifications. For example, under "snack foods" in the USDA Agriculture Handbook No. 8-19 (6), one finds vegetable-based products (potato chips/crisps), grain-based products (corn chips, tortilla chips, popcorn), and fruit or nut-based products (trail mix, banana chips).

Food Grouping Problems

For databases with both food type and food use classifications, there may be some difficulty in placing foods that fit under two or more groups. For example, "French fries" (an American food equivalent to British "chips") could be classified under "vegetables" or "fast foods"; "cookies" (American food equivalent to British "biscuits") could be classified under "grain products" or "desserts"; "bouillon" (American term equivalent to British "beef tea") could be classified under "soups" or "beverages." Such products may be forced into one group or listed in several. The latter solution would result in foods with the same name being in different groups, e.g., some French fries under the fast food group and some under the vegetable group. This makes it difficult for users to locate similar foods and compare their nutrient content.

Within each major food group, similar decisions about how to place foods among subgroups must be made, especially if there are rigid hierarchies. Some foods clearly fit two or more subgroups. For example, "Irish coffee" (American name for coffee with whiskey) is clearly a "beverage," but is both an "alcoholic beverage" and a "coffee beverage". Other foods seem to be transitions between food groups or subgroups. For example, a broth with chunks of meat and vegetables may be a transition between a soup and a stew.

In hard-copy databases with space constraints, subgroups are usually formed by identifying common descriptive terms and using them as subgroup headings. This may lead to some inconsistences in a database as to how subgroups are formed. For example, pancakes and waffles could be subgrouped under grain products first by type (frozen, frozen batter, home-made, liquid batter) and then by flavor (blueberry, cinnamon, plain, old fashioned, strawberry, whole grain) or the other way around. A fast-food fish sandwich might be subgrouped by entree type "fish," by entrée type "sandwiches," or by restaurant name (e.g., "McDonald's").

Decisions about groups and subgroupings are usually made by the database compiler after the data are collected and sorted. At that point, the number of repetitive terms can be determined and minimized. The provision of an index assists users in locating foods that might be placed in multiple groups or subgroups or that have inconsistent subgroup structure from group to group.

In computerized databases, one might view only one food name (and its descriptors) at a time without benefit of seeing the other foods and descriptors in the classification hierarchy. It is necessary to repeat descriptive terms in this case. For example, the terms "breakfast cereal," "cookie," and "frozen dinner" would need to be repeated with each listing for which it is appropriate.

■ Terminology Systems

Terminology systems refer to the systematic methods of applying descriptive terms to foods. These terms, which provide information about color, flavor, maturity, preparation, preservation, brand names, etc., are important because the nutrient contents of foods vary according to such terms. For example, the USDA database for the 1987-88 NFCS (7) lists 18 entries for string beans, each of which has different nutrient values based on descriptive terms for color, preservation, cooking, and/or added ingredients. Descriptive terms also provide insights about food safety (storage, preservation) and nutritional quality (fortification, processing).

The simplest type of terminology system is one which orders the descriptive terms (as appropriate) around the food name (linear descriptors). Descriptors for most food names could be ordered in several ways. Database compilers generally try to use consistent terms and ordering of linear descriptors to facilitate the use of the database.

Faceted terminology systems assign descriptive terms for each food for specific characteristics (facets). The terms are not necessarily a part of the food name, but are linked to the food name in a manual or computerized system. Faceted systems allow for different characteristics of food to be considered independently. To develop such a system, one must identify the facets, collect the descriptive terms belonging to each facet, and define the terms.

Faceted systems for foods are based largely on the faceted system developed in 1971 by the International Network of Feed Information Centers (INFIC) for international exchange and dissemination of information about feeds (10). Approximately 21,000 feeds have been described according to the facets: origin, part, process, growth stage, cut, and grade. The descriptive information (in English, French, and German) and numerical data associated with various feeds can be stored, summarized, retrieved, and printed in various formats.

Three unique terminology systems are briefly discussed: Eurocode 2 (1), a food classification/coding/terminology system; Langual/Interface Standard (8,11,12), a faceted description system with standardized vocabulary; and the INFOODS system (13), a free-text faceted description system.

Eurocode 2

Eurocode was originally developed in the early 1980s as a common European system for coding foods consumed by participants in dietary surveys (14,15). In this case, "coding" refers to the assignment of alphanumeric codes to foods in databases. The codes link the food name to the data (e.g., composition or consumption data) associated with it and allow for computer manipulation of the data. The Eurocode 2 manual (1) provides

Table II. The Eurocode system[a]

Eurocode Fields with Examples

Field 1. Field 2. Field 3. Field 4
Main group.Subgroup.Food name.Recipe (optional)

Meat and meat products (3)
    Mutton (3.4)
        Mutton, carcass meat (3.4.1)
            Mutton recipe prepared in Ireland (3IE.4.1.2)[b]

Grains and grain products (6)
    Wheat breads (6X.1)[c]
        Rusks (6X.1.8)

Vegetables and products (8)
    Cabbages (8.2)
        Kohlrabi (8.2.6)

Eurocode Descriptors	Examples
T Thermal treatment at consumption	T7 (deep fried)
N Non-thermal treatment	N4 (mashed)
P Preservation method/packing medium	P19 (frozen)
A Component added	A10 (fiber added)
R Component removed	R4 (skin removed)

[a] Information adapted from Poortvliet and Kohlmeier (1)
[b] IE indicates a recipe prepared in Ireland. The "2" in the fourth field indicates a specific recipe for a dish based on mutton, e.g., Irish stew
[c] The X in the first field indicates that this food has been coded as a mixed food

rules for coding single foods, mixed foods, and foods as recipes. The codes (as described in the manual) may to be applied to foods in manual or computerized databases.

The food codes have four fields (Table II). The first field identifies one of 13 main food groups, the second field identifies the food subgroup, the third field identifies the food item, and the fourth field, which is optional, provides reference to a recipe. For example, in the code for rusks, 6X.1.8, 6 represents grain products and 6X.1 represents wheat breads. The "X" in the first field indicates that a food is coded as a mixed food (i.e., a multi-ingredient food). A two-character country code replaces the "X" to identify the country for a national recipe. For example, 3IE.4.1.2 is the code for a mutton recipe prepared in Ireland (3 is for meat and meat products, IE if for Ireland, 3.4 is for mutton, 3.4.1 is for mutton carcass meat, and the 2 at the end refers to the recipe).

Eurocode 2 provides an optional terminology system with descriptive terms for five facets: thermal treatment, non-thermal treatment, preservation and packing, components added, and components removed. Descriptors are identified with alphanumeric codes (e.g., T7 for the thermal treatment "deep fried"), and definitions are provided for consistent coding. The authors of the Eurocode 2 manual indicate that the descriptors are designed for dietary surveys and do not attempt to

Table III. Langual factors and examples of factor terms

Langual Factors		Examples of Factor Terms
1.	Product type	Breakfast cereal
2.	Food source (plant or animal)	Leafy vegetable
3.	Part of plant or animal	Organ meat
4.	Physical state, shape or form	Semisolid
5.	Extent of heat treatment	Partially heat-treated
6.	Cooking method	Cooked by dry heat
7.	Treatment applied	Hydrogenated
8.	Preservation method	Pasteurized by heat
9.	Packing medium	Packed in gelatin
10.	Container or wrapping	Paperboard container
11.	Food contact surface	Plastic
12.	Consumer group/dietary use	Human food, low calorie
13.	Geographic places and regions	
	a. Area of origin (grown/produced)	Zimbabwe
	b. Area of processing	Italy
	c. Area of consumption	Tennessee
14.	Cuisine	Chinese
15.	Adjunct characteristics of food (examples)	
	Color of poultry meat	Dark meat
	Grade of meat, US	Choice grade
	Plant maturity	Ripe or mature
	Location of preparation	Restaurant/fast food prepared

satisfy the degree of technical detail used in food technology (1).

Langual

Langual is a faceted food description language that has been under development by the US Food and Drug Administration (FDA) since the early 1970s (8). It is a software system that may be applied to food-related databases such as those of food composition and food consumption. Each food is assigned a set of descriptors, using standardized language, from the following facets: product type; food source; part of plant or animal; physical state, shape, or form; extent of heat treatment; cooking method; treatment applied; preservation method; packing medium; container or wrapping; food contact surface; consumer group/dietary use; geographical places and regions; cuisine; and adjunct characteristics (Table III). If the factor term for a food is not known or does not apply for a food, the terms "unknown" and "not applicable" may be used. For internal storage and processing, factor terms are assigned alphanumeric codes. Langual is currently used on a mainframe computer at FDA, but has been adapted for personal computers in other locations.

Foods in various databases may be searched or retrieved by one or more of the Langual descriptive terms. The more accurate the descriptions of the foods, the more informative are the searches and retrievals. To facilitate retrieval and aggregation, the descriptors within each facet are arrayed in a hierarchy from broader to narrower terms. The vocabulary includes definitions for the terms and explains when and in what contexts they should be used. The Langual thesaurus includes cross references for synonyms and Latin names, and for preferred, broader, narrower, and related terms.

An European Langual Working Group was established in the early 1990s to be the focal point for Langual use in Europe and to communicate needs to the US Langual Committee. In May 1992, Langual was evaluated for use in European databases. Several European dietitians/nutritionists were trained in Langual and were asked to code a number of foods to determine the applicability of Langual to European foods. The results of this test indicated that Langual is an appropriate terminology system for European foods (16).

The concept of an interface standard (a common communication link based on the food name and descriptors) to allow international exchange of food-related data arose at a meeting of the Committee on Data for Science and Technology (CODATA) in March 1990 in Maryland, USA. Criteria for an international interface standard were drafted at this meeting, and FDA used those draft ideas to formulate an interface using Langual (11). The interface was further refined under a FDA contractual effort (Figure 1) (12), and the computer software for the interface standard is expected to be completed in April 1995.

The aspects of the interface standard, which are linked to the food names, include food name synonyms, Langual factor terms, other food descriptors (agricultural and storage variables), other descriptive coding systems, ingredients and recipes, food standards, and reference files. The reference files allow for the identification of substances administered or applied during production and storage, the organization that produced or prepared the food, and the source of the data.

As much information as possible is provided about the food without making questionable assumptions. Only those descriptors that pertain to a food need to be used. Once the foods in a database are described according to the interface, databases may be queried and information may be retrieved. The system will also allow for matching (or finding the closest matches) of foods in different databases.

INFOODS

The International Network for Food Data Systems (INFOODS) was organized to improve the quality and accessibility of food composition databases. It was funded by US government agencies from 1984 to 1987 with headquarters at the Massachusetts Institute of Technology. The Food Nomenclature and Terminology Committee (one of the three INFOODS committees) was charged with developing a proposal to standardize the nomenclature and description of foods to allow for useful exchange of food composition data among countries (13).

The Committee met at several international meetings and worked via mail to develop and refine a system for describing foods. The report that resulted from this work (13) provides for free text descriptors for specific characteristics of foods. The system, which was not specifically designed for computer implementation, includes six major facets (Table IV): source of food name and descriptive terms; name and identification of the food; description of "single" foods; description of "mixed" foods; customary uses of food (optional), and sampling and laboratory handing of food. The INFOODS system was not intended to supersede or replace systems currently in use, but to support and be compatible with them (13).

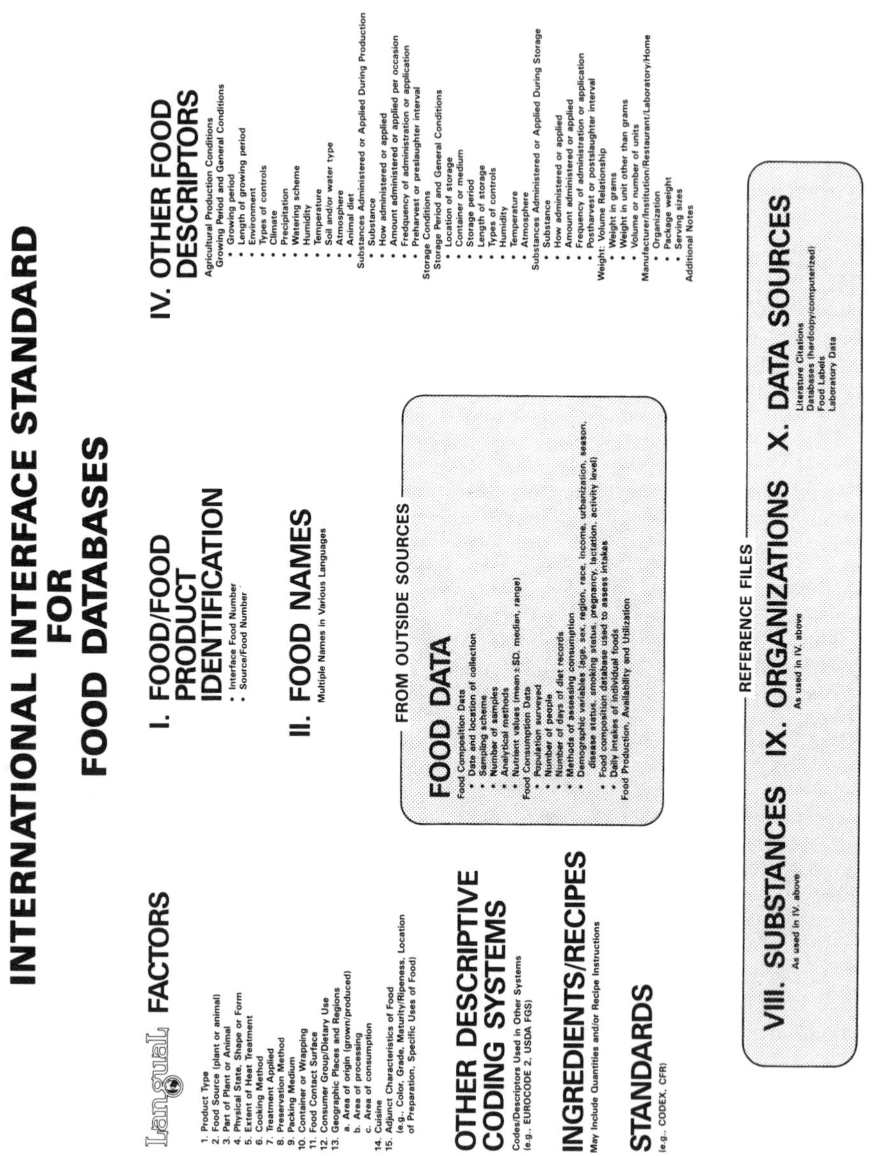

INTERNATIONAL INTERFACE STANDARD
FOR
FOOD DATABASES

I. FOOD/FOOD PRODUCT IDENTIFICATION
- Interface Food Number
- Source/Food Number

II. FOOD NAMES
Multiple Names in Various Languages

III. Langual FACTORS
1. Product Type
2. Food Source (plant or animal)
3. Part of Plant or Animal
4. Physical State, Shape or Form
5. Extent of Heat Treatment
6. Cooking Method
7. Treatment Applied
8. Preservation Method
9. Packing Medium
10. Container or Wrapping
11. Food Contact Surface
12. Consumer Group/Dietary Use
13. Geographic Places and Regions
    a. Area of origin (grown/produced)
    b. Area of processing
    c. Area of consumption
14. Cuisine
15. Adjunct Characteristics of Food
    (e.g., Color, Grade, Maturity/Ripeness, Location of Preparation, Specific Uses of Food)

IV. OTHER FOOD DESCRIPTORS
Agricultural Production Conditions
  Growing Period and General Conditions
  • Growing period
  • Length of growing period
  • Environment
  • Types of controls
  • Climate
  • Precipitation
  • Watering scheme
  • Humidity
  • Temperature
  • Soil and/or water type
  • Atmosphere
  • Animal diet
Substances Administered or Applied During Production
  • Substance
  • How administered or applied
  • Amount administered or applied per occasion
  • Frequency of administration or application
  • Preharvest or preslaughter interval
Storage Conditions
  Storage Period and General Conditions
  • Location of storage
  • Container or medium
  • Storage period
  • Length of storage
  • Types of controls
  • Humidity
  • Temperature
  • Atmosphere
Substances Administered or Applied During Storage
  • Substance
  • How administered or applied
  • Amount administered or applied
  • Frequency of administration or application
  • Postharvest or postslaughter interval
Weight: Volume Relationship
  • Weight in grams
  • Weight in unit other than grams
  • Volume or number of units
Manufacturer/Institution/Restaurant/Laboratory/Home
  • Organization
  • Package weight
  • Serving sizes
Additional Notes

V. OTHER DESCRIPTIVE CODING SYSTEMS
Codes/Descriptors Used in Other Systems
(e.g. EUROCODE 2, USDA FGS)

VI. INGREDIENTS/RECIPES
May Include Quantities and/or Recipe Instructions

VII. STANDARDS
(e.g. CODEX, CFR)

FROM OUTSIDE SOURCES

FOOD DATA
Food Composition Data
  • Date and location of collection
  • Sampling scheme
  • Number of samples
  • Analytical methods
  • Nutrient values (mean± SD, median, range)
Food Consumption Data
  • Population surveyed
  • Number of people
  • Number of days of diet records
  • Methods of assessing consumption
  • Demographic variables (age, sex, region, race, income, urbanization, season, disease status, smoking status, pregnancy, lactation, activity level)
  • Food composition database used to assess intakes
  • Daily intakes of individual foods
Food Production, Availability and Utilization

REFERENCE FILES

VIII. SUBSTANCES   IX. ORGANIZATIONS   X. DATA SOURCES
As used in IV. above   As used in IV. above

Literature Citations
Databases (hardcopy/computerized)
Food Labels
Laboratory Data

Figure 1. International interface standard for food databases

Table IV. Major facets of the INFOODS system for describing foods [1]

A. Source of food name (5) and descriptive terms
B. Name and identification of the food
  1. Name in national language
  2. Local name
  3. Nearest equivalent name in English, French, or Spanish
  4. Country/area where obtained
  5. Food group and code in national database
  6. Food group and code in regional database
  7. Codex Alimentarius indexing group
C. Description of "single" foods
  1. (a) Food source
    (b) Scientific name (Latin)
    (c) Variety, breed, strain
  2. Part of plant or animal
  3. Country/area of origin
  4. Manufacturer's name and address (batch or lot number)
  5. Other ingredients
  6. Food processing and/or preparation
  7. Preservation method
  8. Degree of cooking
  9. Agricultural production conditions
  10. Maturity or ripeness
  11. Storage conditions
  12. Grade
  13. Container and food contact surface
  14. Physical state, shape, or form
  15. Color
  16. Other descriptors
  17. Availability and location of photograph/drawing of food
D. Description of "mixed" foods
  1. Ingredients and quantities
  2. Recipe procedure
  3. Place where prepared
  4. Availability and location of photograph/picture
  5. Manufacturer's name and address
  6. Container and food contact surface
  7. Preservation method
  8. Storage conditions
  9. Final preparation
E. Customary uses of food (optional)
  1. Typical portion weight and measure
  2. Availability (frequency and season of consumption)
  3. Role of food in the diet
  4. Food users
  5. Specific purposes of the food; special claims
F. Sampling and laboratory handling of food
  1. Date of collection
  2. Weight(s) of sample(s)
  3. Percentage edible portion; nature of edible portion
  4. Percentage of refuse; nature of refuse
  5. Place of collection
  6. Handling between supplier and laboratory
  7. Handling on arrival at laboratory
  8. Laboratory storage and subsequent handling
  9. Strategy for analyses
  10. Reasons for doing analyses

[1] Adapted from Truswell et al. (11).

■ Importance of Terminology Systems

Terminology systems allow for descriptive information about foods in a consistent, standardized way that extends beyond the food name. Many food names are not sufficient by themselves to identify foods. Descriptors are especially useful for implicit food names; different foods that have the same name; foods that have different names; and vague, generic names. Terminology systems can address these problematic food names through descriptive terms relating to food source, food group, Latin name, language of food name, maturity, geographic region, cuisine, synonyms, preferred terms, and/or other facets.

Implicit Food Names

There are several types of implicit food names. Some convey no meaning without prior familiarity and do not translate meaningfully to other languages. Examples include bubble and squeak (British), kaerlinghedskranse (Danish "love rings"), hete bliksem (Dutch "hot lightening"), himmel und erde (German "heaven and earth"), scottadito (Italian "burning fingers"), himmelsk lapskaus (Norwegian "heavenly potpourri"), brazo de gitano (Spanish "gypsy's arm"), putt i panna (Swedish "tidbits in a pan"), and the American foods baked Alaska, red flannel hash, pigs-in-a-blanket, and succotash. Most of the commercial names for alcoholic mixed drinks (Bloody Mary, Rusty Nail, Screwdriver), ready-to-eat breakfast cereals (Frankenberries, Froot Loops, Pebbles), and candies (Baby Ruth, M&Ms, Now'n'Later, Payday) are fanciful, implicit names.

Some food names are implicit misnomers, i.e., the literal translation may lead to the wrong food. If one is not familiar with these food names, the wrong conclusions may be drawn. Examples of American food names that are implicit misnomers are corn dogs, grasshopper, hush puppies, rocky mountain oysters, and sweetbreads. Examples of implicit misnomers from the UK are Scotch woodcock, spotted dog, toad-in-the-hole, and Yorkshire pudding.

Some implicit geographic food names imply an area of origin (Brussels sprouts, Danish (pastry), English muffins, Lima beans, and London broil), but have little to do with the identified areas.

Same Name, Different Foods

Some foods share the same (or nearly the same) name, but are different foods. "Tuna" in American English is a fish; in Mexican Spanish, the term refers to a prickly pear. "Rape" is a plant oil used in Mid-Eastern cookery, a Spanish fish, or a French cheese. In England and France, "flan" is an open fruit tart in sponge cake or pastry crust; in Mexico or Spain, it is a baked caramel cream custard. A terminology system which defines the language of the food name and the cuisine is useful for distinguishing the correct usage of a food name.

There are many examples of the "same name, different food" problem among American and British names for foods. "Half-and-half" in the UK is a beverage of half porter and half pale ale; in the US, the food name refers to a mixture of cream and milk. "Mince" could be chopped ground beef or chopped fruit in the UK, but is chopped, dried fruit (mainly raisins) in the US. "Silverside" is a beef cut in the UK and a fish in the US. A cordial is a soft drink in the UK, but is a concentrated alcoholic beverage in the US. A terminology system which identifies the language of the food name and specifically distinguishes between different forms of the same language (i.e., English in the UK, the US, Canada, and Australia) would assist the data user.

Common usage of food names (usually a tendency to shorten the name) may result in names that refer to several different foods. For example, the term "chili/chile" may refer to a chili pepper (vegetable or spice), to chili beans (beans with a chili pepper sauce), or a mixed dish made with beef, beans, and a chili pepper sauce. The term "curry" may refer to the spice or to a rice dish made with the spice. The term "dressing" refers to salad dressing as well as to poultry stuffing (breading). A terminology system can help clarify these many uses of a food name through food groups, food source, and homonym definitions.

Some foods share the same name, but are prepared with different ingredients and are not really the same foods. For example, cocoa (hot chocolate) is usually made with milk, but some of the instant, dry cocoa products are reconstituted with water and contain little or no milk. Similarly, "lemonade" may be made from lemons or with artificial flavoring. The nutrient data associated with various cocoas and lemonades show clear differences in these products. Main dishes, soups, salads, and desserts may share the same food name (e.g., lasagne, gazpacho, carrot cake), but have different recipes. A terminology system should allow for information on ingredients and recipes (how the ingredients are put together) and information on place of procurement (e.g., restaurant, homemade, grocery store).

Some foods have the same commercial product name (Kellogg's Corn Flakes, McDonald's Big Mac), but are made from different ingredients in different countries. Different formulations may be due to different food standards, different nutrient fortification levels, the local availability of ingredients, or local taste preferences. A terminology system may help by providing information on ingredients and geographic descriptors.

Food standards (e.g., the definitions for what constitute milk, butter, margarine, beer, wine, ice cream), nutrient fortification levels, and nutrient claims (e.g., low fat) are established by government regulations and vary among countries. A terminology system should allow for descriptive information relating to food standards, nutrient fortification levels, and claims and identify the country associated with these legal terms.

Same Food, Different Names

The "same food, different name" problem can be handled by synonyms in a terminology system. In many cases, the preferred food name varies by geographical location or culture. There are different names for the same food within a country, e.g., ocean perch is known regionally in the US as rosefish, redfish, snapper, sea perch, and redbeam (17). There are different names for the same food in the same language among countries, e.g., American molasses and British treacle; American oatmeal and British porridge; American raisin bread and British currant loaf; American gelatin dessert and British jelly, and American jelly and British jam.

Vague, Generic Names

Food descriptions in databases are often lacking for basic, traditional foods such as fruits, vegetables, animal flesh, and grain products (breads, etc.). For example "oranges" and "white bread" could be described by year of production and/or market share of cultivars and brands, respectively. Such descriptors are especially important when database compilers are aggregating data from various sources and filling in missing values by matching food names. A terminology system could allow for these types of descriptions through agricultural variables and information on sampling designs.

Database users need to know if "generic" foods are market basket samples and/or mixtures of cultivars or maturity levels. If generic foods are not adequately described, inappropriate or misleading conclusions may be drawn about the data associated with them. For example, the vitamin A content of 1/2 grapefruit (120 g) is 318 IU for pink and red and 12 IU for white (6). The weighted vitamin A value of 149 IU for the US market share product (6) does not reflect either the pink or white product.

▮ Current Status and Future Goals

Food classification systems are developed by database compilers according to the number and types of foods in the database, cultural uses of foods, and/or intended users of the database. Thus, each food composition database tends to have its own system. The importance of food group classifications in databases depends on the types of terminology systems that are present, i.e., what other sorting or retrieval mechanisms are available. If there are no other mechanisms to describe or locate foods in a database, then classifications are very important, and must be carefully structured to place foods logically and consistently in the hierarchy. If there are other means by which to describe (and hence retrieve) foods, then the classification system is of less importance.

Because food classification systems are culture dependent, they are probably best designed to assist immediate (local) users of the database. A universal classification system is not necessary for the exchange and sharing of information in food-related databases.

Faceted terminology systems, especially those with standardized vocabulary, have specific advantages for use with food composition databases. These advantages include consistency in the use of defined terms; access to a hierarchy of terms with information on narrower, broader, and preferred terms and synonyms; retrieval of food names based on descriptive terms across food groups; and ability to match foods in various databases based on identical or similar descriptive terms.

Terminology systems must keep up with foods available in the marketplace which are changing to meet consumer preferences for convenience, appreciation of ethnic foods, and increased interest and knowledge of nutrition. Several types of foods in the marketplace are presenting challenges for food description

systems. They include products from newer or changing plant cultivars and animal breeds; foods previously used only by select population groups that are becoming available in different geographic areas (e.g., ugli fruit, jicama); synthetic foods made of mixtures of refined ingredients (formula-type meal replacements, medical foods); meat analogues; traditional foods made with fat and sugar substitutes; and traditional foods that have been reformulated to meet special dietary claims.

The type and level of descriptive information needed about foods vary among database users (i.e., researchers, epidemiologists, government agencies, educators). However, it is possible that a terminology system can serve multiple needs. It is important to note that current systems are not incompatible and that much knowledge and experience have been gained by the development of several different systems.

Foods in databases must be clearly and accurately described so that we can better use the data associated with them. Descriptive information associated with foods prior to laboratory analysis (e.g., information about sampling, preparation, and cooking methods and information from labels), should be recorded and carried with the food composition data to the database. Countries need to work together toward flexible and compatible food description systems for databases to increase the capability to capture, exchange, share, and retrieve information about foods.

▮ References

(1)   Poortvliet, E.J., & Kohlmeier, L. (1993) *Manual for Using the Eurocode 2 Food Coding System*, Federal Health Office, Institute for Social Medicine and Epidemiology, Berlin

(2)   Souci, S.W., Fachmann, W., & Kraut, H. (1989) *Food Composition and Nutrition Tables 1989-90*,

Wissenschaftliche Verlagsgesell-schaft mbH, Stuttgart

(3) *Fettsyratabeller for Livsmedel och Matratter* (1989) Statens Livsmedelsverk, Produktion Informako AB, Stockholm

(4) English, R., & Lewis, J. (1992) *Nutritional Values of Australian Foods*, Australian Government Publishing Service, Canberra

(5) Holland, B., Welch, A.A., Unwin, I.D., Buss, D.H., Paul, A.A., & Southgate, D.A.T. (1991) *McCance and Widdowson's The Composition of Foods*, 5th Ed., Royal Society of Chemistry, Cambridge

(6) US Department of Agriculture (1976–   ) *Composition of Foods: Raw, Processed, Prepared*, Agric. Handbook No. 8 series, USDA, Washington, DC

(7) US Department of Agriculture (1993) *USDA Nutrient Data Base for Individual Food Intake Surveys*, Release 6, National Technical Information Service, Springfield, VA

(8) McCann, A., Pennington, J.A.T., Smith, E.C., Holden, J.M., Soergel, D., & Wiley, R.C. (1988) *J. Am. Diet. Assoc.* **88**, 336-341

(9) Food and Agriculture Organization (1982) *Food Composition Tables for the Near East*, Rome

(10) Haendler, H., Neese, U., Jager, F., & Harris, L.E. (1980) in *International Network of Food Information Centers*, Pub. 2, L.E. Harris, H. Haendler, R. Riviere, & L. Rechaussat (Eds.), International Feed Databank System, Utah State University, Logan, UT

(11) Pennington, J.A.T., & Hendricks, T.C. (1992) *Food Add. Contam.* **9**, 265-275

(12) Pennington, J.A.T., Hendricks, T.C., Douglass, J.S., Petersen, B., & Kidwell, J. *Food Add. Contam.* (in press)

(13) Truswell, A.S., Bateson, D.J., Madafiglio, K.C., Pennington, J.A.T., Rand, W.M., & Klensin, J.C. (1991) *J. Food Comp. Anal.* **4**, 18-38

(14) Arab, L., Wittler, M., & Schettler, G. (Eds.) (1987) in *European Food Composition Tables in Translation*, Springer-Verlag, Berlin, pp. 132-154.

(15) Kohlmeier, L. (1992) *Eur. J. Clin. Nutr.* **46** (Suppl. 5), S25-S34

(16) Deary, J. (1993) *Langual Coding Experiment*, MAFF, London

(17) FDA (1988) *The Fish List. FDA Guide to Acceptable Market Names for Food Fish Sold in Interstate Commerce*, US Government Printing Office, Washington, DC

Nutritional Metrology: The Role of Reference Materials in Improving Quality of Analytical Measurement and Data on Food Components

James T. Tanner

Center for Food Safety and Applied Nutrition,
Food and Drug Administration, Washington DC 20204, USA

Wayne R. Wolf

Food Composition Laboratory, Beltsville, Human Nutrition Research
Center, ARS, US Department of Agriculture, Beltsville MD 20705, USA

William Horwitz

Center for Food Safety and Applied Nutrition,
Food and Drug Administration, Washington DC 20204, USA

This paper discusses the role of reference materials (RMs) in improving analytical results in order to complement existing quality control procedures focused on processes such as standard methods and collaborative trials. Activities to improve the range of RMs available, and their incorporation into standard methods are also discussed.

Analytical measurements of the content of food components are the foundation of nutritional science. Knowledge and application of the principles of *metrology* (the science of measurement) are essential to improve and assure the quality of the data generated by these measurements. In the past, analytical methodology for nutrient measurements had focused primarily on the *process* of these analytical measurements, i.e. the emphasis on use of Official Methods of Analysis which have been collaboratively studied and evaluated through procedures established by AOAC INTERNATIONAL (formerly the Association of Official Analytical Chemists). These collaborative studies show the capability to achieve agreement of results among analysts using specifically defined analytical procedures.

More recently metrology in general has focused on the *result* of the analytical measurement process, i.e. the accuracy of the data generated by the specific application of the procedure. There is a well recognized need to build a foundation for data validation through establishment of accuracy based measurement systems (1). In these systems "routine" or "field" methodologies are linked and traceable through Reference Materials (RMs), Reference Methods, Certified Reference Materials and Definitive Methods to the basic measurement systems of national and international bodies. The use of RMs in conjunction with Official Methods is necessary to build this foundation, not only for establishment of an accurate database of food composition data, but also for the monitoring of appropriate regulations dealing with these types of data.

This concept of "traceability" is essentially important in nutritional science because many of our essential nutrients are not single chemical entities, but are families of related components. Chemical families ordinarily can not be analyzed by methods designed for specific analytes. They require tailor-made methods that try to include only components of nutritional interest. Therefore, many nutrient measurements are method specific, requiring that the procedures be followed in exact detail to obtain repeatable answers.

Such methods are even more dependent on reference materials than are methods based upon chemical stoichiometry. The assignment of reference values by a certifying organization, based upon validation by experienced laboratories faithfully following the details of the same method, produces the value which is to be reproduced by laboratories supplying analytical values to nutritional science. Only if a reference value can be duplicated by an analytical laboratory can any degree of confidence be ascribed to values produced by that laboratory for the same nutrient in other foods.

Indeed the foundation of the U.S. Food and Drug Administration (FDA) regulatory process is a tested, reliable method combined with a reference material to validate accuracy of the resulting analytical data. This is a basic requirement of Good Laboratory Practices (GLP) and the corner-stone of good science. In its regulatory programs the FDA requires use of the analytical methods of AOAC INTERNATIONAL, which have been validated through interlaboratory methods performance studies to ensure that they are capable of providing acceptable accuracy and precision. This requirement does not eliminate use of other analytical methods which have been evaluated through similar studies. Indeed the *Code of Federal Regulations* (2), which specifies that AOAC methods will be used for regulatory purposes, requires that: ". . . if no AOAC method is available, by reliable and appropriate analytical procedures." Other methods developed by such organizations as the American Association of Cereal Chemists, the American Oil Chemists Society, the International Standards Organization (ISO), or other organizations may in some cases also be useful for regulatory purposes.

However, all of these methods provide only half of the requirement. In addition to a well-studied method, some means of determining that the method was performed correctly is also necessary. Obtaining acceptable results with validated methodology for a reference material that has a known concentration of the analyte and is similar in composition to the material being analyzed is presumptive evidence that the method was performed correctly and that the results obtained for the test materials are correct. RMs, for which the true values are known, are important for this validation. From a regulator's point of view, the use of appropriate RMs is desirable for determining compliance with existing regulations.

Unfortunately, RMs are not available for many products and analytes. Dating back over 80 years, standard reference materials (SRMs) have been developed by such organizations as the National Institute of Standards and Technology (NIST, formerly National Bureau of Standards, NBS) for products such as steel, in which the content of trace elements is very important. Building on this expertise, RMs have been developed within in the past 20 years for biological products such as flour, spinach, oysters and other food products for which the main focus has been the major and trace elements rather than the various organic compounds comprising the major components of food. One reason for this focus has been that some organic components may change with time and are not shelf stable, therefore, the exact "true" concentration at the time of use cannot be assigned. Another reason is that analytical expertise for organic components has not progressed at the same pace as for inorganic components.

Reference materials are also necessary to determine the systematic error of new methods. Previously, some AOAC methods had used standard additions for checking for the presence of method bias, when a reference material of known concentration was not available. Although this technique is useful under some conditions, it really only measures the analyst's ability to recover analyte added at the measurement stage and not the ability to determine the analyte that was endogenous to the matrix. For this reason, the technique of standard additions sometimes gives unreliable information. The determination of precision or reproducibility is frequently used as a measure of the success of a method because of the ability of a laboratory to obtain the same values as well as to replicate the results of other laboratories. This is an important part of method evaluation but does not address the accuracy question. The International Standards Organization (ISO) has now broken down the concept of "error" as deviation from the true value into three parts: 1) "Accuracy" is the deviation of a single value; 2) "Trueness" is the deviation of the average set of values; and 3) "Bias (or systematic error)" is the deviation of the long term average (3).

AOAC INTERNATIONAL recently formed a task force to address the problem of the methods available to enforce regulations stemming from the Nutrition Labeling and Education Act of 1990 (NLEA)(4), which made nutrition labeling mandatory as of March 1994 for retail foods distributed in the United States. The purpose of the task force was to determine what methodology was available and whether existing methods were adequate for the purpose of nutrition labeling (5). In addition to methods questions, the task force also examined the availability of RMs. It found a serious deficiency in the availability of RMs for organic nutrients and recommended that action be taken to improve that situation (6).

Several problems must be addressed before reference materials for organic nutrient content can be made available. The first is the selection of matrix materials to represent many different kinds of foods; the second is the packaging and storage of these materials to provide a useful shelf life. Third is the characterization or assignment of the "correct" or "best estimate" of the value for the components of interest.

The AOAC task force addressed the question of matrix materials for different foods in a creative way (7). Food is composed of the basic components: protein, carbohydrate, fat, water and ash. Frequently, analysis of a food is not successful because of interference or interaction from one or more of these components with the analyte of interest. In any analytical procedure, water can usually be added or subtracted to suit the requirements of the method. Ash, in general, does not have a great impact on the performance of analytical methods for organic material in foods. Thus, the behavior of a given food in an analytical method is primarily determined by the relative proportions of protein, fat, and carbohydrate.

A scheme has been proposed to represent foods by first normalizing content of these three components to 100 per cent of their sum (7). This normalized food composition can then be plotted within a triangle with 100 per cent fat, 100 per cent protein, and 100 per cent carbohydrate at the respective vertices with the concentration of each component decreasing to zero approaching the opposite side. This schema can then be divided into nine different sectors, each encompassing a range of concentrations of the three components (protein, carbohydrate, and fat) (Figure 1). If a method of analysis were successful for foods falling in each of the nine different sectors, then it should be applicable to all types of food. Such an approach would also be useful to AOAC Associate Referees and AOAC Official

Methods committees in minimizing the effort required for collaborative studies while maximizing the value of the resulting data to AOAC Official Methods users. For example, the prospect of coordinating a collaborative study involving 40 or more different foods may discourage many researchers from fully exploring the scope of applicability of a particular method. As a result, researchers may limit the scope of their study to a few food groups to reduce the analytical burden on the participating laboratories. However, as demonstrated by the triangle, many of the 40 or more foods selected to represent foods for a collaborative study may be very similar to one another on a dry basis, and may behave chemically, and, thus, analytically, in a very similar way.

If a diagram such as Figure 1 were to be used to select samples for a collaborative study, two samples from a sector could be selected to account for variation in the type of protein, fat, or carbohydrate that may have an impact on the performance of the method. Examples of these variations within carbohydrates are high fiber foods versus high sugar foods. Other variations include fats containing significant amounts of short chain fatty acids versus those containing predominantly long chain fatty acids, or foods containing more hydrophilic proteins as opposed to those containing predominantly hydrophobic proteins. In addition, two foods may be selected within a sector that vary according to the extent of processing each has undergone.

The logical extension of this same approach would be to provide appropriate reference materials for a food type or category representing each of the nine sectors. By using the different types as part of a method-performance study and having a reference material for each type, all foods would have a method and a reference material, similar to the actual food, that could be used for regulatory purposes. These RMs could be produced and made available through an organization such as NIST. The first priority

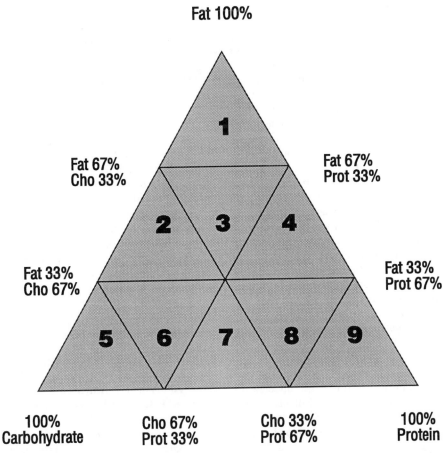

Fat 100%

Fat 67%
Cho 33%

Fat 67%
Prot 33%

Fat 33%
Cho 67%

Fat 33%
Prot 67%

100%
Carbohydrate

Cho 67%
Prot 33%

Cho 33%
Prot 67%

100%
Protein

Figure 1. Schematic layout of food matrices by which all foods can be organized according to their relative proportions of protein, fat, and carbohydrate; the points of the triangle represent 100 per cent of the normalized content of these three major classes of food components (moisture and ash are excluded).

would be to produce reference materials for the nine food sectors named above and for products in areas where a critical need exists for reliable analyses, such as medical foods.

A reference analytical method of known reliability together with a stable RM to monitor analytical performance is the most important requirement for a regulatory agency. With results produced by using this combination, the agency can proceed with appropriate regulatory action that is based on sound analytical science.

This type of verification is part of the infant formula program. Methods for the

analysis of infant formula have been developed and collaboratively studied because infant formula is the most highly regulated food in the United States today. It represents the sole source of nutrition for a large segment of the population, namely, infants. As part of the *Infant Formula Act* of 1980, companies are required to manufacture formula within specified limits, and FDA is required to monitor the formulas to ensure that they are within those limits. Because of differences in methodology, many questions have arisen as to the "true" concentrations of some analytes in the products. Currently, there are analytical methods for infant formula that both industry and FDA have agreed are to be used for regulatory analyses. These methods are now part of AOAC's *Official Methods of Analysis* (8) and have been collaboratively studied by FDA, infant formula manufacturers, and several commercial laboratories. However, no reference material is currently available for validating method performance in each laboratory. One on-going NIST project is the development of a spray dried Infant Formula material (SRM-1846) which is being characterized for organic nutrient content. SRM-1846 will serve as a reference material for Infant Formula, and will also provide a least one reference material for validating measurements that determine conformity with the requirements of NLEA. An infant formula has been prepared, spray-dried, and packaged under nitrogen in individual packets weighing approximately 30 g each. These packets have been stored for about two years and analyzed at specific intervals. They appear to have been shelf stable for that time period. Further testing is still under way. If successful, this method of packaging could be applied to other potential RMs to ensure that the nutrient content is stable for a reasonable time.

An AOAC international Technical Division on Reference Materials has been established in order to facilitate availability and use of RMs in the validation, implementation and use of AOAC Official Methods of Analysis. In addition this Technical Division will coordinate activities to assist in characterizing RMs and will conduct the International Symposia Series on Biological and Environmental Reference Materials (BERM)(9).

■ References

(1) Uriano, G., & Cali, J.P. (1977) in *Validation of the Measurement Process,* ACS Symposium Series No. 63, J.R. Devoe (Ed.), ACS, Washington DC, pp. 114-139

(2) *Code of Federal Regulations,* (21 CFR 101.9(e)(2))

(3) *International Standards Organization* (1994) ISO Standard 5725

(4) Ellefson, W. (1993) in *Methods of Analysis for Nutrition Labeling,* D.M. Sullivan & D.E. Carpenter (Eds.), AOAC INTERNATIONAL, Arlington, VA, pp. 3-26

(5) Sullivan, D.M., & D.E. Carpenter (Eds.) (1993) *Methods of Analysis for Nutrition Labeling,* AOAC INTERNATIONAL, Arlington, VA

(6) Wolf, W.R. (1993) in *Methods of Analysis for Nutrition Labeling,* AOAC INTERNATIONAL, Arlington, VA, pp. 111-122

(7) Ikins, W., DeVries, J., Wolf, W.R., Oles, P., Carpenter, D., Fraley, N., & Ngeh-Ngwainbi, J. (1993) *The Referee* **17,** 1, 6-7

(8) *Official Methods of Analysis* (1995) 16th Ed., AOAC INTERNATIONAL, Arlington, VA

(9) Heavner, G. *Fres. J. Anal. Chem.* (in press)

Strategies for Sampling:
The Assurance of
Representative Values

Joanne M. Holden, Carol S. Davis

Food Composition Laboratory, Beltsville Human Nutrition Research
Center, ARS/USDA, BARC-East, Beltsville, MD 20705, USA

Current interest in the relationship of diet to the maintenance of health has stimulated the demand for representative food composition data. Values for nutrients and other food components are required to calculate dietary intakes, to determine food policy, to monitor food safety, to formulate new products, and to facilitate trade. A specific estimate must be statistically representative of the population of all values for a component in the food product of interest. Serious bias in the estimate can lead to erroneous conclusions about diet-related issues. The Food Composition Laboratory has conducted research to develop statistically based strategies for sampling the US food supply to determine estimates for components in many foods. To determine a strategy for food sampling it is necessary to define project objectives and to determine analytical priorities for foods and components. Foods to be sampled should be described in terms of the product type, ingredients, preservation state, source, cultivar, and other factors which may influence component levels. Demographic and marketing data can be used to identify parameters which are potential sources of variability. In addition, protocols for sample handling and chemical analyses should be standardized to minimize the impact of errors which may arise during the measurement process. Results of sampling research for selenium, total fat, and cholesterol in several foods are presented and the impact of sampling results on the calculation of national estimates is discussed.

S ince 1960 the assessment of food consumption patterns and their impact on health status has evolved, requiring food composition data for more foods and components (1). The recognition of food intake as one factor in the longitudinal development of complex, multi-factorial diseases has occurred more recently (2, 3, 4). Not only are food composition data used to identify and monitor dietary trends but they are also used for hypothesis testing (5). Other uses of food composition data are equally important (e.g. trade, food safety, food manufacturing) (6). This increased interest in food composition data has stimulated the demand for improved data, including an indication of the number of analyses, the sampling plan, and the magnitude and sources of variability, as well as descriptive and quantitative information about the analytical method and quality control (7). The lack of data for foods and ingredients impedes the assessment of diet-health relationships and impacts on the production, regulation, and use of foods. Increased demand for more data can be attributed, in part, to the development of sophisticated instrumentation which permits the measurement of minute quantities of components in foods and in biological matrices more rapidly than ever before. Similarly, the development and accessibility of computers for data processing has improved the ability to manipulate large data files to investigate new hypotheses. In view of the importance of foods as vehicles for nutrients and other components, the generation of food composition data is not an isolated exercise but, rather, an integral part of the assessment of human health status and dietary effects.

Possible specific objectives for generating food composition data include:

- development of a national food composition database
- determination of aflatoxin levels in a rail container of grain
- determination of pesticide levels in a food product
- quality control of food manufacturing
- determination of significant differences in the vitamin content of different animal muscles
- brand to brand (or region to region) comparisons of component levels.

The generation of these data should be based on a statistical sampling plan specific to the objective which will indicate what to sample, where to sample, and how many units to select to represent the food of interest. The definition of the objective provides the focus for the study and helps to determine the most appropriate sampling strategy. According to Horwitz a statistically based sampling plan should guide the selection of representative units from the population to provide component estimates "within a specified degree of variability with a stated degree of confidence" (8). The objective of this paper is to discuss the development of sampling strategies to provide estimates of central tendency and variability for component levels in foods to be used in food composition databases and national dietary assessment projects.

The average daily diet may contain 20–25 different items. It has been estimated that 4,000 different generic products (e.g. beef, white bread, pizza) can be found in the American marketplace. Since a nation's food supply is a complex mixture of processed and non-processed products each food item represents many brands, formulations or styles, and geographical sources. There may be as many

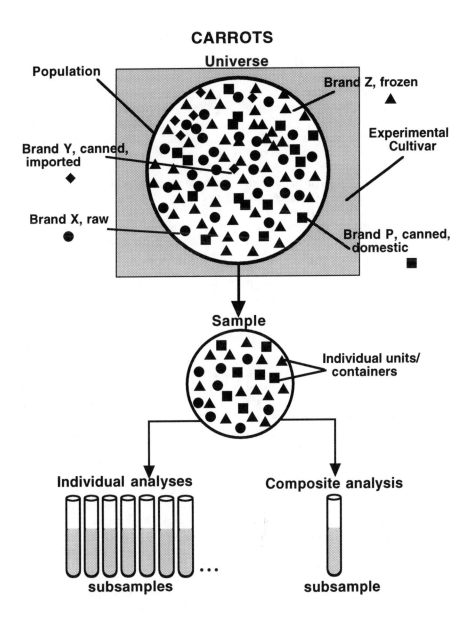

Figure 1. Population and sample: the definition of representativeness

as 50,000 products if one considers different brand names. For example, in the US there are hundreds of brands of white bread (9). Similarly, the diversity of the population, personal preferences for foods, and the availability of sophisticated manufacturing and marketing schemes stimulates the nationwide distribution of new and unusual products. Due to the complexity of a national food supply, the generation of accurate food composition data is a difficult and expensive task.

Figure 1 illustrates the statistical concept of the sample and its relationship to the population of all forms, brands, and units of a food (10). The term population describes the collection of relevant objects from which a subset is chosen for analysis. Generally, the population of interest is very large and can be considered infinite relative to the size of the subset which is to be selected. For example, in Figure 1, the population consists of all forms of carrots usually consumed by individuals. In this same example experimental cultivars of carrots lie outside of the population but are part of the larger universe of all carrots. When estimating levels of a nutrient contained in carrots consumed in the US one would probably not sample such cultivars since they are not widely consumed. While it is not possible or desirable to analyze every package, unit, or lot of a food, the analysis of a subset of carefully selected units will provide the required data to draw inferences about the population of all available units (10) (Figure 1).

Using traditional survey sampling theory, the term sample refers to that subset or *group* of items or units which are selected from the population of interest to represent that population (10) (Figure 1). If the objective is to develop a nationally representative database of food composition values, then the sampling strategy must be carefully planned to construct a sample to include typical items or units in shares proportional to the sales volume or consumption properties of the population of those foods. The sample will include units of predominant brands, manufacturing locations, cultivars, etc. relevant to the specific food as consumed by the individuals of interest.

If one were to analyze all containers or units for all available brands or cultivars defined as the population for a food, e.g. carrots, then one could construct a frequency distribution of all analytical values. The distribution may or may not be Gaussian or normal. Since all units of a food which constitute the population cannot be analyzed without destroying that population the concept of sampling, i.e., selecting a representative subset of the population based on the probabilities of various types has developed (10). The analysis of all units in the subset will yield a collection of values which can be used to construct a frequency distribution for that subset. If the sample is representative of the population than that distribution will be similar in its statistical characteristics and subsequent "shape" to the distribution for the population. If one were to take multiple samples, i.e., multiple subsets of units, of the same size from the same large population one could expect that the statistical characteristics of each sample would be similar to those for the population. However, they will not be identical since the collection of mean values for all samples taken from the population will form a frequency distribution themselves. The degree of similarity of the statistical characteristics between the population and the sample defines, in part, the degree of representativeness of that sample for the population. While, in most cases, the true statistical characteristics of the population can never be known statistical sampling theory can be applied to the generation of food composition data to yield estimates of population parameters. Although the discussion of mathematical sampling theory is beyond the scope of this paper it provides the framework and point of reference for comments about the selection of foods, the number of units, variability, etc. It is important to note that the usual statistical techniques which are used to evaluate the statistical characteristics of the sample subset and to provide estimates of statistical parameters for that subset assume normality of the distribution of all possible analytical values in the subset. In some disciplines various mathematical transformations of the data are possible to permit the evaluation of scientific hypotheses. However, it is difficult if not impossible to use transformation techniques to estimate such parameters as the mean and variance. More research is needed for many components and foods to determine the statistical distributions for food composition data and to evaluate the robustness of statistical techniques as applied to such data.

In general, most values for components and foods in a database are calculated means of two or more individual values. For analytical sources or files the data may have been generated in a single laboratory or in several laboratories. Individual values may be the product of the analysis of an aliquot of a single unit or of a composite of several units. Each mean value in a database is a point in the distribution of sample means mentioned above and, yet each mean also represents a distribution of individual values or points for the sample subset from which it was derived. Since a mean database value represents a sample subset selected from the population a new analytical value for another individual unit chosen at random from the food supply may not fall within the confidence limits of the database value. However, the probability of any new value falling within limits defined by representative sampling and analysis will be high (10). Thus, it is important to estimate the mean composition and some parameter of variability for the most important food/component combinations in a database.

Recently, Greenfield and Southgate have published a discussion of the importance of sampling, including important definitions and approaches for obtaining the representative sample set (11). Analyses may or may not include aliquots of all brands, types, or cultivars present in the population. In keeping with fiscal and physical constraints, it may be necessary to take a subset of the brands or types available. One should seek statistical advice during the development phase of the sampling plan. Aliquots of single units (primary samples) may be analyzed. Conversely, units can be combined or composited by brand name, geographic location, cultivar, etc., as appropriate, before aliquots are taken to minimize the number of analytical measurements and yet represent the contribution of that unit to the estimate of central tendency. The formulation of composites should be based on the statistical data about the collection of units representing brand names, geographic locations, etc. which have been obtained from a pilot study or previous independent investigations. The impact of compositing on the magnitude of variability should not be overlooked. The number of analyses to be conducted will be determined by the desired statistical power of the estimate, the observed variability in pilot tests, and such practical considerations as physical and fiscal resources. More detail will be provided later in the text.

If the objective is to develop a national food composition database, then two major questions need to be answered: "What nutrient(s)/component(s) should be determined?" and "What foods should be selected for analysis?" Food analysis projects can be driven by the need to estimate levels of a single component (e.g. selenium, β-carotene, total fat) in foods consumed by a population of individuals. Conversely, the focus may be on a single food (e.g. beef, milk, carrot) and its major components.

■ What Components Should Be Analyzed?

The components of interest may be nutrients (e.g. protein, vitamin A, iron), additives, biological agents, or contaminants. Each component or class of components represents a unique sampling challenge.

However, the choice of components should be guided by the particular priorities or emphasis of the project or agency. In general three factors determine the selection of components:

- the component should rank highly relative to actual or suspected public health effects

- available analytical methods for the component(s) of interest should be robust, valid, capable of producing accurate data, and economically feasible

- in view of fiscal and personnel limitations, analytical priorities should include those components for which available data are unacceptable or previously unavailable (12, 13).

As an example, the scientific community has become interested in the possible effects of carotenoids intake on health, specifically the development of certain cancers (14). Since the 1930's, several carotenoids (α- and β-carotene, and β-cryptoxanthin) have been known to have significant vitamin A activity (15). While vitamin A deficiency is still prevalent in many areas of the world, the broader role of carotenoids in human metabolism has become the object of interest. However, until recently, no comprehensive assessment of carotenoid data for foods had been conducted (16, 17). In fact, for many foods carotenoid data are lacking. Analytical methods for measuring additional individual carotenoids in simple forms of foods have been developed in recent years (18). While more work needs to be done in this area to release a robust field method, some centers are using liquid chromatography (LC) while other centers are using valid open column chromatography (OCC) methods (19). Finally, carotenoids are good candidates for further analyses because sufficient high quality data are lacking (16, 20). As other less familiar components (e.g. isoflavonoids, flavonoids) have become the objects of research, and as robust methods have become available, their determination in foods will become important. Furthermore, as improved methods for recognized important components (e.g. folates) are developed, new analyses will be needed. As new, more specific, analytical methods become available it is necessary to generate new data to replace the older outdated values. Data for fiber content of foods is an example. Crude fiber analysis has been replaced by other methods, including total dietary fiber (21). Today, carbohydrate values calculated by "difference" have been replaced by analyses of specific fractions since carbohydrates, as a class, contain diverse forms with different molecular weights and chemical structures and, therefore, different metabolic effects. Frequently, newer methods make it possible to determine some components for the first time. A large nationwide study of fast-food chicken included the determination of levels of starch contained in the seasoned flour coating (22).

■ What Foods Should Be Sampled?

The selection of foods is equally important. Stewart et al. (11) and Beecher and Matthews (12) have stated that priorities for analyses should be based on three considerations: First, although many foods may contain the component of interest, the foods selected should be the major contributors of that component to the diet. Frequently, a limited number of foods (5–100) contribute 50–90 per cent of a single component to the diet of the population of interest (23, 24). Existing data and/or pilot studies can provide preliminary estimates of the levels of components in foods. Food consumption survey data and/or data from food balance sheets can be combined with preliminary food composition data to provide a ranked list of the major contributors of specific components (20, 24).

Second, foods for which data are unacceptable or unavailable should be selected. As an example, tomato products are the most important source of lycopene, an abundant carotenoid in the US diet. However, after the assessment of carotenoids data quality for multi-component foods by Chug-Ahuja et al. (20), the authors determined that analytical carotenoid data for popular commercial, tomato-based soups, sauces, and spaghetti sauce were nonexistent. A nationwide sampling plan for three cities was developed to select samples of these products to be analyzed for five of the most important dietary carotenoids (25). New forms of foods are appearing in the markets of many countries and are gaining in popularity. Food composition data for many of these foods are nonexistent. For example, the influx of many previously unknown fruits and vegetables into the US food supply requires that these foods be sampled and analyzed to determine their composition. Initially, new foods may be imported from other countries, prior to commencement of their local production (e.g. kiwi fruit, Granny Smith apples). Since climate, soil conditions and geography affect levels of some components, geographical source and variety/cultivar may be relevant to the sampling plan. Therefore, it would be necessary to compare data for imported fruits with data for fruit from domestic sources; values would be revised, if necessary. For a recent study of human carotenoid metabolism, a single production lot of frozen broccoli was needed to assure uniformity of the product for all subjects over the entire course of the study. When a small regional company was contacted to procure the broccoli it was found that the product was grown and processed in Guatemala. Analyses of carotenoid levels in the frozen broccoli revealed that values were significantly different from those for fresh broccoli procured in the retail market (26). This revelation emphasized the importance of using analytical values for critical components in single lot foods used in human metabolic studies.

A third consideration is the need to analyze foods as eaten. As new forms of important foods become popular they should be analyzed to generate up-to-date data more appropriate to eating habits (12, 13). In many countries the use of fully prepared commercial foods instead of home-prepared commodities has increased rapidly. Estimates for those prepared foods are more representative of what some segments of a population are eating than estimates for foods prepared from the basic ingredients. Formulated foods may contain different levels of fat, sodium, or other components than domestic recipes. A recipe calculation technique can be used for some components. However, formulations for commercial products are generally unavailable and are frequently different from home-prepared products. Therefore, the composition of important commercially-prepared foods will need to be determined by analysis. New ingredients such as fat substitutes, gums and sweeteners alter the formulations of familiar foods, necessitating the need for new analyses. Finally, advances in animal and plant breeding will require new analyses to estimate changes in targeted components. For example, in the US, recent advances in breeding and marketing practices have dramatically reduced the separable fat trim on beef and pork. Nationwide retail studies were planned and conducted in collaboration with meat science departments at Texas Agricultural and Mechanical (A & M) University and the University of Wisconsin to assess the impact of these changes on the composition of beef and pork (27, 28).

■ Food Description Effects

After the foods and components have been determined, the individual and specific products which represent a food must be identified. For a single food (e.g. beef, pizza, or eggs) the investigator can define the characteristics of the product which may influence the composition and variability for the component(s) of interest. Relevant characteristics will include the primary food source and scientific name for a product (e.g. wheat v. corn, coconut v. sunflower, beef v. pork), the part of the plant or animal used, preservation state, food processing treatments, added ingredients, etc. For some components, geographical source (e.g. broccoli, above) and ripening practices will be important. As mentioned, carotenoid values for broccoli cultivars grown in Guatemala were different than values for fresh broccoli grown in California (24). For others, packaging type, pH, or storage conditions will be sources of variability. In recent years, several food description systems have been developed which provide classifications of important descriptors (29, 30). The specific products and components of interest will determine the preliminary list of descriptors for the products.

Following the definition of relevant descriptors for a food, it is necessary to identify the specific major sources of that food which are consumed by the population of interest. In addition, the distribution and marketing schemes need to be identified. For branded products, sales volume data and product information are important to the selection of representative units (9). For commodity products, such as meats, eggs, milk, etc., it is possible to identify the major breeds or cultivars, as well as major commercial purveyors of the products and an approximation of their sales ranking (31). In regions where food production is localized the major outlets for products (butcher, bakery) or ingredients (flour mill, refineries) can be identified. Some products may be manufactured in one location and distributed nationwide while others may be formulated in many regions from different sources of raw ingredients. In a recent study of selenium levels in bread, ninety samples of white bread were selected in nine major population areas across the US (32). Bread is baked in regional or local bakeries in or near cities and towns. Yet most of the wheat in the US is grown in the north central plains area, an area of relatively high selenium levels, and then transported to major metropolitan areas to supplement smaller regional supplies grown near those areas. Selenium levels

in bread in several of the cities varied as the local source of the flour was supplemented by the supply grown in the north central area. The study demonstrated that selenium levels in bread were more closely related to the source of wheat levels of selenium in soil where the grain was grown than to the selenium levels in soils where the bread samples were purchased. By defining the form of the product and its sources, the investigator can begin to determine which specific products will need to be selected as well as the time and location for sampling.

■ Food Consumption Patterns

After marketing and distribution variables have been defined, consumption patterns should be assessed to determine where to select the samples. If the objective is to determine estimates for foods in a national database then it is necessary to sample food products on the basis of the population distribution and product use. Several questions should be answered: Is the food consumed frequently and in significant amounts by the population of interest? In which regions or populations is the food consumed? Is the food consumed more in rural areas than towns? If the food is widely consumed by many sub-groups, what is the distribution of the population in the country or region of interest? Major population centers within a country can be identified and used as locations for sample selection. In the US the majority of the population is concentrated in a number of metropolitan areas called Metropolitan Statistical Areas (MSAs) and defined by the US Office of Management and Budget as cities which have at least 50,000 persons or an urbanized area of at least 50,000 with a total population of at least 100,000 individuals (33). The top ten cities, their percent of the population, and their respective proportion of grocery sales are given in Table I. The percent of the population represented by the top 100 MSAs as well as the number of supermarkets is also given. In most major cities two

Table I. Top 10 US MSA[a] markets by population[b]

Rank	Market Area	% of US Totals	
		Population	Supermarkets
1	Los Angeles–Long Beach, CA	3.59	2.39
2	New York	3.38	2.19
3	Chicago	2.40	1.76
4	Philadelphia	1.93	1.41
5	Detroit	1.72	1.41
6	Washington, DC–MD–VA	1.61	1.25
7	Houston	1.35	1.12
8	Atlanta	1.19	1.21
9	Riverside–San Bernadino, CA	1.14	0.90
10	Dallas	1.07	1.01
–		–	–
–		–	–
–		–	–
100	Youngstown–Warren, OH	0.23	0.28
	Top 100 MSA Market	59.86	50.86
	All Other U.S.	40.14	49.14
	U.S. Total Figures	254,926,669	30,552

[a] Metropolitan Statistical Area
[b] Adapted from Progressive Grocer's Market Scope (40)

to four supermarket chains dominate each city. Most are significant regional vendors.

While many sample mixes are self-weighted—that is, the available products are similar to the number and kind needed to mimic sales volume, it is possible to weight the sample estimates after analysis of equal numbers of individual units/per brand or region by applying pre-determined weighting factors (10). In view of the nationwide distribution and market share of many products and the concentration of the population in major MSAs the USDA and others have selected representative units of foods from retail grocery stores and/or restaurants in three to ten cities across the country (22, 27, 28, 34). For example, for the recent study of selenium in approximately 200 foods, sample units were purchased in two major supermarkets in each of nine cities (Holden, unpublished data). Two to three cities were selected in each of four regions of the country; two major supermarkets were sampled in each city. For each of the major contributors of dietary selenium (beef, white bread, pork, chicken, eggs) approximately 100 analytical samples were randomly selected and prepared. For minor contributors five to 25 analytical samples were chosen. By choosing units of the highest volume brands within the largest supermarkets in major metropolitan areas it was assumed that the most frequently consumed and representative products were selected for a specific food.

To determine selenium in beef, it was necessary to determine the major categories of beef products in the US diet. Marketing and production data obtained from the US Livestock and Meat Board, the private sector trade association for the meat producers, indicated that the per capita consumption of beef was 72.7 lbs. Fresh beef cuts including steaks and roasts, and ground beef, including bulk ground beef purchased in supermarkets as well as hamburger sandwiches sold in fast food restaurants were the major forms of beef consumed (35). Using this information a sampling plan was developed. Ninety four units of five primal beef cuts were obtained from a larger study of beef composition conducted by Texas A & M (27). The samples had been collected from major retail stores in ten cities. In addition, 58 samples of ground beef collected from a USDA nationwide study were analyzed (34). Finally, 27 samples of hamburger sandwiches were collected in nine cities from each of three prevalent chains (Holden, unpublished data). Mean values and standard deviations were calculated and published in the recently released USDA Provisional Table of Selenium in Foods (36).

How Many Sample Units Are Needed?

The number of sample units analyzed will determine, in part, the statistical power of the estimate. Although statistical models for calculating the required number of units can be complex and multi-tiered, the following equation indicates the most important facets of the computation for homogeneous populations (10):

$$n \leq (ts)^2/(r\bar{y})^2$$

The appropriate number of units is based on four parameters. The first is "t", the abscissa of the normal curve that cuts off an area "a" at the tails of the distribution, indicating the desired confidence level. The standard error of the estimate is denoted by "s" while the sample mean is denoted by "$\bar{y}$". This mean and standard error can be obtained from previously published data or pilot studies, if available. Some existing handbooks of food composition data publish standard deviations or standard errors of the mean and can be used as rough estimates of sample

size. Previously published estimates and the scientific objectives for the study should serve as the basis for sample number calculations. The reader should note that the coefficient of variation, if known, can substitute for $s/\bar{y}$. The limit of the desired relative error in the estimate is indicated by "r." That is, the proximity of the estimate to the "true" mean, e.g. within 10 per cent, is represented by "r." The calculation of the appropriate number of samples is an iterative process which begins with an approximation of the number of samples determined by the investigator as a "guess." The "guess" can be based on preliminary cost estimates or capabilities of the analytical laboratory. After the initial calculation the estimate of number of samples is further refined by recalculation until successive trial values of "n" yield similar values. The cost of sampling can be included in the equation as well. Table II demonstrates the effect of increasing the coefficient of variation on the number of samples required to obtain the same level of confidence. The "t" value was set at 2.00 while r=0.1 for the purpose of the illustration. Further information is given by Cochran (10).

In the past, the mean or average value has been used as the estimate of the level of a component in the food. However, the use of the mean presumes that the statistical distribution of all values for that component in a specific food follows the Gaussian or normal distribution (37). Recently, the USDA Food Composition Laboratory, in collaboration with the US National Cancer Institute, compiled and published a food composition table of the levels of five carotenoids in important fruit and vegetable contributors (16). The values were collected from published and unpublished analytical sources. Due to the apparent skewed distribution for several foods and the limited amount of available data (one to 14 acceptable sources per food) the median value was used in the table. However, the use of the median precludes the calculation of a variance indicator. More research is needed to evaluate the characteristics of

Table II. Effect of increasing the coefficient of variation on sample size[a]

If CV equals	then n equals
12.5%	9
25%[b]	9
50%	100
100%	400

[a] $\alpha = .05$, $t = 2.00$, $r = 0.1$
[b] If $\alpha = .10$ then $n = 19$

statistical distributions which result from broad-based original sampling as well as those which result from compilations of data from different sources. Furthermore, the robustness of traditional statistical techniques should be evaluated to determine how appropriate these techniques are for food composition data. The impact of using means v. medians in food composition databases on conclusions drawn from dietary studies, must be tested. In particular, caution is required when estimating food composition values from small data sets.

After the sample is defined individual items or units within the sample can be identified and procured to be prepared for analysis. Once the units, packages, or containers arrive in the laboratory their handling (e.g. preparation, homogenization) and the selection of aliquots must be carefully planned to maintain the representativeness and integrity of the material. Since the developer of the project design and sampling strategy may not be the laboratory analyst the importance of communication between these individuals or groups cannot be overestimated. At this point it is important to emphasize the use of standardized nomenclature with regard to sampling at the laboratory level. According to the 1990 recommendations for nomenclature for sampling in analytical chemistry submitted to the International Union of Pure and Applied Chemistry (IUPAC) Horwitz defines the "sample" as "a portion of material selected in some manner to represent a larger body of material. The result obtained from the sample is merely an estimate of the quantity ... of constituent ... of the parent material." Previously, the term sample has often been used to refer to the portion (e.g. extract, diluted or not) being analyzed at various points in the analytical process. Other terms such as "test" or "analytical" should be used to describe those portions to avoid inconsistencies or ambiguities and subsequent misinterpretation of the results. The reader is referred to reference (8) for further information.

▮ How Good Do The Data Have To Be?

Food composition data must be "good enough" to permit the careful assessment of food consumption patterns and their impact on the health of population groups and subgroups. Similarly, the data must be "good enough" to accomplish other scientific and economic objectives defined by investigators. The quality of a specific estimate is based, in part, on the accuracy and precision of the measurement process. The generation of accurate food composition data requires that variability inherent to the food be accurately quantified while variability inherent to the measurement process be minimized. In general, the major sources of statistical variability in dietary estimates are the food consumption data captured by the dietary assessment tool, and the food composition data. Variability for food composition data includes all variability attributable to sampling plans, sample handling, analytical method, and analytical quality control. Each of these sources can be partitioned into the sources of variability and can be quantified by an analysis of variance (37). The assessment of the sources and magnitude of variability for food composition data can indicate areas where improvement in the measurement process needs to be made (38). While sampling is only one source of variability, the lack of representative sampling can increase the degree of bias in the estimates of central tendency and cause errors in the estimates of variance. As previously mentioned, for a specific component, a small number of foods may contribute the majority of that component to the diet of the population. Therefore, it is recommended that sampling resources be dedicated to obtaining statistically sound estimates for those major contributors.

■ Acknowledgments

The author wishes to express her appreciation to the First International Food Data Base Conference for generous financial support to attend the conference.

■ References

(1) Life Sciences Research Office (1989) *Nutrition Monitoring in the United States: An Update Report on Nutrition Monitoring*, US Dept. of Health and Human Services, Hyattsville, MD

(2) Steinmetz, K.A., & Potter, J.D. (1991) *Cancer Causes and Control*, **2**, 427-442

(3) Hegsted, D.M., & Ausman, L.M. (1988) *J. Nutr.* **118**, 1184-1189

(4) Katan, M.B., Van Gastel, A.C., de Rover, C.M., van Montfort, M.A.J., & Knuiman, J.T. (1988) *Eur. J. Clin Invest.* **18**, 644-647

(5) Judd, J.T., Clevidence, B.A., Muesing, R.A., Wittes, J., Sunkin, M.E., & Podczasy, J.J. (1994) *Am. J. Clin. Nutr.* **59**, 861-868

(6) Vanderveen, J.E., & Pennington, J.A.T. (1983) *Food Nutr. Bull.* **5**, 40-45

(7) Holden, J.M., Schubert, A., Wolf, W.R., & Beecher, G.R. (1987) in *Food Composition Data: A User's Perspective*, W.M. Rand, C.T. Windham, B.W. Wyse & V.R. Young (Eds.), UNU Press, Tokyo, pp. 177-193

(8) Horwitz, W. (1990) *Pure Appl. Chem.* **62**, 1993-1208

(9) Nielsen, A.C. Co. (1990) *Nielsen Scantrack Data*, Northbrook, IL

(10) Cochran, W.G. (1977) *Sampling Techniques*, 3rd Ed., Wiley, New York, NY, pp. 1-78

(11) Greenfield, H., & Southgate, D.A.T. (1992) *Food Composition Data: Production, Management and Use*, Elsevier Applied Science, London

(12) Stewart, K.K. (1981) in *Beltsville Symposia in Agricultural Research IV Human Nutrition Research*, Allenheld, Osmun Publication, Totowa, NJ

(13) Beecher, G.R., & Matthews, R.H. (1990) in *Present Knowledge in Nutrition*, 6th Ed., International Life Sciences Institute, Washington, DC

(14) Le Marchand, L., Yoshizawa, C.N., Kolonel, L.N., Hankin, G.H., & Goodman, M.T. (1989) *J. Nat. Cancer Inst.* **81**, 1158-1164

(15) Moore, T. (1957) *Vitamin A*, Elsevier, Amsterdam

(16) Mangels, A.R., Holden, J.M., Beecher, G.R., Forman, M.L., & Lanza, E. (1993) *J. Am. Diet. Assoc.* **93**, 284-296

(17) West, C.E., & Poortvliet, E.J. (1993) *The Carotenoid Content of Foods with Special Reference to Developing Countries*, USAID/VITAL, Washington, DC

(18) Khachik, F., Beecher, G.R., Goli, M.B., & Lusby, W.R. (1992) *Methods Enzymol.* **213**, 347-359

(19) Rodriguez-Amaya, D.B. (1989) *J. Micronutr. Anal.* **5**, 191-225

(20) Chug-Ahuja, J.K., Holden, J.M., Forman, M.R., Mangels, A.R., Beecher, G.R., & Lanza, E. (1993) *J. Am. Diet. Assoc.* **93,** 318-323

(21) Schneeman, B.O., & Gallaher, D.D. (1990) in *Present Knowledge in Nutrition*, 6th Ed., International Life Sciences Institute, Washington, DC

(22) Li, B.W., Holden, J.M., Brownlee, S.G., & Korth, S.G. (1987) *J. Am. Diet. Assoc.* **87**, 740-743

(23) Hepburn, F.N. (1988) *Proceedings of the 12th National Nutrient Data Bank Conference*, The CBord Group, Inc., Ithaca, NY, pp. 31-33

(24) Schubert, A., Holden, J.M., & Wolf, W.R. (1987) *J. Am. Diet. Assoc.* **87**, 285-299

(25) Tonucci, L.H., Holden, J.M., Beecher, G.R., Khachik, F., Davis, C.S., & Mulokozi, G. (1995) *J. Agric. Food Chem.* (in press)

(26) Micozzi, M.S., Brown, E.D., Edwards, B.K., Bieri, J.G., Taylor, P.R., Khachik, F., Beecher, G.R., & Smith, J.C. (1992) *Am. J. Clin. Nutr.* **55**, 1120-1125

(27) Savell, J.W., Harris, J.J., Cross, D.S. Hale, D.S., & Beasley, L.C. (1991) *J. Anim. Sci.* **69**, 2883-2893

(28) Buege, D., Held, J.E., Smith, C.A., Sather, L.K., & Klatt, L.V. (1990) *Research Bulletin R-3509*, College of Agriculture and Life Sciences, University of Wisconsin, Madison, WI

(29) McCann, A., Pennington, J.A.T., Smith, E.C., Holden, J.M., Soergel, D., & Wiley, R.C. (1988) *J. Am. Diet. Assoc.* **88**, 336-341

(30) Kohlmeier, L., & Poortvliet, E. (1992) *Report of the FLAIR Eurofoods-Enfant Project Second Annual Meeting*, Wageningen Agricultural University, Wageningen

(31) Honikel, K.O. (1994) *Report, FLAIR Eurofoods-Enfant Project Third Annual Meeting*, Wageningen Agricultural University, Wageningen

(32) Holden, J.M., Gebhardt, S., Davis, C.S., & Lurie, D.G. (1991) *J. Food Comp. Anal.* **4**, 183-195

(33) *Progressive Grocer's Market Scope* (1993) Progressive Grocer's Trade Dimension Division, Maclean, Hunter Media, Inc., Stamford, CT, pp. 18, 348-549

(34) Holden, J.M., Lanza, E., & Wolf, W.R. (1986) *J. Agric. Food Chem.* **34**, 302-308

(35) Knutson, J. (1989) *Meatfacts 88*, American Meat Institute, Washington, DC, p. 17

(36) Gebhardt, S.E., & Holden, J.M. (1992) *Provisional Table on the Selenium Content of Foods,* USDA, Washington, DC

(37) Sokal, R.R., & Rohlf, F.J. (1981) *Biometry*, 2nd Ed., W.H. Freeman and Company, San Francisco, CA

(38) Beaton, G.H., Milner, J., Corey, P., McGuire, V., Cousins, M., Stewart, E., de Ramos, M., Hewitt, D., Grambsch, P.V., Hassim, N., & Little, J.A. (1979) *Am. J. Clin. Nutr.* **32**, 2546-2559

Assuring Regional Data Quality in the Food Composition Program in China

Guangya Wang, Xiaolin Li

Institute of Nutrition and Food Hygiene, Chinese Academy of Preventive Medicine, 29 Nan Wei Road, Beijing 100050, China

A nationwide collaborative project on the analysis of food composition for China was organized and conducted by the Institute of Nutrition and Food Hygiene between 1987 and 1990. In order to assure the quality of analytical data from all 20 participating laboratories, a quality assurance system was conducted involving five procedures: a written manual of analytical methods; technical training courses for laboratory technicians; the use of identical methodological protocols for sampling and handling of food samples; analytical duplicate or replicates for unknown samples; standard reference materials and quality control materials. The results were monitored by means of a control chart to check the reliability of technical performance. Data were evaluated by logic and statistical tests and then compiled into new Chinese food composition tables. The total number of food items is 1358, comprising 3280 separate food samples.

A nationwide collaborative project to revise and update the food composition data of China was organized and conducted by the Institute of Nutrition and Food Hygiene (INFH) in 1987–1990. In order to assure the quality of the analytical data provided by each of the 20 participating laboratories, an analytical quality assurance system was designed and carried out. The data obtained in this project were the basis of the new edition of the Chinese food composition tables (FCT) published in 1991.

■ Background

The first edition of the Chinese FCT published by INFH in 1952 included only 12 nutrients, crude fiber and energy value for about 300 food items. In the following years, INFH updated the FCT with three editions having been published. The last printing was in 1981 and its English version was published in 1990 (1). A new edition of the food composition tables has been needed since the early 1980s, because food composition may have changed, due to the changes in crop cultivation and animal husbandry as well as food storage, transportation and marketing during the recent decades; also newer and better analytical methods are now available; and data on a number of important micronutrients (vitamins, trace elements) were missing from the previous editions. In this project, both the nutrients and food items were increased. The food items were selected based on the knowledge of frequency and amount of food consumption obtained from several national dietary surveys, and newer methods were used in the laboratory analyses. All the nutrients were analyzed by AOAC methods (2) and official Chinese methods (3, 4). The analytical data were categorized as follows: proximate composition (moisture, energy, protein, fat, carbohydrate, dietary fiber and ash); vitamins (ascorbic acid, thiamin, riboflavin, niacin, retinol, carotenes, and tocopherols); minerals (calcium, iron, magnesium, phosphorus, potassium, sodium, zinc, copper, manganese and selenium); lipids (fatty acids and cholesterol); and, amino acids. Foods items were divided into 28 groups including cereals, dried legumes, fresh and sprouted legumes, roots, tubers and stems, fresh leafy vegetables, melons, squashes and gourds, fruit-bearing vegetables, pickled, salted and preserved vegetables, fungi and algae, fruits, nuts and seeds, meats, poultry, milk and milk products, infant foods, eggs, fish, molluscs and crustaceans, fats and oils, confections and snacks, tea and beverages, alcoholic beverages, sugars and sweets, starch and its products, condiments and spices, edible Chinese medicinal herbs, and miscellaneous items. The total number of food items analyzed in this project was 1358. Food composition analysis was performed by 20 laboratories located in 15 provinces. Among them, there were 11 provincial and five municipal Institutes of Food Safety Inspection, three provincial Medical Institutes and one provincial Medical College. These provinces and municipalities covered half of the areas of China and more than two-thirds of the total Chinese population (Figure 1).

■ Working Procedures

The following system was introduced to assure the quality of data generated by all the participating laboratories.

Validation of Analytical Methods

A written manual of analytical methods including food sampling and handling was prepared by INFH to ensure laboratories adhered to the same methods. All the methods were validated for accuracy and precision according to published guidelines (5, 6). Each analytical method was evaluated by three to six selected laboratories using standard reference materials (SRMs), i.e. bovine liver (National Bureau of Standard, USA), bread crumbs (a gift from Dr. Harry G. Lento, Campbell Institute for Research Technology, USA), and pig liver (China National Standard Bureau), as well as quality control materials (QCMs) prepared by the central laboratory in INFH, i.e. wheat flour, whole milk powder and carrot paste. Accuracy and precision of analytical methods between laboratories were determined daily to validate the methods. The three QCMs were used to measure the level of precision and recovery. The detectability and correlation coefficient of standard curves were used as additional indices for method validation.

Training Courses for Participating Laboratories

In order to assure that the analytical procedures would be carried out correctly and consistently by all the participating laboratories, several technical training courses were organized by INFH. The first training course was conducted in 1986 and attended by more than 50 technicians from the 20 laboratories. The methods for determination of six vitamins, amino acids, fatty acids, dietary fiber and selenium were demonstrated by instructors and then practiced by the trainees in the training laboratories. The second course was conducted in 1987. Two specialists in food analysis, Dr Gary R. Beecher and Dr Joseph T. Vanderslice from USDA, were invited to give lectures and to introduce new technologies in food nutrient analysis. During 1988 to 1989 secondary training courses were organized at the local level to train more technicians with the instructors from INFH.

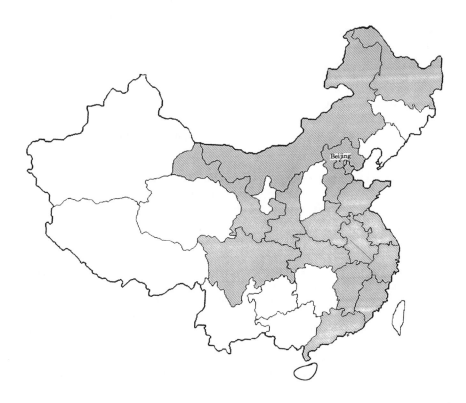

Figure 1. Outline map of China showing provinces included in food composition program (shaded)

Sampling and Handling of Food Samples

It was critical to ensure that identical protocols of sampling and handling of foods for analysis were used in each participating laboratory in order to eliminate both intrinsic and extrinsic sources of variation which could affect the measured levels of nutrients in foods. The sampling scheme was designed to reflect representativeness of the food with regard to the brand or cultivar and geographic origin of the food as well as the differences in food consumption in the different areas. Foods were collected according to the priority of quantity consumed. The sample size for each collection was 1.5 kg by weight or by pieces. If the weight of each piece was over 500 g, three pieces were collected. The same variety of food was collected in three places located in an urban district and/or county area. After the food was homogenized, one-third of each homogenate was pooled into one analytical sample. The analyses for vitamins were carried out as soon as the foods were collected. A set protocol for homogenization, temperature control and other aspects of sample preparation was followed.

Interlaboratory Quality Control

Any interlaboratory variation will affect the variability of the compiled data. The values produced by each laboratory were evaluated by using quality control materials (QCMs). The maximum acceptable relative standard deviation (RSD or CV) was between 5 per cent and 10 per cent. The coefficient of correlation of the regression curve for each standard curve of an analytical method should ideally be 0.999. Recovery tests of fortified QCMs were used as an index of accuracy. Recoveries between 90-110 per cent were defined as satisfactory. The analyzed mean value was expected to fall within plus or minus one standard deviation of the certified value. For the QCMs used in this program a mean certified value and

standard deviation was determined by six of the selected laboratories. In general, values within two standard deviations from the mean were acceptable. Data of QCM analyses produced by participating laboratories were evaluated using the Youden pairs method (8, 9) to test whether the value fell within the 95 per cent confidence interval. The outlier data were examined in order to identify problems. Sample exchanges, replicate analyses, calculation checks and further training of technicians in INFH were carried out to improve analytical accuracy and precision. For unknown samples the results of duplicate analyses had to be within 10 per cent of their mean. Otherwise, a third or further replication was required to re-determine the mean.

Assessment of Analytical Data Reported from Different Laboratories

The analytical data for foods from each laboratory were evaluated with respect to their reliability. Some statistical tests were used such as the Dixon and Grubbs test to reveal the outlier values. The t test was used to determine whether data were significantly different, and the F test was used to determine whether the variances of the data were different (8, 9). Validated values were compiled into the new FCT.

∎ Results and Discussion

SRMs are ideal tools for analytical quality control, but they are too expensive to be used throughout an entire project. Therefore, QCMs prepared by INFH were used by each laboratory. Whole milk powder and wheat flour were easy to obtain in large amounts and very homogeneous, so they were suitable for use as QCMs. On the other hand, carrot paste proved to be difficult to stabilize and was readily spoiled during transportation and storage. Results from carrot paste showed large variations, and are not included in this paper. The certified values of the

Table I. Certified nutrient values of quality control materials per 100 g (mean ±SD)

	Whole Milk Powder	Wheat flour
Moisture (g)	3.1±0.2	12.0±0.5
Protein (g)	24.8±0.8	11.7±0.6
Fat (g)	27.2±3.0	1.6±0.2
Ash (g)	5.8±0.1	0.84±0.02
Dietary fiber (g)	–	2.4±0.2
Thiamin (mg)	0.18±0.05	0.35±0.02
Riboflavin (mg)	0.90±0.11	0.08±0.02
Niacin (mg)	0.80±0.11	2.12±0.19
Retinol (µg)	135±43	–
Vitamin E (mg)	0.44±0.02	1.56±0.39
K (mg)	1010±115	202±17
Na (mg)	350.1±12.5	1.3±0.1
Ca (mg)	847±115	14.0±0.7
Mg (mg)	107±9	69±6
Fe (mg)	0.6±0.2	1.9±0.4
Zn (mg)	3.53±0.48	1.57±0.13
Cu (mg)	0.06±0.01	0.27±0.04
Mn (mg)	0.07±0.02	1.92±0.12
Se (µg)	8.90±0.73	28.7±1.10
P (mg)	770±45	195±16

– = not applicable

QCMs were the mean values calculated from the individual values from six laboratories. Each individual value produced by a laboratory was the mean value calculated from six duplicate determinations on different days. These six selected laboratories passed the quality control test. The certified nutrient values of the QCMs for wheat flour and whole milk powder are shown in Table I.

Bovine liver, bread crumbs and pig liver SRMs were used to validate the analytical methods. The accuracy and percent recovery of analyses were used as indices for evaluation. For example, the accuracy of the fluorometric method for selenium (Se) analysis is shown in Table II. The reported mean values were close to the certified values and the coefficients of variation (CV) of the analytical values were between 2.7 per cent and 6.3 per cent. The percent recoveries of the analysis were between 95.2-99.1 per cent and the CVs of the results were between 2.8 per cent and 6.2 per cent. The data in Table II indicate that the fluorometric method was a valid method for Se.

Other indices for evaluating analytical methods were also used and the results are shown in Table III. Using the data collected from the selected laboratories, all the methods were evaluated. The recoveries of these methods ranged from 87 per cent to 110 per cent, most of them being in the range 90 per cent to 110 per cent. The analytical precision of the methods shows that the CV of repeatability within each laboratory was around 2-7 per cent and the CV of reproducibility between each laboratory was larger (Ta-

Table II. Accuracy of the fluorometric method for determination of selenium

Standard reference material	Certified value	Reported mean value		Reported recovery	
	(X±S,μg/g)	(X±S,μg/g)	CV%	(X±S,%)	CV%
Bovine Liver 1577a	1.1±0.1	1.04±0.03(11)	2.7		
Pig Liver	0.940±0.028	0.960±0.028(8)	2.9		
Milk Powder	0.089±0.007	0.094±0.003(6)	3.1	99.1±2.8	2.8
Wheat Flour	0.287±0.011	0.298±0.019(6)	6.3	95.2±4.6	5.0
Rice Flour	0.083±0.007	0.082±0.005(6)	6.0	95.9±5.9	6.2

Numbers in parentheses are the total number of determinations

Table III. Indices and results for methods validation

Method	Nutrient ananlysed	Recovery		Repeatability	Reproducibility	Linearity of std curve	Limit of detection
		%	CV%	CV%	CV%	(r)	
Atomic absorption spectometry	Ca	93.7-108.3	3.8-5.1	2.0-5.7	1.1-5.7	0.9996	0.1μg/ml
	Fe	95.0-108.5	3.4-5.3	5.2-7.2	4.6-11.0	0.9996	0.2μg/ml
	Mg	94.9-105.1	2.8-4.7	3.8-7.0	1.8-7.9	0.9998	0.05μg/ml
	Mn	94.1-109.0	4.5-6.1	6.4-9.6	2.4-8.2	0.9991	0.01μg/ml
Flame photometry	K	97.9-104.8	2.6-2.8	1.4-2.8	0.3-10.4	0.9998	0.05μg/ml
	Na	96.4-103.8	2.4-3.1	2.6-5.1	2.0-5.8	0.9997	0.3μg/ml
Microbiology	Riboflavin	98.3-110.0	2.6-2.8	2.2-5.2	11.3-11.9	NA	0.05μg
	Niacin	93.6-110.0	3.3-4.7	2.4-4.0	6.4-8.3	NA	0.05μg
Paper chromatography	Total carotenes	88.8-102.9	5.2	1.7	5.9	0.9996	0.1μg
Fluorometry	Thiamin	91-100	7.4	6.8-8.5	17-22	0.9993	0.05μg
	Riboflavin	92-109	3.2-6.2	4.5-5.7	11.7-15.1	0.9998	0.002μg
	Ascorbic acid	99.5-107.1	6.0	2.7-7.3	–	0.9996	0.022μg
	Selenium	87.4-104.5	2.8-6.1	3.1-6.2	9.6-10.2	0.9998	3 ng
LC	Retinol	92-105	9.0	11.0	5.7-8.8	0.9981	0.04μg/μl
	Tocopherol, α	92-105	9.0	10.0	5.4-8.7	0.9996	4.59ng/μl
	γ+β	97-108	3.6	13.0	3.1-7.4	0.9918	1.83ng/μl
	ζ	87-107	4.1	11.1	11.1	0.9910	1.03ng/μl
Spectrometry	Phosphorus	94.9-105.4	4.4-4.8	2.1-6.4	1.1-6.4	0.9999	1.5μg/μl
Gravimetry	NDF	NA	NA	2.5-7.6	3.8-15.5	NA	1.1mg

NDF = Neutral detergent fiber
–   = Not determined
NA   = Not applicable

Table IV. Percentages of acceptable values from participating laboratories

Nutrient	Wheat flour			Whole milk		
	No. of labs	No. of labs accepted	Acceptability %	No. of labs	No. of labs accepted	Acceptability %
Moisture	17	16	94.1	16	13	81.2
Protein	17	17	100	18	17	94.4
Fat	16	16	100	19	19	100
NDF	16	15	93.8	–	–	–
Ash	15	13	86.8	16	14	87.5
K	18	17	94.4	16	15	93.8
Na	16	14	87.5	17	16	94.1
Ca	17	10	58.8	16	15	93.8
Mg	17	15	88.2	16	15	93.8
Fe	18	18	100	17	17	100
Zn	18	17	94.4	17	16	94.1
Cu	17	17	100	17	15	88.2
Mn	16	15	93.8	16	16	100
P	17	17	100	16	15	93.8
Se	14	13	92.8	12	11	91.7
Thiamin	16	8	50.0	16	16	100
Riboflavin	15	15	100	17	15	88.2
Niacin	12	12	100	13	13	100
Retinol	–	–	–	12	12	100
Tocopherol	12	12	100	–	–	–

NDF = Neutral detergent fibre
–   = Not applicable

ble III). The CV for proximate analyses (not shown in Table III) was between 1 per cent to 8 per cent, but for vitamin analyses there were larger variations. In general, the methods for vitamin determination had somewhat lower precision than mineral and proximate analyses. The above results showed that all the methods were satisfactory. In order to monitor analytical performance, the data for nutrient analyses of QCMs were collected and evaluated using three statistical tests. A simple method was the control chart test (10). All the QCMs data from each laboratory were plotted on the control chart. The certified value (X) of a given nutrient was assigned as the central line (CL), the mean value plus or minus one standard deviation (S) as the upper and lower auxiliary lines (XS), respectively, the mean 2S as the upper and lower warning limit line, and the mean 3S as the control or confidence limits. Because the QCMs are biological materials and are unstable, their composition could change with time and be affected by factors such as oxidation, temperature and light etc. So we preferred to use the mean value 3S as the largest acceptable limit. The percentages of acceptable values from the participating laboratories are shown in Table IV and Figures 2 and 3.

Some laboratories failed to submit the results to INFH in time and their data

QCMs-Wheat Flour

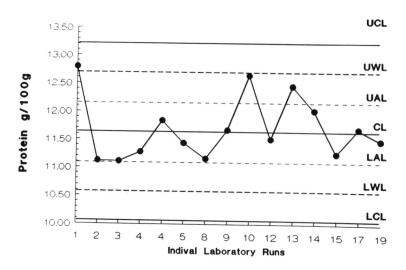

QCMs-Whole Milkpowder

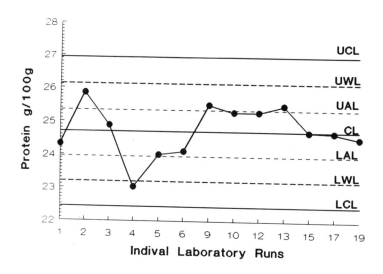

Figures 2 and 3. Examples of a quality control chart for two QCMs with different mean values of protein obtained from collaborative laboratories

were not included in Table IV. According to the results in Table IV, 87-100 per cent of the laboratories passed the quality control tests, except that around half of the laboratories failed in the determination of thiamin and calcium. Most of the calcium values of wheat flour were much higher than the certified values. The errors came from technical mistakes such as not adding the 8-hydroxyquinoline to eliminate interference from reagents. Some thiamin values of wheat flour were higher and some were lower than the central line. Problems included low recovery after column filtration or interfering substances from reagents. Most of the niacin and protein values of both wheat flour and milk powder fell within UWL and LWL (X2S) (shown in Figures 1 and 2). The over-range data were questioned and the problems identified by means of replicating the analyses, making new standard curves and checking the calculations. To calculate the representative value for each analyte in each food item, two standard deviations from the mean value after deleting the suspect data were used to eliminate the values outside the range limits and then the mean value was recalculated. This mean value was used for the food composition table. Some results considered as unreasonable were checked for the causes. In some cases, re-analysis of foods was carried out through exchanges with other laboratories or IFNH. Some unreasonable data which could not be validated were eliminated during data compilation. In practice, some values were difficult to judge based on the current knowledge of food and nutrition, and were, therefore, retained in the FCT.

Conclusion

Quality control is costly and time consuming, but it is essential. We have conducted an efficient analytical quality assurance system in a nationwide project of food composition analysis of 1358 food items, and involving 20 collaborating laboratories. According to our experience, the critical parts in this analytical quality assurance system were the validation of analytical methods, the availability and use of reference materials and the training of the technicians. Large variations existed in the conditions of the collaborating laboratories as well as in the technical background of the technicians. There were some inadequacies in this approach, for example, analytical methods for minerals were not included in training courses, except for selenium, and a few technicians were not familiar with the LC and GLC techniques. The question of how to ensure the comparability of the Chinese food composition data with those of other nations is still an unresolved problem.

Acknowledgments

This project was supported by National Science Foundation of China and Ministry of Public Health and Jia Li Bao company.

References

(1) Ershow, A.G., & Wang, Chen, K. (1990) *J. Food Comp. Anal.* **3**, 191-442

(2) *Official Methods of Analysis* (1984) 14th Ed., AOAC, Arlington. VA, secs 14.002-14.004, 31.005-31.008, 7.009, 43.275-43.277, 24.037-24.040, 7.093-7.103, 43.024-43.038, 43.069-43.081

(3) People's Republic of China Standard GB 12388-12399-90 (1990) *Methods for Determination of Nutrient Composition in Foods* (in Chinese), Chinese Standard Publishing House, Beijing

(4) Institute of Nutrition and Food Hygiene (1990) *Methods of Food Analysis,* 3rd Ed. (in Chinese), People's Medical Publishing House, Beijing

(5) Uriano, G.A., & Cali, J.P. (1977) in *Role of Reference Materials and Reference Methods in the Measurement Process*, J.R. DeVoe (Ed),

ACS Symposium Series 63, American Chemical Society, Washington, DC, Chap. 4

(6) Holden J.M., Schubert A., Wolf, W.R., & Beecher, G.R. (1987) *Food Nutr. Bull.*, Suppl. 12, 177-193

(7) People's Republic of China Standard G.B. 6379-86 (1986) *Precision of Test Methods for Determination of Repeatability and Reproducibility for a Standard Test Method by Interlaboratory Tests* (in Chinese),

Chinese Standard Publishing House, Beijing

(8) Pan, X.R. (1989) *Assurance and Evaluation of the Accuracy of Chemical Analysis* (in Chinese), Chinese Measurement Publishing House, Beijing

(9) Gerrit, K., & Frans, W.P. (1981) *Quality Control in Analytical Chemistry*, John Wiley & Sons Inc., New York, NY

Quality Control for Food Composition Data in Journals — A Primer

Kent K. Stewart, Margaret R. Stewart

Virginia Polytechnic Institute & State University,
Blacksburg, VA, 24061-0308, USA

Scientific journals are a primary vehicle for the transmission of original food composition data and critical reviews of food composition data to the scientific community. Publication of composition data in a scientific journal implies that the data are accurate, precise, and meaningful. To publish data meeting these attributes it is necessary to establish criteria for data quality control. Quality control is achieved by critical evaluation of all aspects of a scientific manuscript by expert reviewers. The key attribute of a good quality control in a manuscript is adequate documentation. In a good publication, those items that should be documented include the purpose of the study; description of the sampling plan for selection of the food items to be assayed; descriptions of the food items; descriptions of the sample preparation, homogenization, and storage; description of the analyte extraction; descriptions of the identification and measurement of the analyte; and description of the analytical quality control measures used to validate the data sets. Reviewers also evaluate the quantitative data including their statistical components and the discussion of how the new data relate to existing knowledge on the composition of foods.

It is almost an article of faith in the scientific community that "good" data will aid in the development of wise decisions and that "bad" data will lead to the development of unwise decisions. In cases of conflicting data, the perceptions of which are good data and which are bad data may well be as important as the actual fact of the quality of the data.

These are not just issues of academic concern to those working on food composition data. The current public concerns about the impact of diet on health will inevitably lead to the promulgation of new policies and regulations on the composition of foods. The public in many countries is concerned about the possibility of inadequate intakes of essential nutrients, problems related to inadequate or excessive intake of energy, the possibility of intakes of toxic levels of man-made chemicals such as pesticides and herbicides, and the perceived dangers of the use of biotechnology in the production and processing of the food supply. Given the current level of knowledge on the composition of foods, a great deal of new food composition data will be needed if wise policies and regulations on the issues of diet and public health are to be made.

The discussions in this paper about quality control for food composition data in scientific journals are extensions of opinions from editorials originally published in the *Journal of Food Composition and Analysis* (1–10). Scientific journals are a primary vehicle for the transmission of original food composition data and critical reviews of food composition data to the scientific community. Publication of composition data in a scientific journal specifically implies that the data and their attributes have been evaluated and reviewed prior to publication by independent experts in the field. The responsibilities of publishing credible, good quality composition data are spread among the authors of the manuscripts, the reviewers of the manuscripts, and the editors of the journals. It is the authors' responsibility to carry out the study properly and then to provide adequate documentation on how the study was done.

While the editor selects the reviewers and ensures that conflicts between authors and reviewers are resolved, it is the reviewers who are the key to quality control of journal articles through critical evaluation of all aspects of a scientific manuscript. Given the chemical complexity of foods and their matrices, the enormous size of the food distribution system, and the frequent technical complexity and difficulty of modern analytical assay techniques, reviewers of food composition data need special expertise as well as significant knowledge of a broad range of subjects.

The reviewers' first responsibility is to determine whether or not adequate documentation (a key aspect of food composition data quality control) was provided in the manuscript reporting the study. Without adequate documentation there can be no critical evaluation of the science, and its lack is a fundamental failure of manuscript quality control and, if not rectified, should ultimately result in rejection of the manuscript.

Once the reviewers ascertain that the documentation is present, then they should determine that the appropriate techniques were used for the acquisition of the food composition data. A review of the appropriateness of various techniques for food composition data acquisition is very complex and requires a great deal of technical discussion beyond the scope of this paper. Finally, it is the reviewer's responsibility to determine whether or not the composition data are accurate, precise, novel, and credible. These are primarily issues of quality control and are the main topic of this paper.

The editor's primary responsibility is to ensure to the readers of a journal that the data published therein are accurate, precise, and meaningful. The goal of a journal is to have the data review and publication done in an authoritative manner so that the burden of proof will be on those who challenge the published assay data of the composition of specific foods. Thus in many ways, while authors are the source of scientific knowledge, scientific journals can be viewed as "gates" for transmission of knowledge, and the reviewers and editors can be viewed as "gatekeepers".

The primary focus of this paper is documentation needed in a food composition paper. The underlying theme is that adequate documentation is required for good quality control of published food composition data.

▋ Documentation Needed in Manuscripts

The documentation for a food composition data manuscript includes the sampling plan, a description of the foods and the laboratory samples, a description of the assay methodologies, the actual composition data, the quality control information for those data, and a comparison of the data presented with those in the published scientific literature.

Sampling Plans

A primary goal in the analysis of food samples is the description of the nutrient content of the foods that are encountered in the real world. This seemingly trivial and almost tautological statement is unfortunately not often followed to its logical conclusion: that the design of the analytic protocol (especially the choice of food items and the number of analyses run) should be directed towards gathering as much information as possible about the distribution of the nutrients in food in the real world. Users of food composition data need information about the average or "usual" level of that nutrient and the

range of values that would likely be encountered.

A key issue is thus which food item should be assayed? Another way to put this is the question "Were the assayed items representative of the foods for which composition information is presented?" It should be intuitively obvious that representative composition data can only be obtained from the assay of representative lots. Thus the determination of which lots to assay may well be the most important of all the questions facing the analyst in the design of a food composition assay program. The goal of a good sampling plan should be to have a protocol which indicates how many lots should be sampled and when and where they should be obtained, and which provides other details on how individual food items should be selected.

Once a good sampling plan is selected and documented, then the means used for distinguishing the sources of variability in analytical data, i.e., those arising from inherent biologic variability that reflect differences in genotype, phenotype, environment, processing, etc., and those arising from analytic variability, introduced in the process of preparation and assay of the laboratory sample, should be documented. In most cases the total number of analyses to be performed is strongly influenced by economics and each laboratory sample should be assayed a minimum number of times. It might seem that a general implementation of this design strategy would be to assay each laboratory sample only once. However, in general, the need for protection against major blunders in the assay of an individual sample leads to the suggestion that each sample be assayed in duplicate.

Food Descriptions

There are a very large number of foods in international and domestic market places. Different species are used as food sources; various growing conditions are used; the processing, packaging, and storage technologies vary. Cultural differences in food recipes are common. At the same time, there is a great commonality within some foodstuffs due to the worldwide availability of some brand name items (e.g., soft drinks and fast foods). Given the complexity of the world food supply, the readers of papers on the composition of foods need to be given the information to identify the foods for which the composition data are being presented. For even with the best of analytical techniques, food composition data are no better than the description of the products or foods being analyzed. The analyst should describe the foods so that another professional in the field can identify the foods. The sources and unique descriptions of the foods should be given. Those foods which were enriched and/or fortified should be so identified. Identification of market share can be useful. The analysts should specify numbers of items collected and the number of units in a composite. The dates of food acquisition should always be given. Frequently, most of the needed description of manufactured foods can be provided by identifying the brand name and place and date of purchase. The post-selection transportation and storage of the food items should be described. Any further fractionation of samples such as trimming and draining should also be described. When the food is cooked, the cooking processes should be described. References to published cooking procedures should be given whenever possible.

Compositing and Homogenizing

Compositing is the process of preparing a single representative composite sample from several food samples. Homogenization is the process of reducing a food sample to equally distributed particles of uniform size. Compositing and homogenization are the invisible components of food assay systems. Homogenization is almost always necessary to transform the large bulk of heterogeneous foods and diets to homogenous representative material suitable for sub-sampling. The proc-

ess has been described as transforming a 5 pound meat roast into an analytic sample which can be introduced by a 5 mL syringe into a chromatograph. The procedures used for compositing/homogenizing can have a significant impact on the accuracy and precision of the final results. The issues inherent in compositing and homogenizing are crucial to the production of accurate, representative, and precise food composition data. It is important that adequate documentation of these processes be given in food composition papers.

In these homogenization processes there is potential for analyte loss due to non-enzymatic oxidation, to various enzymatic actions and to other destructive reactions. Many homogenizing techniques do not yield homogenous material with mixed foods and diets. In such cases, representative sub-sampling is difficult and the precision of the results deteriorates. Much more work is needed on the techniques for validation of the appropriateness of homogenizing techniques.

Even when many samples are used to make a composite, once they have been composited, the analyst has only one test sample. Thus a primary feature of compositing is that all information on the variation between lots is lost once the individual samples are composited. There are several other issues that need resolution when doing compositing. For example, given the purposes of the assays: How many units should be used in a composite? How much information on real variance is lost when a given compositing procedure is used?

Assay Methods

A generalized diagram of an ideal food composition assay system is shown in Figure 1. The key feature of this schema is that a food composition assay should be viewed as a whole. Each part of the assay system must fit with the rest of the assay system. Inappropriate use of any one technique can invalidate the accuracy and/or precision of the entire assay. Basi-

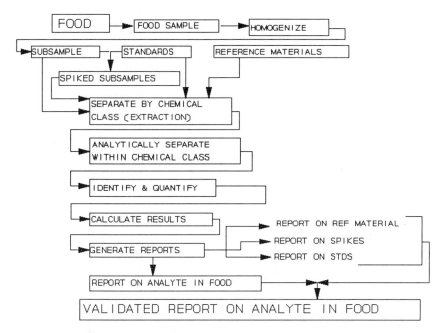

Figure 1. An ideal assay system

cally what is needed is a holistic approach to food composition assays.

Published Assay Methods

In most cases published assay methodologies are used for food composition assays. The authors should provide complete references to published assays. In those cases where methods manuals are used, e.g., an AOAC methods manual, the edition of the book and the assay number should be given. Some indication should be given as to how the selected methods were determined to be appropriate for the assays at hand. Most published methods are not appropriate for the assay of every food matrix. If there are known potential interferences in a given matrix, then the authors should use the method of standard additions to verify that the assay is appropriate for the food matrix. Failure to demonstrate quantitative recovery should raise serious concerns of the appropriateness of the choice of assay.

New Assay Methods

When new food assay methodologies are presented, it is important that these methods be validated for their use in obtaining food composition data. What follows is a general description of what is necessary to validate the use of a new assay methodology for a given matrix. The underlying premise is that the validation of an assay method is a process by which the assay method is demonstrated to be capable of producing the desired analytical results when used with the matrix of interest (i.e., assay methodology validations are matrix specific). Usually such a validation is done in some authoritative manner so that the burden of proof will be on those who challenge the assay method or the data from such a method. For most assay methods, the desired results include acceptable accuracy, precision, and sensitivity. The definition of acceptable accuracy, precision, and sensitivity of an assay is a function of the end use of the assay results. Different end uses will change the perception of what is acceptable. The following criteria are presented as an idealized list for assay validation. While it is understood that not every criterion will be met in every new method validation, each individual criterion should be considered when doing new assay method validations. The idealized assay validation criteria are:

- the entire assay method must be consistent with the chemical properties of the analyte and the matrix
- it should be demonstrated that there are no obvious matrix interferences for any stage of the assay method, or that subsequent or previous stages have eliminated the interferences
- the method should give quantitative recovery of pure standards carried through total assay method
- the method should give quantitative recovery of analytes to matrices of concern
- the method should give acceptable results on composition of standard reference materials of matrices similar to the foods to be assayed
- the method should give acceptable precision of replicate assays (five replicates) of the analyte in matrices of concern
- the limit of detection (LOD) for analyte determination in matrices should be defined and acceptable
- the linear range for analyte determination in matrices should be defined and acceptable
- the method should give the same results as a validated (or accepted) method or there should be an adequate explanation for the observed differences
- more than one analyst and more than one laboratory should be able to produce the same results with the method
- the individual data set validation processes should be made an integral part of any method description.

Analyte Extraction

Recent research studies in analytical chemistry have focused on the development of new instrumentation for the separation and measurement of analytes. Similar significant advances have been made in analytical biochemistry and molecular biology in the development of highly selective and sensitive probes such as immune-reagents and DNA and RNA probes. Significant improvements have been made in the use of enzymes as reagents. Almost all the advanced techniques described above require clean extracts free of interfering compounds. For the most part, it is best if the analytes are dissolved in solutions which are themselves compatible with the separation and measurement components of the assays. These advanced techniques are perfect for the assay of pure standards or the assay of mixtures of pure standards. Unfortunately, most foods do not come in tidy packages free of assay interferences. Rather, most foods are complex mixtures of multi-phase materials with extremely complex chemical matrices. Analyte levels are often low and assay interferences are common. If analysts are to properly use today's marvelous array of analytical tools for the assay of most food components, they first should isolate the analyte from the food matrix.

In an ideal extraction procedure the analyte is quantitatively removed from the food, no analyte remains with the residue, and no analyte is altered by the extraction procedure or by the inherent biochemical and chemical activities of the matrix. The extract should not contain compounds that would interfere with the separation and measurement components of the assays. For example, if chromatographic separations are used, the extract should not contain components which coelute with the analytes or those which alter the chromatographic behavior of the analytes. If immune reactions and/or enzyme measurement systems are used, components which alter those enzymatic and/or immune reactions are unacceptable. Given the complexity and variability of food matrices, quality control procedures for the extraction steps should be required parts of most assays. Certainly, the analyte isolation procedures should be carefully documented and critically reviewed before they are used or published in reputable scientific journals.

Analytical Separation of the Analyte

The current state of the art in analytical separation techniques such as gas liquid chromatography (GLC), and liquid chromatography (LC), super-critical fluid chromatography, and capillary electrophoresis is impressive. These sophisticated separation tools have the capability of separating very complex mixtures in relatively short time periods and as such each of these techniques can be very useful for the food analyst. Accompanying the power and sophistication of these techniques is their complexity. Reproducing assays using these techniques requires detailed information on the entire analytical system including the manufacturer and model of the instrumentation, the column used, the solvents or carrier gases used, the flow rates of solvents or carrier gases, and the temperatures used at the injection port, the column oven, and the detector. Adequate evaluation of any given analytical separation system requires extensive documentation of the system. Each sub-discipline in analytical separations has developed its own shorthand mode of presenting the necessary documentation for system evaluation.

Chromatography systems have several common problems including drift, difficulty in confirming peak identifications, and the difficulty of obtaining reproducible sample injections. The use of internal standards helps to reduce the problems of drift and sample injections. The use of internal standards is now considered to be almost mandatory and the lack of their use is considered to be a serious flaw in the methodology and often leads to rejection of a manuscript. Peak

identification can be difficult in some food matrices and care should be taken to document the proper identification of the analyte peaks convincingly.

Analyte Identification, and Quantification

Today's analyst has an enormous array of detection techniques for analyte quantification including atomic absorption and plasma emission spectrophotometry, mass spectrometry, diode array spectrophotometry, various electrochemical detectors, fluorescence detectors, the highly selective and sensitive probes such as immune-reagents, DNA and RNA probes, various chemical detection systems, the use of enzymes as reagents and of enzyme amplifier systems, and enzyme-linked-immunosorbant-assays. Many of these assay systems have been automated through the use of continuous flow systems, flow injection systems, and robotics. Recently, there have been significant advances in the use of hyphenated techniques such as GLC-mass spectrometry or other combinations such as enzyme-linked-immunosorbant-assays (ELISA) systems using electrochemical detection automated through the use of flow injection analysis. All of these systems are powerful and the analyst has an impressive array of quantification tools to draw upon. However, as in the case of analytical separations, the sophistication is usually accompanied by significant increases in complexity. Reproducing given assays using these techniques requires detailed information on the entire analytical system. The analyst needs to provide significant detailed documentation on the quantification system. Many detection systems do not provide unique identification; verification of analyte identification is often necessary. Even the highly selective assay systems such as immune-reagents and enzymes do not give totally unique identifications and are often quite sensitive to interferences in the quantification reactions. Verification of the ap-

Computation of Results

Unfortunately, computational errors are still one of the most common sources of errors in food composition data (or any other assays for that matter). The introduction of computerized computation systems, such as spreadsheets and black box analytical instrumentation, has not alleviated these problems. Thus it remains important for analysts to check the process by which they do their computations. Since computational errors are still so common, it is prudent for authors to document their quality control procedures for the computation of the analytical results.

Composition Data

Authors should report the means and standard deviation of the composition values and the number of lots assayed. Replicate assays on one test sample or one composite yield a single value and as such are usually not sufficient for journal publication. The significant digit convention (reporting of only all digits known with certainty and the first digit of uncertainty) should be used in reporting all data. Most food assays yield results with no more than three significant digits.

The moisture contents of individual foods are highly variable and thus most composition data should be presented on a dry weight basis. The composition data for beverages are obvious exceptions. Many believe that data presented on a dry weight basis should be accompanied by a moisture value to enable calculation to "as consumed" basis.

Data Set Validation

It is our observation as editors, that mistakes in composition data are a relatively frequent occurrence. Their frequency should be substantially reduced. The challenges in the production of good data

are that while there are a very large number of useful assays, their implementation is often complex and mistakes are relatively easy to make. Even experts can get incorrect results and generate incorrect data when using "good" methods. Therefore, to produce good data that are credible, the food composition community should develop protocols for data set validation. Given the complexity of the problems of assay and the wide variety of methodologies which are available today, we believe that the validation of *individual data sets* is necessary and that all food composition data sets should be individually validated. The concept that each individual data set be validated specifically implies that some type of quality control sample was assayed along with the samples that were assayed. Furthermore, it also implies that the data set results underwent an internal quality assurance check prior to the acceptance of the results. There are many ways to validate data sets including the use of common sense - consistency observation, standard laboratories, standard instruments, certified analysts, certified algorithms, standard reference materials, internal standards, audit trails, and in-house reference samples, (i.e. pool samples). The choice of the data validation procedure depends upon the laboratory, the food samples, and the component being measured. The addition of the concept of validated individual data sets will be of significant help in efforts to provide "good" food composition data that are also perceived to be "good data".

Comparison of the New Composition Data with Existing Information on the Composition of Foods

One aspect of almost all data quality control operations is a comparison of the new data with the existing body of knowledge. There are very few totally unique food composition data and reviewers will normally evaluate a new set of data by comparing it to the existing knowledge on food composition. Extreme departures from existing knowledge are usually rejected by reviewers unless significant justifications are presented for the acceptance of the new data. Authors are well advised to make such comparisons within the manuscript and provide a rationale for those data which appear to conflict with previously published data.

■ Future Actions

While significant improvements in the quality control of food composition data published in journals have been accomplished in the recent years, a great deal of work still needs to be done. A comment by Jorhem and Sundström in a recent paper (11) made the point clearly:

> During the last decade the application of analytical quality control measures has gradually been intensified. However, since analytical quality control activities are not yet in general use or standardized, it is often still difficult to compare results from different studies.

Significant efforts by journal editors, reviewers and authors are needed if we are to improve the comparability of data between studies.

More composition data need to be published in refereed journals. The current practice of directly publishing the results of food composition studies in databases rather than refereed journals means that the documentation behind those new composition data are usually not placed in the public domain. Thus the end users can not evaluate the appropriateness of the analytical quality control used in those studies. The failure to publish composition data in refereed journals prior to placement in a database is a worst case scenario. The data are available but the user has no idea of their quality. Ignorance is not bliss in such cases.

More analysts need to incorporate more analytical control into their assays and to better document those quality control procedures. These actions can be accomplished by both the editors and reviewers having an absolute requirement for documentation of good quality control procedures in all manuscripts accepted for publication.

Currently, almost all textbooks and courses on analytical chemistry, analytical biochemistry, food analysis and nutritional biochemistry contain little, if any, discussion of or instruction in assay quality control. (An exception is the recent book by Greenfield and Southgate (12)). This is a fundamental failure in our training of future analysts and it should be corrected. We strongly advocate that all analytical courses and text books in these areas contain a thoughtful section on the basics of assay quality control.

Adoption of these actions will have several benefits. Authors will increase the documentation of quality control procedures already in use in their laboratories. Authors will increase the use of acceptable assay quality control procedures in their studies. The existence of published papers with appropriate assay quality control will be useful as good examples to those in the field who wish to improve the quality of their own composition studies. Finally, the existence of papers with good quality control procedures will permit the users of food composition data to better evaluate the appropriateness of each food composition data set for the purpose at hand.

■ References

(1) Stewart, K. K. (1987) *J. Food Comp. Anal.* **1**, 1

(2) Stewart, K. K. (1988) *J. Food Comp. Anal.* **1**, 291-292

(3) Stewart, K. K. (1989) *J. Food Comp. Anal.* **2**, 91-92

(4) Stewart, K. K. (1990) *J. Food Comp. Anal.* **3**, 103-104

(5) Stewart, K. K. (1992) *J. Food Comp. Anal.* **5**, 1

(6) Stewart, K. K. (1992) *J. Food Comp. Anal.* **5**, 99

(7) Stewart, K. K. (1992) *J. Food Comp. Anal.* **5**, 183

(8) Rand, W. M. (1992) *J. Food Comp. Anal.* **5**, 267

(9) Stewart, K. K. (1993) *J. Food Comp. Anal.* **6**, 105-106

(10) Stewart, K. K. (1993) *J. Food Comp. Anal.* **6**, 201-202

(11) Jorhem L., & Sundström, B. (1993) *J. Food Comp. Anal.* **6**, 223-241

(35) Greenfield, H., & Southgate, D.A.T. (1992) *Food Composition Data: Production, Management and Use*, Elsevier Applied Science, London, pp. 127-138

▌Additional Reading

General Topics

Beecher, G.R., & Mathews, R.H. (1990) in *Present Knowledge in Nutrition*, 6th Ed., M.L. Brown (Eds.), ILSI-Nutrition Foundation, Washington, DC, pp. 430-443

IUPAC (1978) *Compendium of Analytical Nomenclature*, H.M.N.H. Irving, H. Freiser, & T.S. West (Eds.), Pergamon Press, Oxford

Klensin, J.C., Feskanich, D., Lin, V., Truswell, A.S., & Southgate, D.A.T. (1989) *Identification of Food Components for INFOODS Data Interchange*, UNU Press, Tokyo

Official Methods of Analysis (1995) 16th Ed., AOAC INTERNATIONAL, Arlington, VA

Rand, W.M., Pennington, J.A.T., Murphy, S.P., & Klensin, J.C. (1991) *Compiling Data for Food Composition Data Bases*, UNU Press, Tokyo

Rand, W.M., Windham, C.T., Wyse, B.W., & Young, V.T. (1987) *Food Composition Data: A User's Perspective*, UNU Press, Tokyo

Stewart, K. K. (Ed.) (1980) *Nutrient Analysis of Foods — The State of the Art for Routine Analysis*, AOAC, Washington, DC

Stewart, K.K., & Whitaker, J.R. (Eds.) (1984) *Modern Methods of Food Analysis*, AVI Publ. Co., Westport, CT

Stewart, K.K. (1985) in *Methods of Vitamin Assay*, 4th Ed., J. Augustin, B. Klein, D.R. Becker, P.B. Venugopal, P.B. (Eds.), Wiley, NY, pp. 1-15

Wernimont, G.T. (1985) *Use of Statistics to Develop and Evaluate Analytical Methods*, W. Spendley (Ed.), AOAC, Arlington, VA

Wolf, W.R. (Ed.) (1985) *Biological Reference Materials*, Wiley, NY

Quality Assurance

Garfield, F.M. (Ed.) (1980) *Optimizing Chemical Laboratory Performance Through the Application of Quality Assurance Principles, Proceedings of a Symposium*, AOAC, Arlington, VA

Garfield, F.M. (1991) *Quality Assurance Principles for Analytical Laboratories*, AOAC, Arlington, VA

Taylor, J.K. (1987) *Quality Assurance of Chemical Measurements*, Lewis Publ., Chelsea, MI

Modern Assay Techniques

Becker, J.M., Caldwell, G.A., & Zachgo, E.A. (1990) *Biotechnology, A Laboratory Course*, Academic Press, San Diego

Boehringer Mannheim, GmbH (1987) *Methods of Biochemical Analysis and Food Analysis*, Mannheim, Germany

Borman, S.A. (Ed.) (1982) *Instrumentation in Analytical Chemistry*, Vol. 2, ACS, Washington, DC

Harlow, E., & Lane, D. (1988) *Antibodies: A Laboratory Manual*, Cold Spring Harbor Laboratory, New York, NY

Strobel, H.A., & Heineman, W.R. (1989) *Chemical Instrumentation: A Systematic Approach*, 3rd Ed., Wiley, New York, NY

Information Needs and Computer Systems

This Session was chaired by Ms Karen Cashel of the University of Canberra. A keynote address was presented by C.E. West entitled *The Future Information Needs for Research at the Interface between Food Science and Nutrition.* This was followed by papers on *Food Database Management Systems — a Review* by W. Becker and I. Unwin and *Data Identification Consideration in International Interchange of Food Composition Data* by J.C. Klensin. These papers were followed by a computer demonstration *Food Data: Numbers, Words and Images* by B. Burlingame, F. Cook, G. Duxfield and G. Milligan. These are all published in this Section.

The following posters *Computer Construction of Recipes to Meet Nutritional and Palatability Requirements* by L.R. Fletcher and P. Soden (presented by D.A.T. Southgate) and *Requirements for Applications Software for Computerized Databases in Research Projects* by D. Mackerras are published at the end of this Section.

The Future Information Needs for Research at the Interface Between Food Science and Nutrition

Clive E. West

Department of Human Nutrition, Wageningen Agricultural University, PO Box 8129, 6700 EV Wageningen, The Netherlands and
Program Against Micronutrient Malnutrition, Center For International Health, Emory University School of Public Health, 1518 Clifton Road, NE, Atlanta GA 30322, USA

Nutrition and food science are disciplines at the interface between agriculture and health. Therefore, their information needs encompass both those of agriculture and health, and in addition extend into the realms of other disciplines such as the basic physical sciences, mathematics, the social sciences from economics to anthropology, the behavioral sciences, and history. In this paper, attention will be directed to the narrow interface between nutrition and food science, addressing information needs such as food naming and description, food intake, attributes of foods, and nutritional status.

In order to be certain about the identity of foods being consumed or traded, general agreement about food names is needed backed up by an adequate food description system containing a sufficient number of terms to describe foods in an unambiguous way. For this purpose, several systems, or types of systems, have been developed including Langual (1) the INFOODS system (2) and Eurocode 2 (3) as discussed more fully by Pennington (4).

The most important use of Langual in Europe and in other regions outside the United States may not be in its comprehensive use but in the series of definitions which it provides for the description of food attributes. In order to ensure that the Langual system being used in Europe does not develop independently of that continuing to be developed by the Food and Drug Administration, a joint US-European Committee has been established. The long-term success of Eurocode 2 and/or Langual in Europe depends on adoption in major European-wide epidemiological studies and not just on endorsement by projects such as FLAIR Eurofoods-Enfant.

■ Food Intake

It is possible to measure food consumption or intake at three levels: the national level using food balance sheets; at the household level using household budget surveys; and at the individual level using individual food consumption surveys. The data obtained from these approaches enable the availability or consumption of foods, and therefore of nutrients, to be monitored. They can be used for a variety of purposes such as the development and monitoring of agricultural, food and nutrition policies and for studying the relationship between diet and health. The three approaches for measuring food intake are complementary since all have their advantages and disadvantages. At all levels, challenges are emerging.

National and Regional Level

Food balance sheets provide a picture of food disappearance within a country during a specified reference period. The term "food disappearance" refers to "food available for human consumption" and not to "food actually eaten". It can be calculated not only for the whole population but also on a per capita basis by dividing the quantity of food by the population. Food balance sheet data are useful in monitoring trends in food consumption over time and in making rough comparisons between countries. Often, such data are the only data which can be readily obtained for rapid evaluation of new problems. The continued need for such data was highlighted by the resolutions of the International Conference on Nutrition held in Rome in December 1992 (5). Countries attending gave a commitment to meet the Nutrition Goals of the Fourth United Nations Development Decade:

- to eliminate starvation and death caused by famine
- to reduce malnutrition and mortality among children substantially
- to reduce chronic hunger tangibly
- to eliminate major nutritional diseases.

The first three goals are directed essentially to problems in developing countries, while eliminating nutritional diseases also refers to the problems associated with the excess consumption of particular foods and nutrients. Food balance sheets will be one instrument in monitoring the food and nutrition situation in countries throughout the world and reacting to it. There are a number of challenges associated with the provision of food balance sheet data which are peculiar to various areas of the world.

European Union. Ways have to be found to collect data, at the national level in countries in the European Union after the creation of the single market. Traditionally, national food balance data have been compiled largely from data collected for customs purposes. However, with the creation of the single market, customs data are no longer available. Unfortunately, this has also come at a time when statistical offices in Europe are undergoing reorganization and budget cuts. The problem will be exacerbated with the enlargement of the European Union. The FLAIR Eurofoods-Enfant Project has held discussions with the three organizations responsible for publishing food balance sheets up until this time: with Eurostat, which is the Statistical Office of the Commission of the European Union,

FAO and with OECD. The purpose of the discussion is to explore whether other survey techniques can be used to complement or even replace the data collected in the conventional food balance sheets. FAO and OECD are keen to maintain food balance sheets but Eurostat will provide data only for the countries of the European Union as a whole because other Directorates in the Commission have no interest in food intake in individual countries in Europe. This is because the Commission has no direct mandate for health and nutrition matters but only an indirect mandate through its involvement in social issues. Thus the interest of the Commission in food intake will probably be restricted to the household level. It remains to be seen whether FAO and OECD can continue to collect food balance sheet data for the countries of the European Union.

Eastern Europe. The increasing number of newly emerging countries of Eastern Europe and the established countries in transition have an even more pressing problem in providing data on food intake at the national level. Many surveys have shown that the amount of food available in these countries is declining rapidly but the data available to monitor such changes are often poor and not comparable over time or among countries. The situation is exacerbated by the lack of infrastructure for the collection, analysis and dissemination of the data. OECD is providing help to many countries in the region to improve the provision of such data but more needs to be done. This is important in order to maintain stability in the countries and for making international arrangements concerning trade and external assistance.

Developing Countries. In developing countries, especially in Africa where the per capita availability of food remains low, there is a continuing need to collect data. However, often the data are of low quality because of the inherent problems in collecting and analyzing information on food provided through non-commercial channels such as that produced at the household level or obtained by hunting, gathering or fishing. FAO and a number of governments provide assistance to some countries to improve their data collection and analysis procedures and capabilities. However, more needs to be done especially because of the need to plan external assistance when the food situation in countries deteriorates.

Coordination. In addition to maintaining and improving the collection, analysis and dissemination of data from food balance sheets, there should be more coordination of other surveys designed to build up a picture of food consumption at the national level. Such data are often collected at the household or individual level. As mentioned later, there is a need to improve the quality of food composition data associated with food balance sheets.

Household Level

At the household level, there are three main challenges: to improve the quality of the data on food purchases generally; to obtain comparability between countries; and to determine food consumption outside the home. Household budget surveys were designed to measure household expenditure, often for determining retail price indices, and not to measure food intake for nutritional purposes. Although household budget surveys are coordinated among countries of the European Union, the scope for improving the usefulness of data collection for nutritional purposes is somewhat limited because of the priorities of those collecting the data, the need to maintain the comparability of the data over time, and the problem of converting expenditure on food to food consumption. As yet, surveys designed to measure food purchases at the household level are not coordinated within Europe or among other countries. This is unfortunate because, for nutritional surveys, household food surveys will provide better data on household food consumption than will household budget surveys which are designed with another function in mind. However, unless those who wish to coordinate national household food surveys can come up with money to improve or modify surveys, there is very little chance that national household food surveys will be coordinated in the foreseeable future. Measuring food consumption outside the home is very difficult because the person responsible for purchasing food for the family as a whole is often not aware of food purchases by individual household members.

Individual Level

Data at the individual level, particularly if for a sufficient number of people, provide the best information for nutritionists especially for examining the relationship between diet and health or diet and disease. It is not appropriate to discuss here all that needs to be done to improve dietary intake information at the individual level as this topic has been discussed in detail at other meetings such as the Dietary Assessment Meetings, the first of which was held in 1992 (6). However, a number of points should be noted. Firstly, there should be more coordination to improve consistency of data among countries. This can only be achieved when the coordinating agency can offer funds to those carrying out the work. Otherwise countries are reluctant to change their systems because such changes can affect the continuity of the data. Secondly, countries not collecting data at the individual level should be encouraged to do so. This will enable countries to compare themselves with each other. Any coordination will probably have more effect on new surveys than on those already established such as the National Food Survey in the UK (7) and in the food intake components of the NHANES surveys in the US (8). Thirdly, more attention should be paid to collecting data required to answer such research questions as the bioavailability of nutrients and the etiology of cancer and other diseases.

■ Food Composition

One of the first priorities when IN-FOODS was established (9) was to produce guidelines for the production, management and use of food composition data. These guidelines (11), which were published with the assistance of the FLAIR Eurofoods-Enfant project, have now become the definitive work in the area. However, for nutrition research, there are a number of problems which need to receive increased attention in the future.

Data on More Foods

Developed Countries. In developed countries, the main gap in our knowledge is for data on prepared and processed foods, especially those prepared in the home. Much of the information on these foods is derived by calculating the nutrient content from that of the ingredients and the proportion of the various ingredients given in recipes. This can give rise to errors because of the imprecision of the recipe and because of the losses and gains of individual constituents during the process. Often, for example, fat added during preparation is not eaten while the removal of water by evaporation during cooking or drainage after cooking can increase the concentration of many constituents in a food. Minor components such as water-soluble minerals, trace elements and vitamins can be discarded with the cooking water while fat-soluble vitamins can be discarded with cooking oil. Some food components, such as vitamin C are destroyed during food preparation. It is also important to know the degree of nutrification of processed foods.

Developing Countries. In developing countries, data for many nutrients and energy not only for prepared and processed foods but also for unprocessed foods are lacking. If data are available, they are often derived from data from "comparable" foods elsewhere which may not be appropriate.

Analytes of Interest

When deciding which substances to analyze in foods, priorities have to be set because analytical chemists can produce information on a very large number of food components. Thus, it depends on the nutritional problems being investigated. However, this means that a chicken-and-egg situation develops because nutritionists often do not know which food components are important if they do not have information on the concentration of the components in the food. For example with dietary fiber, it was necessary to have data on different classes of fiber before their nutritional significance could be investigated. In the past, one total value for a vitamin or a value for a particular vitamer was regarded as adequate but now, many nutritionists would like separate data on all individual vitamers. Carotenoids are an interesting case in point. In the past, only provitamin A activity was considered with 6 mg of β-carotene or 12 mg of other provitamin A carotenoids being equivalent to 1 mg of retinol. However, it is now thought that carotenoids also have non-provitamin A vitaminoid activity. Thus it is possible to classify carotenoids based on the activities they possess. This is not simple because non-provitamin A vitaminoid activity is not a single function but includes a range of antioxidant activities and activity in modifying the immune response which to some extent is independent of antioxidant function (12). Individual carotenes differ in their ability to carry out the various non-provitamin A vitaminoid activities attributed to them. Thus the following classification based on that of Olson (13) uses singlet oxygen quenching activity as the non-provitamin A activity:

- Type 1: Provitamin A and non-provitamin A vitaminoid activity (β-carotene)
- Type 2: No provitamin A activity but non-provitamin A vitaminoid activity (canthaxanthin)
- Type 3: Provitamin A activity but no non-provitamin A vitaminoid activity (β-apo-14'-carotenal)
- Type 4: No provitamin A nor non-provitamin A vitaminoid activity (phytoene)

It may well be that the non-provitamin A vitaminoid activity of carotenoids is over-emphasized because measurements of carotene intake usually reflect consumption of dark green leafy vegetables and orange/yellow-colored fruits. Other minor components of such foods may have greater nutritional significance. For example, it has recently been reported that quercetin in plants is associated with lower rates of heart disease (14). Such components are generally referred to as non-nutrients, a class of substances with a wide range of structure and function. As discussed for dietary fiber, it will be difficult to set priorities in the analysis of non-nutrients because, without composition data, epidemiological studies will not be able to show whether their intake is important or not.

There are a numbers of ways which food components can be classified. Apart from classifying them as nutrients or non-nutrients, we could also classify them as favorable, neutral or unfavorable components (often depending to a large extent on the content in a particular food or the diet as a whole). However, a more useful classification may be into intrinsic substances, non-intentional food additives and intentional food additives.

Intrinsic Substances. These are absorbed from the environment or produced by the plant or animal from which the food is derived. The content of some of the components is reasonably constant while the content of other components, such as of trace elements (essential; non-essential but non-toxic; and toxic) would depend on their content in the food chain and the environment. Important intrinsic non-nutrients in foods are tannins and phytic acids which affect the bioavailability of iron (15,16).

Non-intentional Food Additives. These are neither intrinsic to the food nor added intentionally. They include microbial metabolites, such as aflatoxin and some B vitamins, hormones, antibiotics, and components derived during storage, preparation and transport including components derived from packing materials. Thus, generally, the content of these components in foods is very variable.

Intentional Food Additives. This group comprises substances added to give the desired physical appearance or structure, organoleptic properties or nutrient value and include emulsifiers, colors, flavors and also nutrients. Generally, but not always, the content of these components is reasonably constant for a given food.

The way in which values on the concentration of components in a database are handled depends not only on the distribution or range of values encountered but also on the general usefulness of the data. If values are tightly distributed, they would be of use to a wide audience but if they are specific to the batch of food in question, they would be of use only to people with an interest in that food. Food naming and description will be very important in determining the degree to which the data can be used more generally. The extent to which the data are widely applicable will be important in determining the policy on making the data available.

Analytical Methods

Many of the basic methods for food analysis were established about one hundred years ago and there has been very little change in the principles of the methods since then, even though the apparatus used may have been automated to some extent. However for some components, the introduction of new techniques has been essential for obtaining reliable data. Such techniques include chromatography, both gas-liquid chromatography and liquid chromatography, and atomic absorption spectrophotometry, a technique which was developed in Australia.

Through their use, it has been possible to generate data on the content in foods of amino acids, fatty acids and a wide range of vitamins and minerals. There are a number of tasks facing analysts today.

Development of Techniques for the Analysis of Food Components for Which No Adequate Methods Exist. Such food components include not only those which are well recognized, such as vitamin K, heme iron and non-heme iron, but also compounds which are just being recognized as having nutritional importance such as the flavonoids (17).

Development of Techniques Suitable for Use in Laboratories in Developing Countries. In western countries, equipment has become sophisticated and sometimes highly automated because of the high cost of labor and the ready availability of funds for equipment and expendables. In developing countries, often labor is relatively cheap but limited funds are available for equipment, parts and reagents. In addition, provision of constant power and water is often a problem. Since the need for data on food composition in developing countries is even more pressing than in developed countries, the development of methods suitable for use is a pressing problem. Such development will have to be accompanied by the establishment of suitable quality control procedures. Since two of the most important nutritional problems in developing countries are vitamin A and iron deficiencies, methods for the determination of provitamin A carotenoids, tannin and phytic acid should receive high priority.

Quality Control of Analyses and Determination of the Quality of Data. The use of reference materials has been discussed by Tanner et al. (18). Their proper use is essential for producing good quality analytical data. Evaluation of data is a difficult task and it needs to be made less subjective. Mangels et al. (19), have made some progress in this area by developing expert systems for the evaluation of data on the carotenoid, copper and selenium content of foods. It is essential if data in databases are going to be widely distributed that uniform criteria for data are adopted.

Levels of Data Required. When nutritionists consider food composition tables, they generally think of them for calculating nutrient intake from food intake (or vice versa) at the individual level. However, as mentioned above, data on food consumption are also collected at the household and at the national or regional level. As part of the FLAIR Eurofoods-Enfant Project, Belsten and Southgate (20) reviewed the so-called "conversion factors" for converting food disappearance data to nutrient data. Up until now, the factors are a combination of nutrient composition values with factors analogous to the extraction rate of nutrients from cereals but the system was not well documented. Thus they suggested that the factors be separated so that each component could be checked and revised if necessary. Preliminary work has also been done on food composition tables for use with household budget surveys.

■ Physical Properties

Although much work has been done on the physical properties of foods, such as on viscosity, elasticity, tensile and shear strength, and water-holding properties, the information is not as readily available as that on the content of various constituents. This is an area which should receive more attention in the future. The data are not only of interest to food processors but should also be of interest to nutritionists especially those involved in bioavailability.

■ Bioavailability

An area which must receive much more attention in the future is the measurement of the bioavailability of food constituents. A start has been made with a number of vitamins and minerals such as calcium, iron, zinc and a number of B vitamins but very little has been done with respect to bioavailability of other nutrients such as

the carotenoids. Since bioavailability depends to a large extent on the meal in which the food constituent in question is consumed, this means that we will need information not only on daily food consumption but also on intake of other constituents at individual meals.

Recently, I have developed a series of *caro*tene *bio*availability indices (or Carbi indices) to correct carotene intake for bioavailability (West, in preparation).

Carbi-1 Index. This provides a measure of the absorption of provitamin A carotene from a given matrix relative to the absorption of the same amount of carotene dissolved in oil. Based on the work of Hume and Krebs (21), the following is a provisional list of Carbi-1 indices:

- β-carotene dissolved in fats/oils, 1.00
- β-carotene in cabbage and spinach, 0.53
- β-carotene in carrots, boiled, sliced, 0.33
- β-carotene in carrots, domestic puree, 0.33
- β-carotene in carrots, homogenized, 0.73.

Carbi-2 Index. This provides a measure of host-dependent reduction in carotenoid absorption and/or conversion to retinol and would be related initially to the intake of fat (Carbi-2a index) and the degree of parasitemia (Carbi-2b index). Based on the work of Jayarajan et al. (22), the Carbi-2a index would be 0.5 when the intake of fat in children was less than 3 g/d. Similarly, based on work from our laboratory on the absorption of iodized oil (23), the Carbi-2b index in *Entamoeba histolytica*-infected children would be 0.25. Other Carbi-2 indices could be developed to take into account factors such as the effect of various types of dietary fibre on carotenoid absorption and of zinc deficiency on the conversion of carotenoids to retinol.

Carbi-3 Index. This provides a measure of the effect of carotene intake on the rate of conversion of β-carotene to retinol as suggested in the FAO/WHO recommendations (24). For the purposes of calculating the Carbi-3 index, carotene intake should first be corrected by applying the Carbi-1 and Carbi-2 indices.

Carbi-4 Index. This provides a measure of the extent of conversion of various carotenoids to retinol. With the Carbi-4 index for β-carotene set at 1.00, the Carbi-4 index for other provitamin A carotenoids is generally set at 0.50 (24). However, the extent of conversion of these carotenoids to β-carotene varies.

The idea of such indices is not new. Monsen et al. (15) have developed a method by which the amount of iron which is bioavailable can be estimated from the intake not only of iron but also of enhancers and inhibitors of iron absorption. It is just as important for the Carbi concept to be used in order to assess whether the intake of carotene-containing foods meets the vitamin A requirements of individuals. For example, a child consuming boiled sliced carrots, with a fat intake of less than 3 g/d, and infected with *Entamoeba histolytica* would need to consume 24 times more of the food in order to meet requirements than the content would suggest.

▮ Nutritional Status

Nutritional status with respect to a particular nutrient depends to a large extent, but not entirely, on the intake of the nutrient in question. Bioavailability, concurrent ingestion of other nutrients, physiological factors, and environmental and genetic factors also play a role in determining nutritional status. Be that as it may, there is a need to examine the relationship between nutrient intake and status and to collect more information on the nutritional status of people especially at the national or regional level. Using such data in conjunction with food and nutrient intake data, it is possible to develop and monitor strategies for controlling nutritional imbalances.

▮ Priorities for the Future

Providing Data on Food Composition for Developing Countries

In developed countries, increased resources for generating data on food composition will require a reallocation of resources within the countries themselves (including via the Commission of the European Union). Forums such as IN-FOODS, FLAIR Eurofoods-Enfant and the National Nutrient Databank Conferences in the US, and meetings such as the present one will play an important role in the exchange of ideas. However in developing countries, Eastern Europe and the former countries of the Soviet Union, the needs for data are being met only poorly and the countries need assistance from outside to improve the situation. For example, in Africa, the most comprehensive source of data on the composition of foods was published by FAO in conjunction with the US Department of Health, Education and Welfare in 1968 (25). This book, as well as those prepared for a number of other world regions, is now hopelessly outdated and inadequate in terms of the number of foods, nutrients and other food components on which data are available, food naming and description, analytical methods used, and the quality control of the data. For example, many of the methods available at the time for the determination of nutrients were poorly developed. This is particularly true for the determination of provitamin A carotenoids so estimates of the amount of vitamin A which can be provided from the diet are overestimated, probably by a factor of two (26). For non-nutrients, practically no data exist. This is particularly important for those factors influencing bioavailability such as phytic acid and tannin referred to above with respect to iron.

Since 1982, a number of groups have been active in stimulating international cooperation on improving the quality and availability of data on food composition. The INFOODS project of the United Nations University has examined the needs of users (27) and developed guidelines in a number of areas such as on the description of foods (2), definition of names of nutrients with appropriate tag names which can be used when transferring data (28), and on procedures for transferring data between nutrient databases (29). In addition, they have made a start in establishing regional centers throughout the world. This effort has been strengthened by INFOODS joining forces with FAO (11). In Europe a similar organization, which has worked closely with IN-FOODS was established. Initially, this was referred to as Eurofoods but was later incorporated into the Food-Linked Agroindustrial Research (FLAIR) Programme of the Commission of the European Union as Eurofoods-Enfant. These organizations have been working towards the improvement of the quality and compatibility of data on food composition and consumption in Europe. There work has led to a marked improvement in the quality, comparability and accessibility of data on food composition in Europe (30). The contract supporting Eurofoods-Enfant finished at the beginning of 1994 but a new project is planned to commence at the end of 1994 through the COST mechanism of the Commission of the European Union. One activity evolving out of the Eurofoods-Enfant Project is the series of biennial Postgraduate Courses on the Production and Use of Food Composition Data in Nutrition. The Second Course, held in October 1994 under the auspices of the Graduate School VLAG (Advanced Studies in Food Technology, Agrobiotechnology, Nutrition and Health Sciences) at Wageningen Agricultural University in conjunction with UNU, FAO and the International Union of Nutritional Sciences was attended by over 30 people from about 20 countries. Such courses will help to increase expertise in the area of food composition tables and nutrient databases worldwide.

There is no doubt that in order to meet the goals of the International Conference on Nutrition, it is essential that a program of action should be instigated to produce and disseminate data on the composition of foods in developing countries and in Eastern Europe. All nutrition-related programs depend on the availability of such data in the same way as traffic depends on maps. This work will require an input of resources from industrialized countries especially the US and those in Europe.

New Developments in Computer Use

Computers are becoming faster and cheaper, data storage is also becoming cheaper and software is becoming more sophisticated. All of these developments mean that computers will be more able to serve the needs of nutritionists and food scientists. However, it is becoming more and more important to develop systems and practices to ensure the quality of both input and output from computer systems. It is all too easy to think that more is necessarily better. Users should remember the computer adage: "garbage in means garbage out". The expert systems described by Mangels et al. (19) need to be improved and extended to nutrients other than copper, selenium and the carotenoids in order to ensure the quality of data being entered into nutrient databases is adequate for the use envisaged. Similar systems will need to be developed for dietary intake data and for ensuring the quality of food names and descriptions as well as for monitoring the quality of data output. There is a lot of pressure for on-line systems to be developed for supplying food composition and consumption data. In my opinion, the need for on-line systems is over-emphasized because most of the food composition data in nutrient databases in the world can be accommodated on one compact disk. Perhaps some entrepreneur would like to consider an annual version of "World Nutrient Data" on compact disk although such a venture may not be economically viable.

As far as computers are concerned, the biggest challenge is to present non-alphanumeric information. A start has been made with pictures of foods being stored on compact disk. Perhaps food texture will be recorded as the sound of a standard person biting into a standard carrot. But what about smell and taste of foods and the ethereal atmosphere in which foods are eaten? Is computer technology up to storing these data yet?

∎ References

(1) McCann, A., Soergel, D., Holden, J., Pennington, J., Smith, E., & Wiley, R. (1980) *Langual Vocabulary, Users' Manual*, US Food and Drug Administration, Washington, DC

(2) Truswell, A.S., Bateson, D.J., Madafiglio K.C., Pennington, J.A.T., Rand, W.M., & Klensin, J.C. (1991) *J. Food Comp. Anal.* **4**, 18-38

(3) Poortvliet, E.J., & Kohlmeier, L. (1993) *Manual for Using the Eurocode 2 Food Coding System*, Wageningen Agricultural University, Wageningen

(4) Pennington, J.A.T. (1995) in *Quality and Accessibility of Food-Related Data*, H. Greenfield (Ed.), AOAC INTERNATIONAL, Arlington, VA, pp. 85-97

(5) FAO/WHO (1992) *International Conference on Nutrition. World Declaration and Plan of Action for Nutrition*, FAO, Rome

(6) Buzzard, I.M., & Willett, W.C. (Eds.) (1994) *Am. J. Clin. Nutr.* **59**, 143S-306S

(7) Ministry of Agriculture, Fisheries and Food (1953–) *Household Food Consumption and Expenditure*, HMSO, London

(8) Briefel, R.R., & Sempos, C.T. (Eds.) (1992) *Dietary Methodology Workshop for the Third National Health and Nutrition Examination Survey*, US Government Printing Office, Washington, DC

(9) Rand, W.M., & Young V.R. (1984) *Am. J. Clin. Nutr.* **39**, 144-151

(10) Greenfield, H., & Southgate, D.A.T. (1992) *Food Composition Data: Production, Management and Use*, Elsevier Applied Science, London

(11) Lupien, J. (1995) in *Quality and Accessibility of Food-Related Data*, H. Greenfield (Ed.), AOAC INTERNATIONAL, Arlington, VA, pp. 3-9

(12) Bendich, A. (1992) *Voeding* **53**, 191-195

(13) Bendich, A., & Olson, J.A. (1989) *FASEB J.* **3**, 1927-1932

(14) Hertog, M.G.L., Feskens, E.J.M., Hollman, P.C.H., Katan, M.B., & Kromhout, D. (1993) *Lancet* **342**, 1007-1011

(15) Monsen, E.R., Hallberg, L., Layrisse, M., Hegsted, D.M., Cook, J.D. Mertz, W., & Finch, C.A. (1978) *Am. J. Clin. Nutr.* **31**, 134-141

(16) Hallberg, L., & Rossander-Hultén, L. (1993) in *Bioavailability '93: Nutritional, Chemical and Food Processing Implications of Nutrient Availability*, Part 2, U. Schlemmer (Ed.), Bundesforschungsanstalt für Ernährung, Karlsruhe, pp. 23-32

(17) Hertog, M.G.L., Hollman, P.C.H., & van der Putte, B. (1993) *J. Agric. Food Chem.* **41**, 1242-1246

(18) Tanner, J.T., Wolf, W., & Horwitz, W. (1995) in *Quality and Accessibility of Food-Related Data*, H. Greenfield (Ed.), AOAC INTERNATIONAL, Arlington, VA, pp. 99-104

(19) Mangels, A.R., Holden, J.M., Beecher, G.R., Forman, M.R., & Labuza, E. (1993) *J. Am. Diet. Assoc.* **93**, 284-296

(20) Belsten, J.L., & Southgate, D.A.T. (1992) *Review of FAO Food Balance Sheet Nutritional Data*,

AFRC Food Research Institute, Norwich

(21) Hume, E.M., & Krebs, H.A. (1949) *Vitamin A Requirement of Human Adults: an Experimental Study of Vitamin A Deprivation in Man,* Medical Research Council Special Report Series No. 264, HMSO, London

(22) Jayarajan, P., Reddy, V., & Mohanram, M. (1980) *Indian J. Med. Res.* **71**, 53-56

(23) Furnée, A.C. (1994) PhD thesis, Wageningen Agricultural University, Wageningen

(24) FAO/WHO (1988) *Requirements of Vitamin A, Iron, Folate and Vitamin B_{12},* FAO Food and Nutrition Series No. 23, FAO, Rome

(25) Wu Leung, W.T., Busson, F., & Jardin, C. (1968) *Food Composition Table for Use in Africa,* US Department of Health, Education and Welfare, Bethesda and FAO, Rome

(26) West, C.E., & Poortvliet, E.J. (1993) *The Carotenoid Content of Foods with Special Reference to Developing Countries,* USAID-VITAL, Washington, DC

(27) Rand, W.M., Pennington, J.A.T., Murphy, S.P., & Klensin, J.C. (1991) *Compiling Data for Food Composition Data Bases,* UNU Press, Tokyo

(28) Klensin, J.C., Feskanich, D., Lin, V., Truswell, A.S., & Southgate D.A.T. (1989) *Identification of Food Components for INFOODS Data Interchange,* UNU Press, Tokyo

(29) Klensin, J.C. (1992) *INFOODS Food Composition Data Interchange Handbook,* UNU Press, Tokyo

(30) Castenmiller, J., & West, C.E. (Eds.) (1994) *Report of the Third Annual Meeting of the FLAIR Eurofoods-Enfant Project,* Wageningen Agricultural University, Wageningen

Information Needs and Computer Systems

Food Database Management Systems — A Review

Wulf Becker

Nutrition Division, National Food Administration, Uppsala, Sweden

Ian Unwin

The Opas Centre, Cambridge CB4 4WS, UK

The use of database management systems (DBMS) for handling food composition data is reviewed, together with some basic concepts underlying database design and current developments in DBMS support for food data. The results of a survey of system users in Europe, USA and Australasia indicated that facilities supporting the identification and description of foods, as well as methods for specifying compositional data, need to be extended and harmonized. Most systems are unilingual, but include synonyms for foods, while some support multiple languages. Generally, a single grouping or classification system for foods is used; it is often based on food source and built into the system of food codes. Facilities for calculating and storing measures of variation in a compositional value, and for describing the quality of a value are frequently lacking. Computer-readable composition data are usually exchanged as text files on floppy disk. Although most food information handling DBMS have been developed for the needs of a specific organization, more sophisticated software tools and international standardization (e.g. INFOODS, FLAIR Eurofoods-Enfant and multinational epidemiological studies) are encouraging collaborative development. The New Zealand Food Composition Database, the Swedish NUTSYS system and the EuroNIMS collaboration are briefly described as examples of recent developments in this area.

An increasing number of countries is compiling and publishing food composition tables. Inventories of food composition tables and nutritional software in Europe (1, 2, Slimani & Poortvliet, unpublished) showed that many organizations responsible for publishing tables use a computerized database management system (DBMS) for the handling and management of food composition data and related information. The systems were either developed in-house or based on commercial software packages, operated in various computing hardware and software environments, and were generally designed for the specific needs of the individual organization. Few of these systems were commercially available for other users. There are high costs involved in the production of high quality food composition data as well as in the development of FDBMS (Food DBMS) for handling the data. In view of this, efforts have been made, during the last decade, to improve the availability of national food composition data and to develop the means to achieve the international exchange of data. The purpose of this review is to outline modern database management techniques, including the relational model, and to give a brief overview of some existing database systems used for handling food composition data and of some recent international developments. More detailed descriptions of the handling of bibliographic information (3) and food composition information (4) using the relational model have been published.

■ Databases — Basic Concepts

Although alternative data structures based on hierarchical or network models may be used in database management software, much attention is at present paid to the relational approach in the design of food information handling systems. The first of two main reasons for this is that commercially available relational DBMS (e.g. Oracle, Sybase, Ingres) provide the software of choice for many organizations. The second is that food composition data appear well suited to the application of relational principles, consisting of data values which relate to a food, a component, and to various other entities such as analytical method, analytical laboratory and literature reference. Therefore very briefly we shall review the main concepts underlying relational DBMS and note some possible limitations which might impinge on food-related information-handling facilities based on them.

Database analysis and design (5, 6) involves, inter alia, the building of a conceptual data model and its translation into a logical data model. For example an Entity-Relationship (E-R) diagram (7) may be used to model the data conceptually. This model may then be implemented using a logical data structure based on the relational model (8, 9). Some attention needs to be paid to the terminology which derives from several origins including "traditional" file processing data description, data modeling methodology such as E-R diagrams, and relational theory. Further care will be required as terminology from object-oriented data modeling becomes wide-spread. In referring to data, whether conceptual or logical, associated with basic data structures, it is convenient to use E-R terminology. Thus in the following description, "entity type" refers to a single data structure and "entity instance" for an individual occurrence of that type of item.

All items of data in a relational DBMS are held in data structures constructed as "tables" (in the more formal literature often referred to as "relations"). Each table deals with a separate subject or entity type, e.g. a nutrient value, journal article or author. In a table each row refers to a different instance of the entity, an individual value, article or author, and each column to a particular property (or "attribute") of the entity for which data are held, e.g. the journal, volume, issue and pagination data for a journal article. Rows are frequently referred to as records and columns as fields.

It is a requirement of the relational model that each row of the table is uniquely identified by the data for one of its attributes (or the combined data of more than one attribute); the identifier is known as the table's "primary key". A primary key may include meaningful data, e.g. food name (or food group) for a food item, or have no meaningful content, being for example a sequentially assigned number. Care must be taken in selecting a meaningful key since it must remain unique over any valid items which may need to be added to the table and must remain constant for the given item; so-called "intelligent keys" are usually avoided. Any identifier whose assignment rules, assignment or use are external to the system under design should be treated with similar caution. For example, neither Chemical Abstracts Registry Numbers nor ISBN (for example as for the 4th Edition of *The Composition of Foods* (10) are unique for substances or books, respectively, at the level appropriate to an FDBMS. Equally for meaningless keys, adequate checks must be made whether incoming data belong to a new row (a new entity instance), or update an existing row. Although this may not be a significant problem for real-life discrete objects and events such as employees and sales, less discretely defined entity instances, as in food items, may provide some difficulty.

The "relationships" of an E-R model are associations between instances of one or more entity types, the "degree" of the relationship being the number of entity types involved. A "unary" or "recursive" relationship is a link from one instance to another of the same entity type. A common example is an entity type in which instances have a hierarchical organization, as with employees in a management structure or in a facet of a food description language. Usually a relationship is between two (binary), three (ternary), or occasionally more entity types. A further property of a relationship is its "cardinality" which expresses the number of instances which can partake from each side of the bidirectional relationship. Cardinalities are often expressed as 1:1 (a "one-to-one" relationship), 1:N (a "one-to-many" relationship) or M:N (a "many-to-many" relationship). However further detail is important, in particular whether the cardinality is mandatory or optional, i.e. whether for a one or many cardinality the minimum requirement is one or zero occurrences. A maximum or minimum number of occurrences may apply to "many" cardinality; this is less significant for data structure but important for data validation.

The relational data model provides the means to eliminate the redundant storage of information in the database which would result in possible inconsistencies during data insertion, deletion and amendment procedures. In the process of "normalization" the structures of tables are subjected to a series of steps in which dependent attributes are removed to separate tables. For example, a table of food component values may include attributes concerning the analytical laboratory. However these details should not be repeated in each row corresponding to a value generated by that laboratory. Instead details of the laboratory such as its name, address and contact person are removed to a separate table linked by a one-to-many laboratory-to-values relationship.

Table I. Component value table

FOOD_ID	COMP_ID	SOURCE_TYPE	SOURCE_ID	VALUE	UNIT_ID
1234	CARTBEQ	L	4321	1540	(µg/100 g)
1234	RETOL	L	4321	16500	(µg/100 g)
1234	VITA	L	4321	16760	(µg/100 g)
1234	VITAA	A	6789	54000	(IU)
1234	VITA-	L	3456	20000	IU

The relationship links between tables are made through a "foreign key", an attribute which records the primary key for a row in (except for a unary relationship) another table thus pointing to related data. A direct link can be made between tables for 1:1 relationships and for 1:N relationships, since more than one table row on the N side of the relationship can hold the same foreign key. Since this can only apply in one direction, an M:N relationship is stored by breaking it into two 1:N links through the insertion of an additional table. This has an attribute column for the primary key of each entity table of the relationship. Although these keys can be repeated as necessary, any one row of the relation table has a unique combination of the keys from the entity tables, and indeed the combination serves as its primary key. In practice, data can be associated with the M:N relationship and stored as attributes in the table. For example the relationship between authors and published papers is M:N, with details on each held in separate tables. However data concerning the authorship of a given paper must be held in the linking table. In particular, the position of a given author must be recorded here if the ordered list of authors needs to be reconstructed, for example in the formatting of references.

A central component of a food composition database, the component value record, can be considered further. A table for such data must include foreign keys at least to identify the food and the component. It will also have actual data such as the value, its units, and perhaps reports of quality, precision, status, etc. Values for the same food-component pairing will need to be differentiated through additional entity types such as literature reference or analytical detail which may include identification of the laboratory. To avoid having separate attributes pointing to literature and analytical source information, a separate attribute could be defined for "source type" to point to different tables (e.g. Literature or Analytical). This is then required in the unique key since duplicate values of the single attribute (SOURCE_ID) might appear in both the literature and analytical information tables. Thus, with the columns constituting the unique key delineated in bold, the component value table might be constructed as in Table I.

In Table I, components are identified using INFOODS tagnames (11, 12). The first three represent β-carotene equivalents, retinol and vitamin A (as retinol equivalents). A separate tagname, VITAA, identifies vitamin A determined by bioassay and another, VITA–, indicates a value for vitamin A whose method of determination is unknown. The attribute UNIT_ID identifies the unit in which the value is expressed. Those in parentheses are default values for the corresponding component. This information could be held for the component and might be omitted in this column. Note the default unit for VITAA is IU. However it is µg/100 g for VITA– and thus the unit of IU must be held explicitly for the final row.

An important aid to the standardization of development in relational database applications has been Structured

Query Language (SQL; often pronounced "Sequel") which is based on work done by IBM in the 1970s. SQL provides a concise set of commands to support the definition, display and updating of relational tables (a broad interpretation of "query"!). These facilities include the handling of "views" providing in a convenient derived table the data based on a subset of rows and columns selected from underlying existing tables. Views are dynamic; changing their data changes the corresponded stored data and any change in the underlying data is reflected in the values displayed in a view.

Basing the design of an FDBMS on the relational model allows similar data structures and data management procedures, using SQL, to be implemented in a wide range of hardware and software environments. However various shortcomings in the use of the relational model for FDBMS have been noted (13) and a more extensive review, particularly with respect to the limitations of SQL for the management of statistical data, has been published (14). The relational model needs each instance of an entity type to be clearly distinguishable from all other possible instances. This is often not the case with entity types required in an FDBMS such as food components, analytical methods and particularly, as we note below, food items. Also relational systems may not be adept at handling the textual information needed to document such entities and the statistical descriptions associated with component values.

A fundamental problem for food information management is the underlying assumption, apparently required if the relational model is to be applied, that a food item must be uniquely defined and distinguished from all other food items. This may provide difficulties, inter alia, with variants of composite foods and when switching contexts, for example between composition and consumption records and between nutrient and non-nutrient studies. A possible alternative staying within the relational model is to avoid predefining items in the data collection at the level normally considered an individual food item. Instead every distinguishable instance or sample could be stored as separate records, with data being aggregated on search criteria (given that an adequate system of food indexing is available) or through links between equivalent items as identified by data managers and stored in a food correlation table. The latter approach would allow separate sets of aggregate items to be maintained, for example to support food table production and non-nutrient work.

Further circumstances where the "all or nothing" separation of food items is unsatisfactory include seasonal data sets which vary in only one or two components and the need to apply taxonomic and alternative names to each item derived from one raw food. Although relational solutions can be envisaged, new developments, in particular an object-oriented model, may provide an approach which more closely represents the real world. In object-oriented programming a key concept is the "class" object which can hold a number of objects of different types (such as various types of variable, data structure and function), together with functions for manipulating the objects and mechanisms to control inheritance and access from other classes. Variables and functions declared for the class are known as class members. A derived class can be declared, inheriting members from one or more base (parent) classes. In the derived class, new members may be declared and existing ones redefined. It may be that an object-oriented data model will handle the characteristics acquired (for example, in processing or cooking) by a derived food item more effectively, including the multiple inheritance from the various ingredients implicit in composite foods.

∎ Facilities of Existing Food DBMS

In order to obtain additional information on facilities available in DBMS imple-

Table II. Food information technology

Food	A general term, sometimes used more specifically for a basic (e.g. unprocessed) food item.
Food item	A specific term for a unique entity which can be differentiated from all other food entities with which it may be compared.
Food identification	The decision whether two food entities can be considered the same food item. This may be achievable within defined objectives or particular data collections, but such decisions may not be valid in any broader context, e.g. data exchange.
Food identifier	Any tag (code, name, etc.) which is unambiguously associated with (but not necessarily unique for) a food item.
Food code	A code (which may be a sequential number based on an ordered list of items or incorporate some degree of hierarchical classification) used to identify a food item unambiguously.
Food name	A name assigned to a food item considered sufficient to distinguish it from all other items which may also occur in the data collection. The names for existing items may need to be made more specific when new, similar items are added.
Food description	Information on a food item which may be relevant to the data (e.g. on composition) associated with it; the information may reside in the food name, in an overlying classification or as additional descriptive detail.
Food descriptor	A term included in a more or less formal set used as a food description system. The system may be *faceted* where the descriptors are organized in subsets according to the attribute described, e.g. preservation method, cooking method.
Food grouping	A categorization of food items based on an individual attribute or a selection of attributes which groups the items usefully within a given (broad or narrow) context.
Food classification	Any grouping system for food items (often using hierarchical categories) which attempts to assign a single "correct" (i.e. unique) location[a] for any food item.
Food Group (note capitalization)	The primary food classification, based on a single hierarchy, which a food information system uses; generally based on food type and/or source.
Parallel _ _ _ systems	Where more than one independent system of either food codes, names, description, grouping or classification coexist in an implementation, these are referred to as parallel systems.

[a] If unique locations are defined down to the level of each individual item, the location may also be considered unambiguous with respect to that item. However this approach to food identification will only be canonical if incontrovertible rules can be defined for assigning items to locations. This is highly improbable for foods.

mented for handling food composition data, a questionnaire was sent to a selection of 20 system users in Europe, USA, Australia, New Zealand and the Pacific. The questionnaire focused on aspects of information handling of foods and components, recipe calculation, and storage of compositional data. The system users were also asked to give examples of improvements they would consider to be most important. The purpose of the survey was to compare how systems differed in the handling of food and component information and thus to identify areas that could be considered problematic in relation to international exchange of food information.

The organizations covered were mainly those responsible for official national food composition data compilations but others mainly involved in dietary surveys and epidemiological research were also included. Answers were received for 17 systems. Fifteen systems were developed in-house using various programming languages or commercial DBMS (e.g. Oracle, Advanced Revelation, dBASE III). No clear preferences were evident for the hardware environment, programming language or DBMS; it appeared these were determined by practise and availability within the organization.

Information Handling of Foods

Food databases contain records on food items and the information detailing these is crucial. Thus the identification, description, grouping and classification of foods, the ways of representing information on the items, are key areas in the handling of food information. However, there are still no universally accepted definitions and taxonomy of these terms, which would be desirable when using them in an international context. Table II shows suggested definitions for a number of terms used in the paper.

According to the questionnaire responses, foods are usually identified by their names and a code. Some systems (one-third of those used for data compilation but none used for dietary survey work) can include several coding systems in parallel. Two systems use Langual (15), and six a less formal but similar type of descriptor, for a more detailed food description. Otherwise the name is used for describing the food, sometimes supplemented with additional free-text description. Most systems can include synonyms for foods but are unilingual, although six systems allow food and component names to be held in multiple languages.

Generally, a single grouping or classification system for foods is used; it is often based on food source and may be built into the coding system. Half of the FDBMS used for national food composition data allow the use of multiple grouping or classification systems in parallel.

Preferably, a FDBMS should allow the use of multiple coding systems, e.g.

parallel management of national food codes and Eurocode 2 (16), and of parallel grouping and classification systems based on different criteria. For the use of international data it is also necessary to be able to handle in parallel multiple food names, including different language versions.

Information Handling of Recipes

A recipe system for calculating the composition of dishes or mixed foods from their ingredients is usually needed in a FDBMS. Apart from calculating the composition of cooked dishes, such a system can be used to estimate the composition of mixed foods from the proportions and compositions of their constituents. A recipe system is included in fourteen of the systems reviewed, especially in those mainly intended for processing of data from dietary surveys. About half of the recipe systems allow for the use of alternative preparation methods, portion sizes, and yield factors for change in weight/water content during preparation but facilities for adjustments in fat content were included in five systems. Ingredient substitution (e.g. between different types of fats) in recipes is possible in some systems. The application of retention factors for components (e.g. vitamins) has been included in the calculations with varying degrees of sophistication in eight of the systems. Although there are many difficulties in accounting for losses and gains during food preparation, facilities to allow for these are in many situations essential.

The ability to break down recipes by ingredient and to calculate the contribution of each ingredient to each component was possible in five systems. Such a function is of importance, e.g. when calculating the contribution of various foods or food groups to various nutrients. Flexibility in input of recipe data is desirable and ideally it should be easy to enter recipes expressed in both household measures and grams. It should also be possible to modify a recipe, e.g. exchange alternative liquids, fats, etc.

Information Handling of Component Data

Various considerations are important in the storage and handling of component data, especially in an international context. These can be subdivided into two main areas, identification of the component reported and the details of the compositional value stored.

In the systems reviewed, components are usually identified by a code and/or by a name or abbreviation. Two systems also use the INFOODS tag system (11, 12) in parallel. The INFOODS tag system was developed to uniquely identify components, especially in data exchange.

Several systems have separate databases for the compilation of "raw" data (the "working" database) and for the "official" values used for publication of food tables, calculation of intakes from dietary surveys, etc. Component data are stored as single analytical results for individual samples (in the working database) or as mean values derived from analytical data or data from other sources. There was generally a lack of facilities for calculating and storing measures of variation in a value as well as for reporting the assessed quality of a value. Component values from other organizations, together with a reference to their source, could be included, but generally the imported values were not stored in the original data format (thus, for example, not necessarily retaining the original precision). Indication of the period for which an official value is or was valid, possible in four systems, is a useful facility, e.g. for reconstructing previous databases used for dietary surveys or earlier editions of food tables.

The compositional data for a given component in a given food can be stored in various forms, ranging from individual results for each individual analytical portion to only a single derived or imputed value. Ideally, a database would contain mainly analytical data based on verified methods. Food analysis is, however, costly and requires large resources. Therefore many organizations also use data from the literature and also alternative methods for calculating or estimating component levels. A comprehensive FDBMS should support facilities for recording literature references and also the means to indicate the quality and method of derivation of a value.

Half of the organizations use their FDBMS for the production of food composition tables. Three systems directly output data formatted for publication of food tables, while six use commercial word-processing software such as WordPerfect or Microsoft Word for editing the data. The underlying principle in using a relational DBMS is that a given item of data is only entered and stored once, but repeated as necessary on output, for example when a food name appears in the main food table and in the food index.

Other Aspects of Information Handling

Exchange of computer-readable composition data was common, with text files on floppy disk being the most widely used format.

User friendliness is important for any software handling complex information like food composition data, a graphical user interface (GUI) being preferable. This should provide the ability to interchange data with commercial software, e.g. spread-sheets, word processing, statistical packages, since each of these support specialist facilities which it is not practical to implement in a DBMS. Another aspect of user friendliness is the inclusion of individual profiles for users so that their working environment is customized when they log on, e.g. by setting their preferred working language, code system.

Suggested Improvements

The systems users were asked to state the three improvements that they would consider the most important if they were about to enhance their system. Responses included improved facilities for the calculation and storage of compositional data (including measures of data quality), for recipe calculation and the handling of multi-constituent foods, and for food classification and aggregation. Better user-friendliness in general was cited, as well as specifically a GUI, and there was a requirement for multilingual support, particularly of food names. A need for greater flexibility was expressed, for example in allowing extra components to be included, the modification of existing recipes and the handling of user-specific data (e.g. "own foods"). In general the results seem to imply a considerable agreement on the overall facilities which are required in a comprehensive system when the resources are available to implement them.

■ Current Developments in International Food Databases

In addition to supporting the facilities required for the handling of food information, a modern FDBMS should be based on modern computing and informatics techniques and standards. This should allow a flexible design which made the system easy to enhance and modify. The interface should be user friendly and preferably be a GUI. The design and operating environment should allow for data exchange, both with other applications such as spread-sheets and with other FDBMS.

Currently the computing techniques most appropriate to FDBMS involve relational databases accessed through SQL, although as noted earlier these may not prove a perfect solution and potentially better alternatives may become available.

They do, however, provide a basic standard, making practical collaborative developments to create transportable systems implementable in the current hardware and software environments of many organizations. Such developments should also encourage the implementation of compatible data structures and the application of standard policies to the food-related data stored, key aspects in improving the effectiveness of data exchange.

Until recently, most FDBMS were developed specially for the needs of an individual organization, in part because the development and use of common software had been limited by compatibility and portability problems. Generally the systems have not been available for purchase on a commercial basis. However there are high costs involved in production of high quality food composition data as well as development of DBMS for handling the data. The sharing of development costs to produce a highly functional system would enable the most effective use to be made of the analytical data obtained. Increased standardization, more sophisticated software tools, and international cooperation (e.g. INFOODS, Eurofoods-Enfant and multinational dietary and epidemiological research) have stimulated interest in a DBMS capable of handling high quality food data, which would allow the use of multiple languages, coding, description and classification systems for foods and components (17–19).

Recent FDBMS developments include the New Zealand Food Composition Database, the Swedish NUTSYS system, and the EuroNIMS collaboration.

New Zealand Food Composition Database

The New Zealand Food Composition Database is designed to handle data from different countries in a flexible way (20). It has been developed in-house using Advanced Revelation DBMS and its programming language Rbasic and is operated on a PC network. It is well suited for easy data interchange with other countries and institutions, while maintaining the ease of information and data output, in both electronic and hardcopy formats. In addition to using various facets for describing and naming foods, the system includes images of foods (color photographs), which are linked to the compositional data. The system is now installed in Latin America (INCAP in Guatemala), the South Pacific Commission (New Caledonia) and for ASEANFOODS (at INMU in Thailand).

NUTSYS

NUTSYS is the name of a prototype FDBMS developed at the Swedish National Food Administration (21). It is the result of a project to develop a modern, flexible DBMS for handling food composition data. A number of functions and modules were identified by a project group that ideally should be included in a fully developed system. Some of the most important were:

- registers for foods, nutrients and other components
- database for nutrients and other components
- recipe calculation system
- system for compositional data source references
- modules for print-out of food composition tables
- system for handling data from dietary surveys
- system for menu planning.

The system was designed to contain functions that allow for:

- storage of an "unlimited" number of foods, recipes, components
- indication of the origin, quality, source, etc. of a value
- indication of the period during which a value is valid
- indication of the origin (country, region) of a food

- indication of the method of preparation and processing of a food
- indication of the density, portion weight, etc. of a food
- grouping of foods and components according to different criteria
- use of different names, synonyms, languages, codes, measures, etc.
- breakdown of recipes to ingredients and exchange of recipe ingredients
- use of yield and retention factors in recipe calculation
- easy communication with other systems.

A data model was outlined with a number of entities and concepts. Based on the model, a prototype was constructed using the Ingres 4GL tool Vision. About 70 programs were generated and completed.

EuroNIMS

Development of a new system (EuroNIMS, European Nutrition Information Management System) began after the start of the NUTSYS project. The EuroNIMS cooperation is a result of an initiative from the Belgian NUBEL Foundation, responsible for the management of national food composition data, and NIMS representatives. NIMS (NUBEL Information Management System) is a software package for management of nutrient composition data currently being used by the NUBEL Foundation in Belgium and was developed by Logimed, a software development company. NIMS supports some of the key functions defined in NUTSYS, e.g. multiple languages, coding and classification systems for foods. Representatives from about a dozen European countries and one international organization (IARC) have participated in the discussions on EuroNIMS.

The design of EuroNIMS is based on a client-server software architecture in which networked PCs or workstations, as "clients", access data held on a central machine, the "server" (although in practice a single, powerful PC could support both the client and server functions). The database is held on the server using a proprietary DBMS such as Ingres or Oracle, perhaps one already installed by the user. EuroNIMS interacts with the DBMS through an ODBC (Microsoft Open Database Connectivity) interface and this uses a single dialect of SQL. At the client end, data exchanged with the server will be processed through an object-oriented DBMS to be presented to the user with a graphical user interface (GUI). In the first EuroNIMS software release (Version 1.0), client machines use Windows 3.X as the GUI and the server runs under Windows NT. As a result, EuroNIMS uses 16-bit Unicode data storage, but with 8-bit images in parallel to accommodate operating environments using current character storage conventions.

EuroNIMS Version 1.0 includes most functions defined in NUTSYS. Features of particular interest include:

- multilinguality both at the user interface and data storage levels
- international food identification (country, organization, sequential and version number)
- parallel management of different coding and classification systems
- registration of food manufacturers and distributors and of analytical laboratories
- registration of items as aggregated or representative foods
- a range of algorithms for the calculation and conversion of values
- recipe storage with link to spreadsheet calculation using yield and retention factors
- facilities for Langual encoding.

Conclusions

The use of up-to-date computing techniques allows FDBMS currently under development to support more comprehensive facilities than hitherto, for example in the handling of documentary information and images, accessed through user-friendly interfaces. In addition to providing an effective operational environment for the compilation of food composition and related data, the systems are increasingly being developed and implemented on the basis of international cooperation. This complements the efforts of the past decade in establishing guidelines for such data collections and should prove to be an important step in facilitating the use and exchange of high quality food composition data.

▪ Acknowledgments

The authors thank the following for kind assistance in completing the DBMS questionnaire and supplying further information: D. Buss and M. Day, UK; M. Buzzard, USA; F. Cook, New Zealand; K. Day, UK; M. Hoke, USA; D. Douglass, USA; J. Ireland-Ripert, France; J. Klensin, INFOODS; J. Lewis, Australia; B. O'Shea, Ireland; J. Taylor, UK; A. Trichopoulou, Greece; A. Turrini, Italy; L. Valsta, Finland; A. Walker, UK; C. E. West, The Netherlands.

▪ References

(1) West, C.E. (Ed.) (1989) *Inventory of European Food Composition Tables and Nutrient Database Systems*, National Food Administration, Uppsala

(2) Loughridge, J.M., Walker, A.D., & Towler, G. (1993) *Inventory of Nutritional Software*, FLAIR Eurofoods-Enfant, Wageningen Agricultural University, Wageningen

(3) Crawford, R.G. (1981) *J. Am. Soc. Inf. Sci.* **32**, 51-64

(4) Feinberg, M., Ireland-Ripert, J., & Favier, J-C. (1992) *World Rev. Nutr. Diet.* **68**, 49-93

(5) McFadden, F.R., & Hoffer, J.A. (1994) *Modern Database Management*, 4th Ed., Benjamin-Cummings, Redwood City, CA

(6) Jennings, R. (1993) *Using Access 1.1 for Windows*, Special Ed., Que Corporation, Carmel, IN

(7) Chen, P.P-S. (1976) *ACM Trans. Database Syst.* **1**, 9-36.

(8) Codd, E.F. (1970) *Comm. ACM* **13**, No. 6

(9) Date, C.J. (1981) *Introduction to Database Systems*, 3rd Ed., Addison-Wesley, Reading, MA

(10) Paul, A.A. & Southgate, D.A.T. (1978) *McCance and Widdowson's The Composition of Foods*, 4th Ed., HMSO, London

(11) Klensin J.C., Feskanich, D., Lin, V., Truswell, A.S., & Southgate, D.A.T. (1989) *Identification of Food Components for INFOODS Data Interchange*, UNU Press, Tokyo

(12) Klensin J.C. (1992) *INFOODS Food Composition Data Interchange Handbook*, UNU Press, Tokyo

(13) Klensin J.C. (1991) *Trends Food Sci. Technol.* **2**, 279-282

(14) Klensin J.C., & Romberg, R.M. (1989) *Lect. Notes Comput. Sci.* **339**, 19-38

(15) Hendricks, T.C. (1992) *World Rev. Nutr. Diet.* **68**, 94-103

(16) Poortvliet, E.J., Klensin J.C., & Kohlmeier, L. (1992) *Eur. J. Clin. Nutr.* **46** (Suppl. 5), S9-S24

(17) Truswell, A.S., Bateson, D.J., Madafiglio, K.C., Pennington, J.A.T., Rand, W.M., & Klensin J.C. (1991) *J. Food Comp. Anal.* **4**, 18-39

(18) Greenfield, H., & Southgate, D.A.T. (1992) *Food Composition Data: Production, Management and Use*, Elsevier Applied Science, London

(19) Simopoulos, A.P., & Butrum, R.R. (1992). *World Rev. Nutr. Diet.* **68**, 1-160

(20) Cook, F., Duxfield, G., & Burlingame, B. (1992) *Proc. Nutr. Soc. NZ* **17**, 204-207

(21) Becker, W. (1993) *NUTSYS — a Food and Nutrition Composition and Information Management System*, National Food Administration, Uppsala

Data Identification Considerations in International Interchange of Food Composition Data

John C. Klensin

INFOODS Secretariat, United Nations University,
PO Box 500, Charles St Sta, Boston, MA 02114-0500, USA

Correct use of food composition tables and databases outside the country of origin requires identification of the values in those tables. In addition to the problems of adequate nomenclature, identification, and classification of foods, problems also exist in adequate description of laboratory samples, identification of the food components being reported, and identification of the accuracy, precision and representativeness of the data values themselves. This paper reviews the procedures for identifying food components developed by INFOODS in collaboration with IUNS and their increasing use around the world. The paper then discusses the issues associated with data value identification and, in particular, methods of reporting accuracy and precision that provide maximum information to sophisticated users and compilers of food composition tables.

When data are exchanged among countries, or even among researchers within a country, the recipients must have adequate identification, or at least description, of those data to make intelligent use of them. Some of that identification is provided implicitly, by the conventions of the field. For example, scientists doing cryogenic studies always use degrees Kelvin to report temperatures. The use of Fahrenheit, or even Celsius, degrees would be odd indeed, so the scale is almost never explicitly reported. A peculiarity of food composition data is that there are so many different aspects of the data that must be identified, and yet few established international conventions that would permit this implicitly.

Adequate identification of the data values depends on the purpose for which they will be used, but typically requires describing:

- the food involved in terms of what it is called, since we typically want to match foods-that-are-analyzed with the foods-that-people-eat or report eating

- the food involved in terms of its biological or recipe origins, since we often need to know how one food is related to another to compare values

- how the food was sampled, stored, packaged, prepared, etc., since these factors can greatly affect magnitudes of nutrient values and the degree to which the values reported actually represent the quantities present in the food as eaten

- how the food was handled after selection but prior to analysis, since this, too, can greatly affect the resulting values

- the nutrient or other food component being reported, since a value given without indication of what it represents is useless

- the analysis method used and how the "nutrient" was defined, since different methods and definitions, and even different conversion factors, where required (energy, protein, vitamins A and E, and so on), can produce different values that cannot be compared directly

- the statistical (distributional) properties of the value reported, since it is useful to know both how similar the values are from different analyses and samples (precision or variance) and, to the degree possible, how closely the value is related to the nutrient levels that would be encountered in the food

as found in nature (representativeness).

In addition to being issues of description, many of these items bear on data quality both the quality of the data values themselves and, in the presence or absence of appropriate description, the overall quality of the tables or databases in which they are embedded.

Many other papers, including some at this conference, have focused on the first of the above elements and particularly on the issues associated with attempting to describe or classify foods accurately. Accurate and standardized description of sampling methods has been discussed a great deal and identified as important (1, 2), but there are no known specific proposals for how to do this that are applicable to food composition data work as actually practiced. The last three elements in the list above the identification of the data values themselves are the topic of this paper.

▋ Identification of Food Components and Analysis Methods

Many of the nutrient values reported in food composition tables actually are the result of (sometimes local) standards for conversion factors, conventions about the relationship of one value to another, or differing assumptions about the relationship of measurable properties to bioavailability, rather than things that can be uniquely and unambiguously determined in the laboratory. For example, while energy measurement by putting people into calorimeters is well-understood, it is rarely done today. Instead, conversion factors are applied to other nutrients, but those conversion factors differ over time

Table I. Some recent additions to INFOODS Food Component Identification Tags

Tag	Description
<BRD>	Bromide
<CYAN>	Cyanide
<F10D1>	Fatty acid 10:1
<F18D1N7>	Fatty acid 18:1ω-7
<F18D1N7>	Fatty acid 18:1 ω-9
<F22D1>	Fatty acid 22:1
<F23D1>	Fatty acid 23:1
<F18D2>	Fatty acid 18:2
<F18D3>	Fatty acid 18:3
<F22D3>	Fatty acid 22:3
<F22D5N6>	Fatty acid 22:5 ω-6
<F24D6>	Fatty acid 24:6
<FIBADC>	Fiber, acid detergent method, Clancy modification
<FIBTSW>	Fiber, total dietary; Wenlock modification
<SB>	Antimony
<TOCPHT>	Total tocopherol
<F10D1F>	Fatty acid 10:1; expressed per quantity of total fatty acids
<F18D1N7F>	Fatty acid 18:1 ω-7; expressed per quantity of total fatty acids
<F18D1N9F>	Fatty acid 18:1 ω-9; expressed per quantity of total fatty acids
<F23D1F>	Fatty acid 23:1; expressed per quantity of total fatty acids
<F18D2F>	Fatty acid 18:2; expressed per quantity of total fatty acids
<F18D3F>	Fatty acid 18:3; expressed per quantity of total fatty acids
<F22D3F>	Fatty acid 22:3; expressed per quantity of total fatty acids
<F22D5N6F>	Fatty acid 22:5 ω-6; expressed per quantity of total fatty acids
<F24D6>	Fatty acid 24:6; expressed per quantity of total fatty acids
<NPR>	Nitrogen-protein ratio

and from one country to another. So having a value in a food composition table labeled "energy" is rarely sufficient to permit comparing that value to others. Similar issues arise for a variety of other commonly-reported nutrients. For others, definitions have changed over time and sometimes remain controversial: a value that is simply identified as "fiber" may be nearly useless. And for still others, differences in methods of analysis produce differences in results, i.e., not exactly the same things are being analyzed.

These issues were examined from the standpoint of food component identification a few years ago. That work resulted in publication of a listing of food components and value-affecting methods for analysis that could be found in the various food composition tables and databases of the world (3). That list also contained abbreviated names for each component-method pair. These names can be used in electronic data interchange and abbreviated table headings and, using the terminology of the International Standard (4) on which the associated data

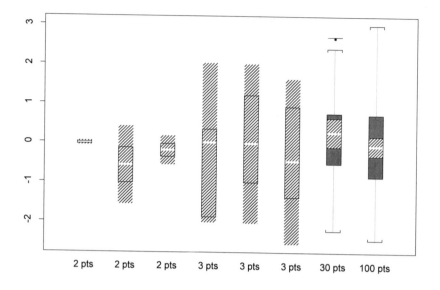

Figure 1. Small-sample normal distributions with 5% confidence intervals

interchange system (5) is based, are called "tags" or "tagnames". The list is now being incrementally updated, using an electronic mail distribution list as the primary mechanism for suggesting and reviewing new proposals. To subscribe to that list, send Internet mail to food-tags-request@infoods.unu.edu. Several new definitions, especially of fatty acids, have been added recently (see Table I). As additional nutrients of interest are identified and incorporated into tables, the list is likely to be extended further.

It is important to note that these food component identification "tags" are not normative and are not associated with any concept of good or desirable practice. There are only two requirements for something being listed: (i) a national or regional food composition table compiler, somewhere, thought that the value was important enough to include in his or her table, and (ii) there is an adequate definition available. The second requirement was waived in the original publication for commonly-occurring under-identified values (e.g., "energy" with no further description, is tagged as

<ener->), but future registrations are expected to be adequately defined.

At the other extreme from "unknown method", some tags have provision, through sub-elements and keywords, for substantially more information than today's food tables and databases provide. This added detail is intended to provide a target for improvement so that no one assumes that the tags represent as much information as might be desired. It should also encourage the recording of more detailed information, as it becomes available and is appropriate in the view of table compilers, in databases.

■ Data Value Description

Just as the choice of analytic methods can have a significant impact on the particular value that is produced for a nutrient, decisions about the statistic to use to represent the result of multiple analyses, estimates, or methods of imputation, may make a considerable difference in the value placed in the table. Means cannot

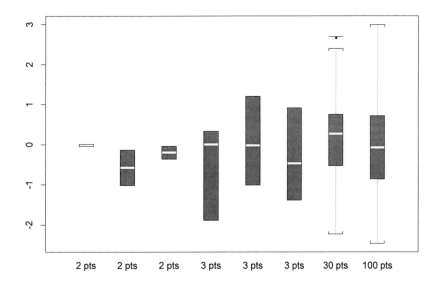

Figure 2. Small-sample normal distributions: medians and fences

be readily compared to medians and, especially with small sample sizes, different estimates of variability are even more difficult to compare in a reasonable way.

To an even greater degree than with nutrient identification, the nature of numeric data values is typically not reported to a degree specific enough to make them usefully comparable (6). Values reported are typically not identified as to whether they are means, medians, or some other estimate of location, nor is the type of data censoring (e.g., "outlier elimination") reported and discussed. Standard errors or variances are often reported with sample sizes as small as two or three. Even with normally-distributed data, such small sample sizes tend to yield confidence limits broad enough to make this type of variance reporting almost useless.

The relationships between sample size and confidence limits are illustrated in Figures 1 and 2. The plots show repeated samples, using a good random number generator, from a Gaussian distribution with the traditional mean of zero and standard deviation of one. Figure 1 shows "boxplots" from these successive

samples, with the white bar representing the median and the shaded area representing the hinges or "fourths" (approximately quartiles—the middle half of the data). The "whiskers" on the two plots to the right extend out to the "fences" or outlier cutoffs, calculated as 1.5 time the hinge-spread past the hinges. These types of plots, widely introduced after Turkey's "orange book" (7) and explained in detail in Hoaglin et al. (8), usually provide a better overview of small-sample data than more traditional scatter plots or histograms.

It is interesting to observe with this group that the second and third random draws produced values all of which fell below the known population mean of zero. While this is clearly a random event, it illustrates the dangers of making statistical estimates that are designed for the large sample case with only two points. The three-point samples are better, as one would expect, but the medians fall well away from the expected mean (especially in the third case), and the hinge spreads are quite wide relative to the standard deviations one would hope for. Things

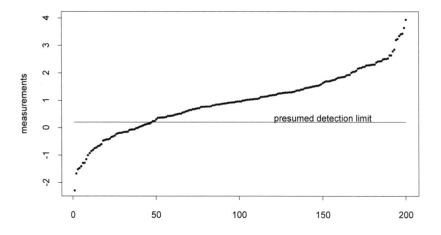

Figure 3. Two-hunderd point sample from Normal (1,1) distribution

begin to stabilize at 30 points (the value at the very top is an outlier when the fences are used to set the criteria) and the 100 point sample looks quite reasonable.

Figure 2 exhibits these same data and plots in more traditional confidence interval terms (shown by crosshatching): while some food composition tables report medians for small samples rather than means, none that INFOODS has discovered report hinge spreads or similar robust measures. The confidence intervals for the sample size of two are artificially small due to the nature of the computation. But those for sample sizes of three illustrate the problem: 5 per cent confidence intervals extending out past two standard deviations of the universe being sampled. It is nearly impossible to make statements about values with these types of confidence intervals: they could be used to "prove" almost anything. Things start to become acceptable at 30 points: the 5 per cent confidence intervals actually fall within the hinge spread.

Some food composition tables try to avoid the difficulties with small samples by reporting the range, i.e. the maximum and minimum values actually obtained. But, since they represent extremes, those values are exceptionally sensitive to sam-

pling and experimental error: it is almost impossible to create a statistical estimate of the reliability of an extreme value.

Worse yet, empirical evidence is accumulating that the distributions of many nutrient values are asymmetric. Rand and Pennington discussed the issues two years ago (9); Pennington provided an update and some additional data in a more recent paper (10). Those efforts attempt to examine variability in foods, but, when quantities of nutrients are being measured that are close to the detection level of the instrumentation, inherent censoring of trace levels also causes asymmetry in the values actually obtained.

Instrumentation censoring occurs when nutrients exist in foods at levels below the detection thresholds of the measurement methods being used. For illustration, one possible situation was simulated by drawing 200 points at random from a Gaussian distribution with mean 1 and variance 1. When those points are sorted into ascending order to make an easy-to-understand plot, they appear as in Figure 3. The corresponding frequency histogram appears as Figure 4. In both cases, it is easy to observe that the distribution is approximately Gaussian with a mean at 1, as one would expect. (If

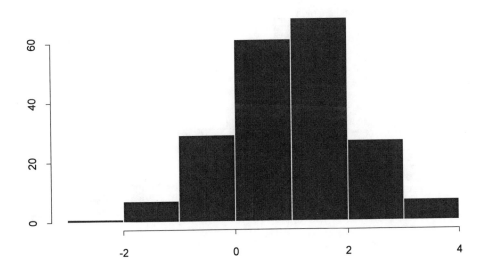

Figure 4. Frequency histogram corresponding to 200 point Normal (1,1) sample: data values

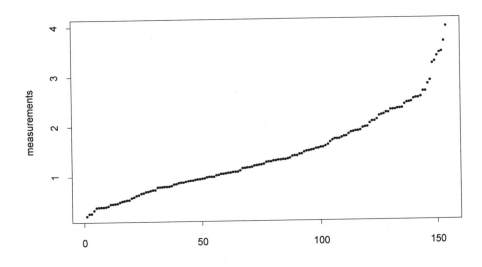

Figure 5. Truncated sample from Normal (1,1) distribution: small values removed at Y=0.2

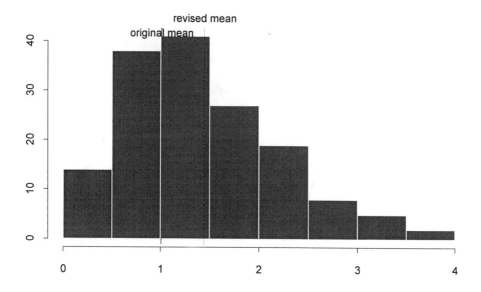

Figure 6. Frequency histogram corresponding to truncated sample: data values

the negative values are bothersome, mentally shift the graphs by adding about 3 to all of the "measurements" in Figure 3 and the "data values" in Figure 4. That shift, of course, has no impact on the analysis.)

Now suppose that the method involved is incapable of detecting any values smaller than 0.2 (marked as "presumed detection limit" in Figure 3). One would then observe plots that look more like Figures 5 and 6 instead of the "true" plots in Figures 3 and 4. The new histogram is especially interesting, since it shows not only significant asymmetry, but the mean of the values actually detected has shifted from 1.0 to about 1.4. A different assumption, that all the undetectable values were actually at the theoretical minimum (somewhat below -2 if one judges from the sample illustrated in Figure 3), would shift the mean considerably in the other direction.

The combination of distributions that represent asymmetric natural phenomena and instrumentation censoring is worse than additive in terms of the degree to which it tends to force measured distributions into non-normal form.

Since the mean value is very sensitive to extreme values and the shape of the distribution, it may not be very useful when the data are severely asymmetric or when trace-censoring eliminates very small values without a corresponding impact on the higher tail. The median is often considered a cure for fussy data problems, but asymmetry due to trace-censoring can distort it even more than the mean, moving it well away from the subjective "center" of the data.

Combination of means and medians in a single table, or comparison of them, is rarely appropriate, especially where central limit assumptions may not apply. Their use together is usually confusing. Neither of them can easily be compared with the more sophisticated measures of location that are appropriate for distributions that are known to be asymmetric. In particular, it is not possible to compute a "weighted average" of a mean from one report with a median from another, even if the sample sizes are known. It is, in general, not even possible to combine two medians this way since substantially all of the distributional information is discarded when half of the data are eliminated from each side, leaving only a single point. When data are to be re-used and re-evaluated by others, as in interchange situations and reference databases, and only the usual small numbers of data points have been determined by analysis or combining values, it is perhaps better to list the actual values themselves, rather than using marginally appropriate, or inappropriate, statistical summaries.

∎ Tagging the Data Values

As with nutrient identification, while doing things correctly is important, it may be even more important that whatever is done be identified accurately so that a recipient or evaluator of data can determine if they are suitable for his or her purposes. Just as it provides for identification of food components and methods by the use of "tags" with exact definitions, the INFOODS interchange system provides tags to identify data values and descriptions of variability. As with the nutrient tags, these tags provide more information than appears in any known food composition table today. At the same time, and again like the food component tags, the data tags are not normative: tags are provided for values that are reported in tables even if they are useless from a statistical point of view. The system for data values extends beyond labeling of simple measures of location (e.g., mean, median, trimmed mean, or the "X percent of RDI" values that appear on food labels in some countries) and variability (e.g., standard deviation, standard error, quartiles, range, or percentage points) to permit description of distribution-based statistical filtering procedures applied to the laboratory data and description of particular challenges encountered in analysis that might bias the results. If much of this type of information were provided, it would pose a serious challenge to database management systems, since few of those are designed to handle data with these types of interrelationships. However, the advantages to those trying to do serious evaluation or quality assessment of data values under consideration for use in studies, calculation of imputed food values, or for inclusion into other tables would make it worth the trouble.

∎ References

(1) Greenfield, H., & Southgate, D.A.T. (1992) *Food Composition Data: Production, Management, and Use,* Elsevier Applied Science, London

(2) Truswell, A.S., Bateson, D., Madafiglio, D., Pennington, J.A.T., Rand, W.M., & Klensin, J.C. (1991) *J. Food Comp. Anal.* **4**, 18-38.

(3) Klensin, J.C., Feskanich, D., Lin, V., Truswell, A.S., & Southgate, D.A.T. (1989) *Identification of Food Components for INFOODS Data Interchange*, UNU Press, Tokyo

(4) *Standard Generalized Markup Language* (1986) ISO 8879

(5) Klensin, J.C. (1993) *INFOODS Food Composition Data Interchange Handbook*, UNU Press, Tokyo

(6) Rand, W.M., Pennington, J.A.T., Murphy, S.P., & Klensin, J.C. (1991) *Compiling Data for Food Composition Databases*, UNU Press, Tokyo

(7) Turkey, J.W. (1977) *Exploratory Data Analysis*, Addison-Wesley, Reading, MA

(8) Hoaglin, D.C., Mosteller, F., & Turkey, J.W. (1983) *Understanding Robust and Exploratory Data Analysis*, John Wiley and Sons, New York, NY

(9) Rand, W.M., & Pennington, J.A.T. (1991) *Proceedings of the 16th National Nutrient Databank Conference,* The CBORD Group, Ithaca, NY, pp. 179-182

(10) Pennington, J.A.T. Albert, R.H., & Rand, W.M. (1993) *Proceedings of the 18th National Nutrient DDatabank Conference*, ILSI Press, Washington, DC, pp. 155-158

Food Data:
Numbers, Words and Images

Barbara Burlingame, Fran Cook, Graham Duxfield, Gregory Milligan

Nutrition Programme, New Zealand Institute for Crop & Food Research, Private Bag 11030, Palmerston North, New Zealand

Food composition databases are generally collections of numeric and descriptive data in various formats with a variety of limitations related to proper documentation. Current technologies make it feasible for databases to go beyond words and numbers now to include images and graphical representations of foods. Presently there are over 130 food images in the New Zealand Food Composition Database, ranging in size from 25 KB to 1.3 MB each, and occupying a total of about 33 MB of disk space. The process at Crop & Food Research involves digitizing photographs of the actual food samples using an optical scanner at 400 dpi resolution. Advanced Revelation 3.0, the development environment system used, does not deal with images yet, but can call DOS-based programs which convert and display digitized images in several different formats such as PCX and GIF. To date, several important uses for food database images have emerged. These include sample validation where common name could relate to several different scientific names; data validation where intensity of the orange color led to accepting β-carotene values outside the expected range; food intake surveys where food descriptors were insufficient due to language or cultural differences or where children were subjects; and for international interchange of food composition data.

Many problems arise as a result of poor, incomplete or ambiguous descriptions of foods listed in databases and as a result of confusion over the interpretation of commonly used names for foods. Many solutions have been recommended to deal with these problems (1,2). These solutions typically rely on words, alphanumeric codes, position-specific facets, etc, and go some way toward alleviating some problems. These systems will never solve all the problems.

A picture is worth a thousand words, as the old adage goes, and technologies have advanced to the stage that all food descriptor files could contain a field or an accompanying file of digitized images or series of images so that barriers of language, culture, and the limitations and subjectivities of our vocabularies are minimized (e.g., how lean is lean meat? how do you describe the depth and intensity of the color of an apricot? and what is a muttonbird?).

■ Documentation by Image

In the New Zealand Food Composition work, the process of documentation begins at the sample preparation stage. Food samples are collected and then prepared in the laboratory. Samples are photographed intact, raw and after consumer-type preparation (e.g. processed by cooking). Each sample is photographed as prepared for consumption and with a scale definition (e.g. metric ruler), and lately with a color index (see Figure 1). Food packaging and labels are also routinely photographed (see Figure 2). All this is done in addition to the recording of word descriptors and detailed text containing the standard documentation details (age of sample, date of sampling, geographic region, common and scientific name, physical state, processing, packaging, etc).

The photos are then digitized into PCX formats (IBM PC Paintbrush Picture File) using an optical scanner at 400 dpi (dots per inch) resolution. Much higher resolution is available, but there is a trade-off between resolution and space required to store the image. Presently, there are 130 PCX images in the NZ Food Composition Database, occupying about 33 MB (megabytes) of disk space. The size of the individual files ranges from 25 KB (kilobytes) to 1.3 MB each. Compression would significantly reduce amount of disk space required.

Disk space requirements vary depending on size of the image, number of colors, and the image resolution. Various manipulations can be done to achieve efficient storage. One NZ beverage record represents a composite of three different brands of powdered drink mix. The packaging scanned in 256 colors occupies 630 KB; this same file compressed with PKZIP (compression format by PKWare) occupies 416 KB; and as a GIF (Graphics Interchange Format) file, 93 KB. The same information contained on the packaging, when entered into the database as text, occupies a mere 30 bytes. Table I shows disk space required by other images and plain text.

More and more software products are allowing the inclusion of digitized images. Advanced Revelation 3.0 (ARev), the development environment used for the New Zealand Food Composition Database, does not incorporate graphics procedures. Presently, however, we associate scanned images of food via other software. ARev is programmed to call DOS-based programs — we use SVGA (Super Video Graphics Adaptor) and ColorView — which can display digitized images stored under various formats.

Using a number of different software package and shareware, images stored in PCX format can be transferred to media as PCX or other less byte-consuming formats such as GIF. This is important because users will have different hardware and software products available to them. GIF and TIFF (Tag Image File Format) have become industry standards, and JPEG (Joint Photographic Experts Group) with the ISO (International Standards Organization) and CCITT (Consultative Committee on Interna-

Table I. Disk space requirements for food record images in bytes compared with non-graphical text

Storage format	Bread bag	Powdered drink packaging	Powdered drink packaging; composite of 3
.PCX (color)[a]	1,925,289	805,234	2,238,904
.PCX (grey)[a, b]	704,053	277,092	780,405
.ZIP[a, c]	1,240,687	471,347	1,327,914
.GIF[a, d]	317,399	110,505	295,897
.JPG[a, e]	116,613	52,925	116,716
Non-graphical text; database descriptors	250	401	946

[a] scanned at 16 million colors; saved as Zsoft PC paintbrush format
[b] converted and stored by PhotoMagic as greyscale Zsoft PC paintbrush format
[c] compressed and stored by PKZIP
[d] converted and stored by PhotoMagic as Graphic Interchange Format
[e] converted and stored by PhotoMagic as JPEG format

tional Telegraph and Telephone) backing (3) is becoming popular for compressing still images for storage. Exchanging of images will be facilitated by having image format flexibility.

∎ The Hardware

The ability to view images is dependent on the hardware available. Images require, as a minimum, a Super VGA (Video Graphics Adapter) monitor which can display 1024 x 768 pixels in at least 256 colors. Some images require a 1 MB video card capable of displaying 32,000 colors from a palette of over 16 million colors. Graphical printers are also now readily available, with as little as 300 dpi resolution and 24 bit color.

Flopticals

Flopticals have been used already in the exchange of images between New Zealand and INFOODS. Floptical drives are inexpensive and can use both floptical disks and normal 3.5" floppy disks. Floptical disks are 21 MB in size, compared to the 1.44 MB size of standard 3.5" disks. This capacity is important because some

high resolution images can be 20 MB and would require fifteen standard floppies for a single image. Most of the images for the New Zealand Food Composition Database are between 25 KB and 1.3 MB each.

Other Media

Third party software will allow integration of compact disks and proprietary technologies such as Photo-CD with food composition databases. Many information systems have been developed using CD-ROM technology. Conventional information retrieval techniques including full-text searching and relational databases were integrated for accessing information stored on the CD-ROM for agricultural extension information (4).

∎ Lossy Compression

Lossy compression is so named because redundant or otherwise unnecessary data are deleted in the compression process. Two compression types that can be used for lossy compression are accepted as current standards for still images: JPEG (Joint Photographic Experts Group) and

Fractal compression. JPEG was designed as a digital image compression standard for continuous-tone, gray scale and color still images (3). It is based on a generic mathematical function known as forward DCT (Discrete Cosine Transform), which basically transforms the image into a different form which takes up less space. Its compression is very fast, but the JPEG-compacted image files are larger for the same quality than files compressed by other methods. Fractal compression uses a mathematical transformation called an affine map which identifies all patterns that can be matched even if it means rotating, stretching or squashing the pattern. It is resolution-independent. Lossy compression used by both these compression types involves a trade off between information and compressed size. Both methods intentionally discard parts of the data (5,6,7).

▪ Limitations

There are some limitations and problems with using images in food composition databases. These include hardware and software restrictions related to storage, compression, decompression, image resolution and faithfulness to the original. Additionally, an image cannot be searched in the same way as text files. For example, the bread wrapper images will identify ingredients, one of which may be potassium bromate. However, the graphics files of bread wrappers cannot be searched for potassium bromate the way a descriptor text file or a Langual file can, and therefore will not substitute for documentation by words or alphanumeric codes.

▪ Uses of Images

Data Validation

Verification of information has become the most valuable use to date of the effort to document by images. Sometimes we have reason to question our own data, and

images have on many occasions allowed us to make the decision about accepting or rejecting the results of some nutrient analyses. For example, we obtained some very high values for β-carotene in apricots in our 1989 work. In some later work we obtained values which were significantly lower. We examined details of methods, compared sampling and sample preparation protocols, and finally resolved the problem by comparing images of the actual samples used. The images showed that the earlier samples had a much deeper, darker, orange color than the more recent samples (see Figure 3). This, of course, raises more issues about the introduction and widespread adoption of modified cultivars, which is often done without consideration of the nutritional implications.

Food Intake Surveys

The NZ Food Composition Database has over 100 beef records. For many of these records, the word descriptors are identical up to the facet containing ratios of separable lean and separable fat (e.g., there are five records for beef, rump steak, grilled, having different ratios of separable lean and fat: 80:20, 85:15, 95:5, separable lean only and separable fat only). Once the database is searched for the words grilled rump steak, and four records are presented, a judgment is required which many people cannot make without the benefit of visual examples. It is far easier for most people, nutrition professionals and lay alike, to select a picture of meat which looks like what they would consume, rather than to say with confidence that their grilled rump steak was 95 per cent separable lean and 5 per cent separable fat.

Language differences present a challenge which is dealt with by including an alternative names facet in each food descriptor file. Still, with international interchange and international trade in agricultural products, some descriptors, however comprehensive and however many language translations are provided, will never be enough. For example, the New Zealand kumara, with the alternative name sweet potato, is quite unlike the North American sweet potato; the New Zealand pumpkin is unlike the typical North American pumpkin. The differences seen in the nutrient composition are not so surprising when the physical differences are shown with a picture of the food (see Figure 4).

Communication barriers exist within countries and with the rest of the world. Language, culture, age, are just a few. In a clinical setting, it is often necessary to determine the nutrient intake of patients. In New Zealand there are several Polynesian languages in use, as well as Maori and English. Children are often subjects in nutrient intake surveys. Food images can assist overcome these communication barriers.

Wildlife Feeding Programs

A recent project involves providing nutrient data to an aquarium in New Zealand. This organization will soon bring in penguins for exhibition which have been successfully bred and reared for many generations on fish from the Northern seas. We are assisting them in determining what locally available foods could substitute for their present diet. The task of matching the nutrient composition of our Antarctic finfish with Arctic finfish would be easier if the nutrient data, a plethora of which is available in the USDA Standard Reference 10 (8), were accompanied by images. This would be particularly useful where the sample numbers are only one or a few, where the information presented does not specify different stages of maturity, different seasons of the year and different catch areas. Image comparisons between the two databases would help us assess the physical similarities of the different species, for example, as size of the finfish would be relevant to the penguin's diet.

In the same area of wildlife nutrition, our supply of nutrient data, coupled with images, will assist others attempting to reproduce the dietary aspect of native habitats. The right nutrients in the right sorts of foods will improve the well-being of the wildlife, including enhancing the potential for reproduction (9). We experience problems even within New Zealand, where endangered bird species must be relocated from their native habitats in the South Island, to small off-shore island sanctuaries. Their traditional foods are not all available, so the nutrient content, as well as physical similarities of the native food, are considered when designing the supplementary feeding program.

International Interchange

What is a feijoa? What is a pukeko? What is a karaka berry? Most people outside of New Zealand would have no idea at all what these foods are. Even the alternative names would be useless, as these are (almost) uniquely New Zealand foods (see Figure 5).

INFOODS has considered the issue of images in food composition databases (10), and an image element is included in the interchange model (11). The structure for interchange using the INFOODS' model requires elements that indicate the picture encoding type as well as providing the actual image. A comment element may also be used. The images are subsidiary to the *classification* element, which is the first immediate subsidiary of the *food* element. Images associated with a cut of meat record might include a carcass diagram showing the position of the cut and a photograph of the cut itself. These would be included in an interchange file as follows (where cmt means comment):

> <image> *the first image itself in PCX format* </pcx/>beef carcass diagram with cut sites identified</cmt/></image>
>
> <image> *the second image itself in GIF format* </gif/>image of cut</cmt/></image>

▮ Acknowledgments

Funding for this work has come from the New Zealand Department of Health and Public Health Commission, and the Foundation for Research, Science and Technology. We acknowledge permission to publish the pukeko photograph from R.B. Morris, Department of Conservation, New Zealand.

▮ References

(1) Pennington, J.A.T., & Butrum, R.R. (1991) *Trends Food Sci. Technol.* **2**, 285-288

(2) Truswell, A.S., Bateson, D.J., Madafiglio, K.C., Pennington, J.A.T., Rand, W.M., & Klensin, J.C. (1991) *J. Food Comp. Anal.* **4**, 1, 18-38

(3) Wallace, G.K. (1991) *Commun. ACM* **4**, 30-45

(4) Watson, D.G., Beck, H.W., & Jones, P.H. (1991) *Am. Soc. Agric. Engin.* **91**, 7017-7024

(5) Carlson, W.E. (1991) *Comp. Graph.* **25**, 67-75

(6) Simon, B. (1993) *PC Magazine*, June 29, pp. 305-313

(7) Simon, B. (1993) *PC Magazine*, July, pp. 371-382

(8) US Department of Agriculture (1993) *Nutrient Database for Standard Reference*, Release 10, USDA, Washington, DC

(9) James, K.A.C., Waghorn, G.C. Powlesland, R.G., & Lloyd, B.D. (1991) *Proc. Nutr. Soc. NZ* **16**, 93-102

(10) Klensin, J.C. (1991) *Trends Food Sci. Technol.* **2**, 279-282

(11) Klensin, J.C. (1992) *INFOODS Food Composition Data Interchange Handbook,* UNU Press, Tokyo

▮ Other Key References on Image Compression

Barnsley, M.F. (1993) *Fractal Image Compression,* A.K. Peters, Wellesley

Storer, J.A. (1988) *Data Compression Methods and Theory,* Computer Science Press, Rockville, MD

Netravali, A.N. (1988) *Digital Pictures: Representation and Compression,* Plenum Publishing Corporation, New York, NY

Russ, J.C. (1992) *The Image Processing Handbook,* CRC Press, Boca Raton, FL

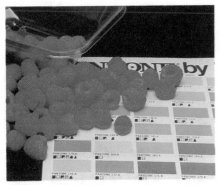

Figure 1. Gold berries (a new cultivar) photographed with a color index.

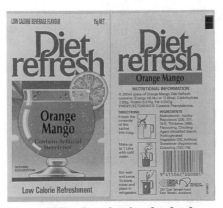

Figure 2. Food packaging for foods recorded in the New Zealand Food Composition database.

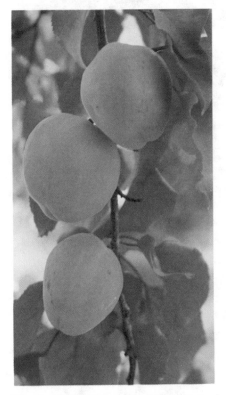

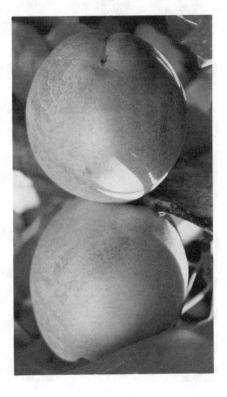

Figure 3. Apricots with different shades of orange

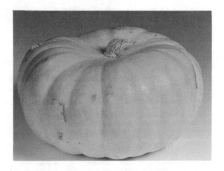
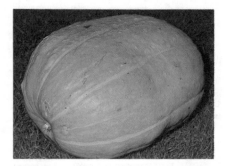

Figure 4. New Zealand pumkin (left): in shape, color and size is very unlike its North American counterpart (right).

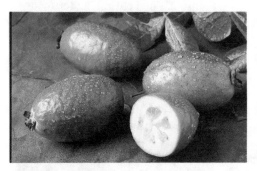
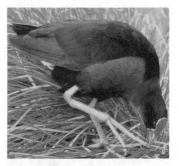

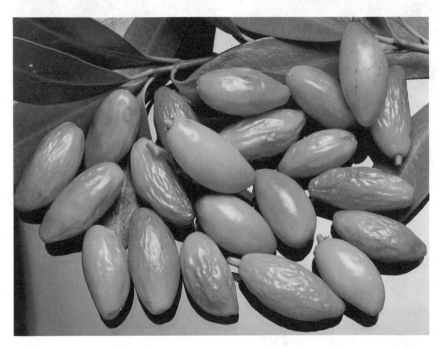

Figure 5. Some (almost) unique New Zealand foods for which descriptors and/or codes would never suffice. From left to right: (top) feijoas, pukeko and (bottom) karaka berries.

Computer Construction of Recipes to Meet Nutritional and Palatability Requirements

Leslie R. Fletcher, Patricia M. Soden

Department of Mathematics and Computer Science,
University of Salford, Salford, Lancs M5 4WT, UK

This paper describes a microcomputer package which carries out the inverse process to dietary analysis — that is, given a list of nutrient targets the software modifies a food list so that its nutritional analysis meets those targets. The initial aim of the work was the development of a decision support system to be used by dietitians, nutritionists and other medical personnel when giving dietary advice to patients with chronic diseases such as diabetes and renal failure. This paper contains a detailed example of another application of the same software, namely the formulation of recipes for acceptable versions of traditional dishes which also meet predetermined targets for some key nutrients.

George Stigler's solution (1) of the classical diet problem — ensuring adequate nutrition at minimum cost — is a celebrated example in optimization and is frequently mentioned in textbooks. However, it is of limited practical significance in human dietetics — the "optimal" solution contains only five foods — and, rather more importantly, the method used is rather inflexible. In particular, given the objective of minimum (monetary) cost and a range of foods from which to choose, the nutrient targets uniquely determine the solution. Adding non-nutritional constraints, limiting the quantities of particular foods in the optimal diet, for example, will ensure that the computed diet is more varied (2,3). Nevertheless, there is still only one solution for each collection of targets and there is no convenient way of taking individual preferences into account.

We have developed, and implemented in microcomputer software, a different model of the diet problem (4,5,6). This generates, in a natural way, varied diets which meet the needs and wishes of individuals as well as nutritional targets. In this paper we describe an application of this same model to the modification of a recipe so that the resulting dish is not only palatable but also has a predetermined nutritional composition.

Solving the diet problem is the inverse of the familiar, and (mathematically) much simpler, process of nutritional, or dietary, analysis. The software implementation of our model is an extension to the dietary analysis package *Microdiet* (7), which is based, in turn, on the authoritative UK food analysis data (8,9,10,11). The new software selects, from all the possible combinations of foods with a predetermined nutritional composition, one which is as close as possible to the wishes of a client or patient. This uses a standard variant of conventional linear programming (12, Chapter 14). Some algebraic details are given by Fletcher et al. (5) and we will report others elsewhere, particularly those relating to our expression of the basic optimization in dimensionless terms. This has proved to be an important technical device, allowing all the targets to be assessed relative to each other when seeking, for example, other ingredients to include in a recipe, and circumvents a possible difficulty mentioned in (2, p. 389). Careful formulation of the algebraic model has also ensured that the solution to the dual problem (12, Chapter 5) provides significant nutritional insight.

∎ Method

A recipe for lasagne verdi was taken from a domestic cookery book (13) and a nutritional analysis carried out. The recipe and some of the corresponding nutrient totals are shown in the indicated columns of Tables I and II, respectively. As a demonstration of the capabilities of the model it was decided to seek a modified version of the recipe which would produce a dish reasonably similar to lasagne verdi but with the modified nutritional composition shown in the column labeled "Target" in Table II. Although these targets are only illustrative, they are also intended to reflect recent expert advice to UK citizens (14) regarding desirable dietary modifications.

The other columns in Tables I and II show the various stages in the modification of the recipe until, at version F, an acceptable version was obtained. The test of "acceptability" was the willingness of the first author's family to consider eating the resulting dish. Ingredients were exchanged, introduced into, or removed from the recipe at various stages in the modification process. A blank entry, denoted by "–", indicates that the particular ingredient was not considered at that stage in the optimization. The reference to "olive oil" in Table II indicates that a (lower) limit was placed on this quantity of this ingredient during the final stages; it is convenient to list this with other, nutrient, targets. There was no target on the quantity of fat in the recipe and it appears in Table II for illustration only. Had the fat content of the diet become too high (or too low) a further constraint could have been added to limit this.

Table I. Ingredients and quantities in lasagne recipe

Food name	Ingredient quantity (g) in recipe number					
	A (original)	B	C	D	E	F
Meat sauce						
Onions, raw	250	250	250	250	250	250
Butter, salted *Removed after stage C*	40	0	0	–	–	–
Olive oil	30	0	0	0	15	30
Beef mince, raw *Reduced to 100g after stage B*	300	115	100	100	100	100
Lentils, boiled *Introduced after stage B*	–	–	100	100	100	100
Haricot beans, boiled *Introduced after stage B*	–	–	100	100	100	100
Garlic, raw	5	5	5	5	5	5
Mushrooms, raw	100	100	100	100	100	100
Bay leaf, dried	2	2	2	2	2	2
Tomatoes, canned	400	747	449	416	417	417
Sugar, white	10	10	10	10	10	10
Basil, fresh	5	5	5	5	5	5
White sauce						
Flour, plain white	25	25	25	25	25	25
Butter, salted	25	0	0	25	6	13
Milk, cows, whole *Exchanged after stage C for*	300	300	300	–	–	–
Milk, cows, semi-skimmed *Exchanged after stage E for*	–	–	–	300	300	–
Milk, cows, skimmed	–	–	–	–	–	300
Topping						
Cream, double *Exchanged after stage C for*	40	16	9	–	–	–
Yoghurt, low fat, natural	–	–	–	40	40	40
Cheese, cheddar type *Exchanged after stage C for*	50	50	50	–	–	–
Cheese, reduced fat, cheddar-type	–	–	–	50	50	50
Lasagne, boiled	225	477	225	225	225	225

▊ Results

The steps in obtaining the displayed results (Table I, Table II) were as follows. Recipe A refers to the original recipe. When the targets were set a software alert pointed out that the fibre contents of garlic, bay leaf and basil were recorded as "unknown". Recipe B represents the smallest change to the quantities of the ingredients in recipe A which will meet the nutrient targets set. Although these quantities do not constitute an acceptable recipe, these results and other subsidiary results from the linear programming show that other ingredients are required

Table II. Nutrient targets and analyses for recipe

Nutrient	Target	A (original)	B	C	D	E	F
			Analysis for recipe number:				
Fiber (g)	>20	13	20	25	25	25	25
Energy (kcal)	<1500	2475	1502	1342	1383	1377	1381
Sodium (mg)	<1100	1444	816	739	1008	843	907
Potassium (mg)	>3500	3453	3882	3501	3499	3499	3500
Iron (mg)	>16	17	16	17	16	16	16
% energy from fat	<35	66	35	35	35	35	35
Quantity of olive oil (g) (in stages E and F)	>15	–	–	–	–	15	15
Fat (g)	–	182	58	52	54	54	54

to complement those already there. The subsidiary result also enabled the pulses introduced thereafter to be selected from amongst the variety of possible new ingredients.

Recipe C shows the beneficial effect on the changes to the recipe of the new ingredients. The subsidiary results from this stage show that the limit on the percentage of energy from fat is causing most of the changes made by the program to the ingredient quantities. Exchanges of existing ingredients for the lower-fat alternatives were made. Recipe D shows the results of making these modifications to the starting recipe and recomputing the smallest changes which will enable the nutrient targets to be met. This still resulted in the removal of all the olive oil so a lower bound of 15 g was imposed on this ingredient. Recipe E represents the smallest change to the modified recipe required to meet the nutrient targets with at least 15 g of olive oil. The consequent reduction in the remaining quantity of butter in the white sauce was judged to be unacceptable so semi-skimmed milk was replaced by skimmed milk. The investigation closed with recipe F which was deemed an acceptable version of the original recipe.

∎ Conclusions

We have demonstrated the use of a linear programming model of food and nutrition in updating a recipe to reflect current dietary expert opinion. The eventual recipe in the example discussed here had limits placed on the totals of various nutrients, on the percentage energy derived from fat and on the quantity of one of its ingredients. Other targets which the software can accommodate include the P/S ratio, the amino acid profile of the protein and the ratios of the quantities of two ingredients. This last target is available to ensure that, for example, the quantities of flour and milk in a computed recipe were appropriate for a white sauce.

The model also allows targeting of nutrient density rather than nutrient totals though some modification of the software would be required to implement this. However, in seeking to minimize the overall change to ingredient quantities in moving to a nutritionally acceptable recipe, the present software tends to maintain the total weight of the recipe approximately constant, leading to a stable relationship between nutrient totals and nutrient density.

■ References

(1)   Stigler, G.J. (1945) *J. Farm Econ.* **27**, 303-314.

(2)   Henson, S. (1991) *J. Agric. Econ.* **42**, 380-393.

(3)   Smith, V. E. (1963) *Electronic Computation of Human Diets,* Michigan State University Press, East Lansing, MI

(4)   Fletcher, L. R., & Soden P. M. (1991) *Diab. Nutr. Metab.* **4**(S1), 169-174

(5)   Fletcher, L. R., Soden P. M., & Zinober, A. S. I. (1994) *J. Oper. Res. Soc.* **45**, 489-496

(6)   Soden, P.M., & Fletcher, L.R. (1992) *Br. J. Nutr.* **68**, 565-572

(7)   Bassham, S., Fletcher, L. R., & Stanton, R. H. J. (1984) *J. Microc. App.* **7,** 279-289.

(8)   Paul, A. A. & Southgate, D. A. T. (1978) *McCance and Widdowson's The Composition of Foods,* 4th Ed., HMSO, London

(9)   Paul, A. A., Southgate, D. A. T., & Russell, J. (1980) *First Supplement to McCance and Widdowson's The Composition of Foods,* HMSO, London

(10)   Tan, S. P., Wenlock, R. W., & Buss, D. H. (1985) *Immigrant Foods: Second Supplement to McCance and Widdowson's The Composition of Foods,* HMSO, London

(11)   Holland, B., Unwin, I. D. & Buss, D. H. (1991) *McCance and Widdowson's The Composition of Foods,* 5th Ed., Royal Society of Chemistry, Cambridge.

(12)   Chvatal, V. (1983) Linear Programming, W. H. Freeman and Company, New York, NY

(13)   Allison, S. (1977) *The Dairy Book of Home Cookery,* Milk Marketing Board of England and Wales, Thames Ditton

(14)   Committee on Medical Aspects of Food Policy (1991) *Dietary Reference Values for Food Energy and Nutrients for the United Kingdom,* HMSO, London

Requirements for Applications Software for Computerized Databases in Research Projects

Dorothy Mackerras

Department of Public Health, University of Sydney, NSW 2006,
Australia

N umerous programs have been written to access nutrient databases using words rather than numeric codes. In general, they have been directed towards the needs of clinical dietitians but many of their features, such as graphs of individual dietary intakes, are irrelevant to the needs of nutrition researchers. A recent dietary survey conducted on a Pacific island highlighted some of the data entry needs of researchers. Survey participants described food intakes using standard volumes and measures (fluid oz, oz, g, mL), household units (bowl, can, slice, tablespoon), small, medium, large (glasses, coconuts, pandanus, donuts, papaya) and locally developed measures (mountain table/teaspoon, small and large tuna steaks, cm of reef fish). Neither the teaspoon nor the tablespoon matched the metric or US standards.

The abilities of two programs, A and B, from two different countries to meet researchers' needs are described. Both these programs, or their earlier versions, have been available for a number of years and are widely used in their respective countries. Both programs were used on a Compaq Deskpro 486/33M computer with a math coprocessor and 8 MB RAM including 558 KB of available conventional memory. Program A was used for surveys involving food frequency questionnaires and diet records and Program B in a survey gathering 24-hour recall data (its food frequency capabilities have not been used).

Facilitating data entry is important. A major goal is to reduce the amount of coding required prior to entry. Every step that has to be coded will also require double coding on at least a proportion of forms to examine the error rate. If the software allows household or common measures as food descriptors, the weight of household measures of each food only needs to be "coded" once into the program and individual diets will not require conversion into grams prior to entry. Both programs allow standard measures (cup etc.) to be used. In addition, Program A allows three household measures to be defined per food and the user can choose from 51 different words to describe the serving. Program B allows only one household measure, called either serving, item, slice or piece, to be defined per food. Abbreviations used for data entry should be standard or intuitively obvious. Program A uses SI units ("g" for gram etc.) and abbreviations such as "oz" for ounce. By contrast, Program B uses "a" for gram, "b" for ounce etc., and this increases the likelihood of data entry errors. Both programs allow the household measures to be altered which is important in cross-cultural studies. However, Program B requires the operator to change each of the nutrient values in the database if the gram weight of the measure is changed whereas this is calculated automatically in Program A. Neither program appears to be capable of converting the assigned volume of cups, pints etc. between the metric, imperial and US systems or of allowing new words to describe serving sizes (e.g. mountain tablespoon) which would have been useful in the study.

After entry, data need to be checked and cleaned. It is also useful to have a code for an unknown food so that incomplete records are flagged until the relevant coding decisions are made. As diet records may contain 25 or more different

food items per day it is useful if the program allows foods to be inserted anywhere in the diet list so that the printout matches the order of the original form. Program A has this feature but Program B does not. Neither program appears to have a range checking facility; this would be particularly useful for food frequency information when the list of foods can be pre-specified.

It is also useful to be able to enter some other data into the dietary program. Both programs allowed long names for the subject and the field will take numbers instead of letters. Thus items such as subject number, date of interview, interviewer code and household number could all be coded and used as the subject's "name". Managing the database needs care, especially if the same program is being used to analyze data from several different surveys at the same time. The programs had different approaches to the data organization. Program A saves the diet files within the database and a separate database of food composition information can be made for each study. This means that some care is needed to prevent the file becoming too large to backup. Program B saves each diet file as a separate file. This makes backup easier, but means that alterations to the database (e.g. deletions) may make the files invalid.

Dietary data are often exported into a statistical program. This can be used for detecting errors in the data, such as outliers etc., and for analysis. Data may need to be cleaned and exported several times prior to the final analysis being done. Most surveys involve large numbers of people and many lines of data per respondent and so batch processing is needed to export a large number of diet files into a single file, generally with a rectangular ASCII format. Program A has this function which is clearly described in the manual. It took approximately ten minutes to export about 9000 lines of data from 45 food frequency files each containing about 200 lines of data. Program B does not have an inbuilt export function although the company will write a program on request. It took three hours to export 4160 lines of data from 369 files and required reconfiguring the computer to free all the conventional memory. These functions will take longer on slower computers.

Particular needs of research in developing countries therefore include:

- programs which allow flexibility in which system of units is used (metric, imperial, US) and which also allow for a mixture of systems and units and for words which describe non-standard units

- programs which allow new (local) serving descriptors to be specified

- programs which can find foods with names of only one and two letters long

- foods may need to have multiple spellings or entries in countries where spelling is not yet standardized.

Attention to some of these details would allow local people greater participation in all phases of the research, and improve the speed and quality of information processing and data output.

Food Composition Data and Population Studies

This Session was chaired by Dr Ian Darnton-Hill of WHO-WPRO and began with a keynote address by A. Møller entitled *Food Monitoring in Denmark* . This was followed by papers on *Food Composition Data Requirements for Nutritional Epidemiology of Cancer and Chronic Diseases* by N. Slimani, E. Riboli and H. Greenfield; *Developing a Food Composition Database for Epidemiologic Studies in the Pacific Islands* by J.H. Hankin, L. Le Marchand, L.N. Kolonel, B.E. Henderson, and Beecher, G.R.; *The Effects of Australian, US and UK Food Composition Tables on Estimates of Food and Nutrient Availability in Australia* by K.M. Cashel and H. Greenfield, and *Quality Control in the Use of Food and Nutrient Databases for Epidemiologic Studies* by I.M. Buzzard, S.F. Schakel and J. Ditter-Johnson. These papers are all published in full in the following pages, along with a poster entitled *Construction of a Database on Inherent Bioactive Compounds in Food Plants,* by A.D. Walker, J.A. Plumb, G.R. Fenwick, R. Preece, & R.K. Heaney.

Posters displayed after the Session were:

- *Relationship Between a Dietary Measure of Antioxidant Intake and Plasma Levels,* Baghurst, K.I., & Baghurst, P.A., CSIRO Division of Human Nutrition, Kintore Avenue, Adelaide, SA, Australia.
- *The UCB Worldfood Dietary Assessment System Utilizing the UCB International Minilist,* Calloway, D.H., & Murphy, S.P., Department of Nutritional Sciences, University of California, Berkeley CA, USA.

- *Use of the Extended Table of Nutrient Values to Assess Nutrient Intakes of Restrained and Disinhibited Women,* Champagne, C.M., & Williamson, D.A., Pennington Biomedical Research Center, Louisiana State University, Baton Rouge, LA, USA.

- *Organochlorine Intake of Victorian Infants from Maternal Milk,* Donohue, D.C., Quinsey, P.M., & Ahokas, J.T., Key Centre for Applied and Nutritional Toxicology, RMIT University, Melbourne, VIC 3001 and National Food Authority, Canberra, ACT, Australia.

- *Aflatoxin M1 in Human Milk Samples for Australia,* El-Nazemi, H.S., Ahokas, J.T., Donohue, D.C., & Neal, G.E., Key Centre for Applied and Nutritional Toxicology, RMIT University, Melbourne, Australia and Medical Research Council, Toxicology Unit, Carshalton, UK.

- *Graile: a Database for Australian Grain Legumes,* Horton, J.D., Petterson, D.S., & Mackintosh, J.B., Cowirrie Computing, Relbia, TAS; Department of Agriculture, South Perth, WA; The University of Western Australia, Nedlands, WA, Australia.

- *A Short Questionnaire and Qualitative Fat Index for the Assessment of Fat Intakes on the Basis of the FINMONICA 1982 Survey,* Kempainnen, T., Rosendahl, A., Nuutinen, O., Ebeling, T., Pietinen, P., & Uusitupa, M., Departments of Clinical Nutrition and Medicine, University of Kuopio, National Public Health Institute, Helsinki, Finland.

- *Heavy Metals in Taiwanese Diets,* Lee, Y.S., & Chou, S.S., Department of Food Science, University of the District of Columbia, Washington, DC, and National Laboratories of Foods and Drugs, Taipei, Taiwan.

- *Variability in Macronutrient Contents of Selected Cereal Products Between Production Batches and Analytical Laboratories,* Mugford, D.C., Bread Research Institute of Australia, Inc, North Ryde, NSW, Australia.

- *Database on Asian Sensory Preferences, Food Markets and Culture,* Ng, F., Bell, G., Prescott, J., Waring, J., & Gillmore, R., CSIRO Sensory Research Centre, Division of Food Science and Technology, North Ryde, NSW, Australia.

- *Impact of Reductions in Fat Content of Australian Pork on Fat Available for Consumption in Australia,* O'Dea, K., Mann, N.J., Sinclair, A.J., & Barnes, J.A., Department of Human Nutrition, Deakin University, Geelong, VIC3217 and Australian Pork Corporation, 174 Pacific Highway, St Leonard's, NSW, Australia.

- *Comparison of the Use of Australian and UK Food Composition Tables for Estimating Nutrient Intake,* Record, S.J., & Baghurst, K., CSIRO Division of Human Nutrition, Kintore Avenue, Adelaide, SA, Australia.
- *The Link Between Defence Food Intake Studies and a Relational Database,* Waters, D.R., DSTO, Materials Research Laboratory, Food Science Branch, Scottsdale, TAS, Australia.
- *Effect of Changes in the Swedish Food Database on Nutrient Estimates from a Food Frequency Questionnaire,* Wolk, A., Becker, W., Ohlander, E-M., & Bergstrom, L., Cancer Epidemiology Unit, Uppsala University Hospital, and the Nutrition Division, National Food Administration, Uppsala, Sweden.

Food Monitoring in Denmark

Anders Møller

National Food Agency of Denmark,
Informatics and Computer Section, 19, Mørkhøj Bygade,
DK-2860 Søborg, Denmark

In 1983 the National Food Agency established a food monitoring system in order to follow the content of nutrients and contaminants in foods in a systematic manner. When the data from this system are combined with the results from the national food consumption survey of 1985 it is possible to calculate the intake by survey participants of both nutrients and contaminants. Also, it is possible to make an estimate of the maximum intake of food additives. Calculations like these are used as a basis for regulating food fortification and the use of food additives as well as establishing safe levels for the content of contaminants in foods.

Food plays a vital role in the Danish economy; the Danish food production amounts to more than US$ 17 billion. Food exports exceed US$ 9 billion, corresponding to around 35 per cent of the country's total earnings from export of industrial manufacture.

In the course of a year each person in Denmark consumes an average of one ton of food, which makes food a central aspect of daily life. In addition, awareness among Danes about the food they eat is increasing.

In Denmark national food legislation is the responsibility of three different ministries, the Ministry of Health, the Ministry of Agriculture and the Ministry of Fishing. Responsibility for the General Food Act of 1973 lies within the Ministry of Health, and the executive functions are carried out by the National Food Agency. The Agency's objectives are to protect consumer health, to protect consumers against misleading information/fraud, to ensure reasonable conditions for retail stores and manufacturers and to promote healthy dietary habits.

The National Food Agency comprises two scientific institutes and four administrative divisions. The institutes, the Institute of Toxicology and the Institute of Food Chemistry and Nutrition, represent the specialist scientific knowledge which forms the basis for the Agency's administration of the *Food Act* and the provision of nutritional guidance to the general public.

The Food Monitoring System

The contents of both nutrients and contaminants in foods on the Danish market have been analyzed by the National Food Agency and associated laboratories for several decades.

Due to the increasing focus on diet and health issues, as well as a desire to ensure that chemical analyses within the individual working areas of the Agency were linked together as a whole, the Agency established a food monitoring system in 1983. The foundation of the food monitoring system was described in a proposal prepared by an internal working group at the Agency (1).

The basic objectives of the Danish food monitoring system are to:

- ascertain whether, over the long term, changes occur in the content of desired and undesired substances in Danish foods
- combine such changes with changes in eating habits
- assess whether changes expose the Danes to nutritional or toxicological health hazards
- obtain background material and a basis for decision-making to remedy any problem that may have arisen.

Therefore, the practical work with the Danish food monitoring system implies:

- watching the content of nutrients and contaminants in selected foods closely
- watching the consumption pattern of the Danish diet closely.

The food monitoring system is designed to supply data about the changes over time in the contents in foods of nutrients and contaminants. It is also designed to be linked with the data from the food consumption survey in order that the nutrient and contaminant intake of the population can be calculated.

As changes in the content of desired and undesired substances as well as changes in dietary habits occur slowly, the monitoring system will run for a long period. The results of analyses of the food monitoring system are reported continuously.

Every five years a major evaluation of the results of the preceding five-year period takes place. The first report for a complete five-year period was published in 1990 covering the years 1983-87 (2).

Selected Areas of Monitoring

The food monitoring system covers nutrients as well as heavy metals/other trace elements, nitrate, pesticides and PCB in selected foods (Table I). With the exception of nutrients, the content of these compounds/substances in most cases originates from influences from the external environment. Components to be monitored are carefully selected on the basis of the existing knowledge about their nutritional importance or toxicity, their occurrence in foods, and the actual consumption of these foods.

Microbiological studies and examinations of radionucleides have until now not been included in the food monitoring system but will be reported in the future. A proposal for a microbiological food monitoring system is in preparation.

In the first five-year period (1983-1987) 10,060 samples were analyzed, in the second period (1988-1992) 9,341 samples, and for the third period (1993-1997) a total of 8,150 samples are to be analyzed.

Table II gives more details about the sampling with regard to nutrients and contaminants.

The expenses of the food monitoring system amount to about US$ 3.3 million per five-year period. During each period a total of approximately 65 full-time persons are devoted to the project, i.e. ap-

Table I. The elements of the food monitoring system

Food category	Nutrients	Trace elements and nitrate	Pesticides and PCB
Fruit and vegetables	Fat, protein, ash, dry matter, fiber, vitamin C (tomatoes: glutamic acid)	As, Cd, Cr, Hg, Ni, Pb, Se In vegetables also nitrate	
Cereal products	Fat, protein, ash, dry matter, fiber, vitamins B_1, B_6, Ca, Fe, K, Mg, Na, Zn	As, Cd, Cr, Hg, Ni, Pb, Se	
Milk, milk products and eggs	Fat, protein, ash, dry matter, fatty acids, vitamins A, B_1, B_2, Ca Fe, K, Mg, Ma, Zn, I	In eggs: As, Cd, Cr, Hg, Ni, Pb, Se	DDT, dieldrin, HCB, α-HCH, β-HCH, lindane (γ-HCH), heptachloroepoxide, PCB
Fish	Fat, protein, ash, dry matter, fatty acids, vitamin D	As, Cd, Cr, Hg, Ni, Pb, Se	DDT, dieldrin, HCB, α-HCH, β-HCH, lindane (γ-HCH), heptachloroepoxide, PCB
Meat	Fat, protein, ash, dry matter. Beef, chicken, pork: Fe, Mg, Zn, vitamins B_1, B_2, B_6		
Offal	Fe, fat, protein, ash, dry matter	As, Cd, Cr, Hg, Ni, Pb, Se	
Animal fat			DDT, dieldrin, HCB, α-HCH, β-HCH, lindane (γ-HCH), heptachloroepoxide, PCB

HCB: hexachlorobenzene; HCH: hexachlorocyclohexane; PCB: polychlorated biphenyls

Table II. Number of samples examined

	1983–1987	1988–1992	1993–1997
Nutrients	1300	920	(900)
Trace elements	4100	3285	(2500)
Nitrate	1200	370	(750)
Pesticides*	3200	3265	(2800)
Mycotoxins	260	1500	(1200)

* The National Food Agency's control programs include approx. 1200 samples/year covering about 120 different pesticides

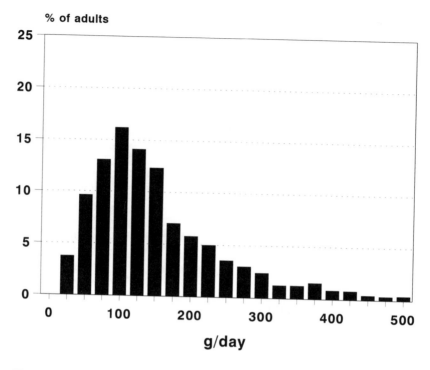

Figure 1. Potatoes, daily intake, Danes, 15–80 yrs

proximately 13 full-time positions per year at the four (formerly five) regional laboratories, as well as several full-time positions at the National Food Agency.

Criteria for selection of samples and analysis

Nutrients. The nutrients included in the system have been selected based on one or more of the following criteria (3):

- the daily intake of the nutrient in Denmark is lower than or around the recommended level, either for the population as a whole or for specially exposed groups of the population

- the nutrient is present only in few foods

- the nutrient shows stability problems

- the nutrient is added to one or more foods, either compulsorily or voluntarily.

The analyses have been given priority based on an overall evaluation according to these criteria and resulted in the substances listed in Table I.

Trace Elements and Nitrate. The trace elements which are included in the system, see Table I, have been selected on the basis of existing knowledge of their toxicity and occurrence in foods compared with food consumption. In the case of nickel, arsenic, chromium and selenium there has also been a desire to gain more knowledge about their occurrence in Danish foods.

Only vegetables have been selected to be monitored for nitrate. The concentration of nitrate in fruit and other foods is so low that they have only minor significance for human intake of nitrate.

Pesticides and PCB. For a number of years combined control and monitoring analyses have been carried out on organochlorine pesticides and PCB in fish, meat, eggs, and milk and milk products. Since

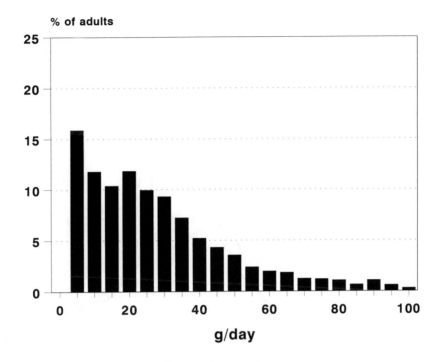

% of adults

Figure 2. Fish, daily intake of cooked edible portion, Danes, 15–80 yrs

1983 these studies have been included in the monitoring system. The analyses comprise persistent organochlorine pesticides. Among industrial chemicals, at present the system includes only the poly-chlorinated biphenyls (PCB).

The Danish Food Composition Data Bank

After careful evaluation of the results of the analyses the relevant food monitoring data are transferred from the Agency's laboratory information management system and stored in the Danish Food Composition Data Bank. The food monitoring system is a substantial data source, due to the systematic and continuous flow of new data from the monitoring system into the databank.

At present the databank comprises information for about 2000 foods on the

Danish market. In the databank information is collected on 255 different compounds.

The National Food Consumption Survey

In 1985 the National Food Agency of Denmark carried out a nationwide food consumption survey (4,5). The objectives of the survey were:

- To identify population groups which are at risk from a nutritional point of view

- To evaluate the significance of fortifying foods with nutrients

- To estimate the exposure of different population groups to contaminants and food additives

- To identify foods which contribute significantly to the nutrient intake in different population groups

% of participants by sex

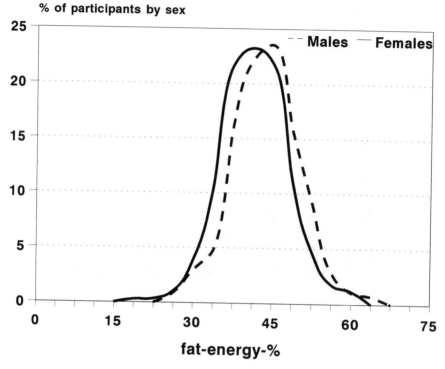

Figure 3. Percentage of dietary energy from fat, Danes, 15–80 yrs

- To contribute to studies of the relationships between diet, health and disease.

The survey included 2242 persons, 15–80 years of age. They constituted a representative sample of the adult Danish population. The participants in the survey were interviewed about their food consumption habits using a dietary history method, which was developed particularly for this survey.

The dietary history method gives information about the usual diet of an individual during an extended period of time. There is no doubt that the method tends to overestimate regularity in the eating pattern. The method itself encourages the participants in the survey to emphasize usual food consumption, because it is easier to remember the usual meal pattern than all the unusual events which interfere with the habitual food intake. The results of the survey are, however, in excellent agreement with the results from other similar data sources, such as food balance sheets, household budget surveys, and other food consumption surveys. The conclusion is that the average consumption found in the survey is very close to the real intake except for a few foods and beverages, such as sugar and alcohol.

The dietary history method used in the present survey enables the ranking of individuals according to their intake of foods, nutrients, contaminants and other known constituents of food.

■ The Food Intake

Two different types of food intake distributions were identified, one for foods eaten by everyone, and the other for foods consumed by only some sectors of the population. As examples, the distribution of the intake of potatoes and fish within

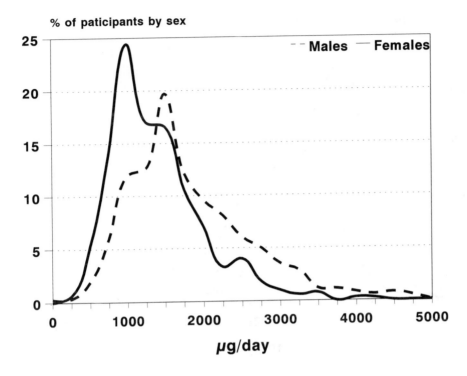

% of paticipants by sex

- - Males ⎯ Females

µg/day

Figure 4. Daily intake of vitamin A, Danes, 15–80 yrs

the adult population is shown in Figures 1 and 2.

The shape of the intake curve for potatoes is typical of foods that are consumed by practically everybody. These foods are cereals, white bread, rye bread, coarse vegetables, meat, poultry, separable fats and eggs. Figure 2 illustrates the shape of the intake curve for foods and beverages which are consumed by some people only. Other examples are cheese, soft drinks, beer and tea.

■ The Intake of Substances from Foods

The Agency has developed computer software that allows the data from the food consumption survey to be combined with the data from the food composition databank. Thus computation of the intake levels of nutrients and contaminants of the individuals who participated in the food consumption survey gives an estimate of the distribution of intake within the adult population.

Nutrients

Figures 3 to 5 are examples of the results of the calculations of nutrient levels. Figure 3 illustrates how the fat-energy-percentage of the diet of Danish women and men is distributed. The fat-energy-percentage seems to be very high when compared to the recommended level of 30 per cent of the dietary energy from fat. In fact almost all Danish adults seem to eat a diet that is higher in fat than the recommendations.

As a result of this, the National Food Agency has intensified its information campaigns on good eating habits with short advertisements on Danish television, written material for schools etc. Re-

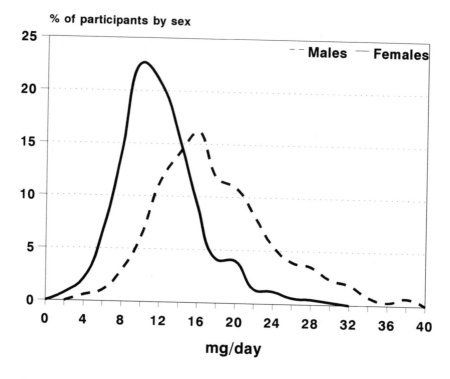

% of participants by sex

mg/day

Figure 5. Daily intake of iron, Danes, 15–80 yrs

cently an extensive campaign for reducing intake of fats, especially butter and margarine, was launched. The motto of this campaign is "Scrape your bread".

Figure 4 indicates that a very large percentage of Danish women and men consume more vitamin A than the recommended level of 800 and 1000 μg/day, respectively.

Figure 5 shows that the same is not the case for iron. The iron intake of most women in Denmark seems to fall below the recommended level of 12–18 mg/day.

The results for nutrient intakes have been used to evaluate the nutritional importance of the fortification of foods. As a result of this evaluation the obligatory fortification of flour and margarines with vitamins and minerals was abolished in 1987, because the contribution of fortification to the total nutrient intake was shown to be either unnecessary or negligible. The evaluations showed that in-

takes of the vitamins and minerals in question (vitamins, riboflavin and thiamin; minerals, calcium, phosphorus) were above the recommended levels. For iron it was shown that the contribution of fortification (inorganic iron) taking bioavailability into consideration was less than 10 per cent of the recommended intake.

A new food consumption survey is at the planning stage. A pilot study was carried out in the autumn of 1993. The main food consumption survey will take place in 1994.

Contaminants

Trace Elements. Table III shows the calculated intakes of mercury, cadmium, lead and arsenic from foods. For mercury, cadmium and lead it appears that intakes from foods are well below the PTWI (Provisional Tolerable Weekly Intake)

Table III. Intake of trace elements, all values in µg per person

Trace element	Daily intake				Weekly intake		
	Mean	p0.50	p0.90	p0.95	Mean	p0.95	PTWI
Mercury	7	5	12	15	55	160	350
Cadmium	20	18	28	32	137	250	490
Lead	42	40	66	76	297	532	3500
Arsenic	118	87	233	313			

PTWI: based on a body weight of 70 kg
p0.50, p0.90, p0.95: 50th, 90th and 95th percentiles

proposed by Joint FAO/WHO Expert Committee on Food Additives (6,7). Special interest has been devoted to the lead content in foods since the dominant source of lead contamination of foods, especially vegetables and crops, is lead emitted from motorcars running on petrol.

During the last decade the lead content of petrol has been lowered substantially and unleaded petrol introduced on the Danish market. The influence of this is clearly seen in the decreasing lead content in many foods, e.g. offal, beverages (wines in particular), berries, certain types of fruits, greens, oat, rye, wheat, rye bread and cod liver. In other food groups no change was discernible. These groups comprise meat, imported fruit, roots and tubers, cabbage, certain vegetables and fish.

For arsenic the total intake of organic and inorganic arsenic is shown in Table III. No PTWI has been proposed for arsenic, but a value of 140 µg/day has been established as PMTDI (Provisional Maximum Tolerable Daily Intake) by a group of experts under FAO/WHO in 1983. This value applies to inorganic arsenic only. Most of the arsenic in the Danish diet originates from fish. This is organic and considered non-toxic to humans. Arsenic is therefore not considered to be a problem in Danish foods.

Pesticides and PCB. So far it has not been possible to calculate the exposure of the population to pesticides and organic pollutants from food in the same manner as for heavy metals. The analyses of pesticide residues in foods have been concentrated on those foods where high levels are most likely. There are too many gaps in our present knowledge about the content in other foods to allow us to make a calculation of the total exposure of the participants in the survey to pesticides from foods.

Food Additives

The use of food additives in Denmark is regulated by the National Food Agency through the so-called positive-list (8). The list specifies the maximum amount of a food additive that can legally be used in individual foods. Although the maximum amount of food additives that might be used is known, there is no complete picture of the actual use by the food industry. Therefore, no calculation can be made of the actual exposure of the population to food additives, but only an estimate of the maximum exposure, which would occur if food producers used all the permitted food additives in their maximum amounts. The calculated exposure will in all cases be higher than the actual, since most foods are manufactured without making full use of all permitted additives. The calculated maximum intake is, however, of considerable interest from a regulatory point of view. It allows a check to be made as to whether the limitations that have been introduced in the use of

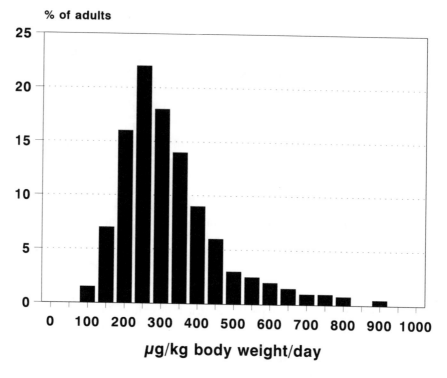

% of adults

Figure 6. Maximum erythrosin intake, Danes 15–80 yrs (ADI: 625 μg/kg body weight/day)

additives in individual foods are realistic in relation to the ADI-values.

Figures 6 and 7 show, as examples, the intake distribution of the calculated maximum intakes of erythrosin and benzoic acid/benzoates. From the figures it appears that while the maximum intake of benzoic acid/benzoates permitted according to the positive-list is well below the ADI-value, the same is not the case for erythrosin.

For erythrosin, however, the ADI-value has been reduced from 625 to 50 g/kg body weight per day recently (7). The distribution curve in Figure 6 was obtained with the erythrosin levels permitted at the time of the survey. Therefore, intake levels have to be compared to the higher ADI-value of 625 μg/kg.

As a whole, the calculations based on actual food intake have shown that the

method used to determine the amounts of food additives permitted in the "positive-list" is applicable. The method is the so-called budget-method (9). It is not a scientific method, but a practical administrative tool to predict the maximum intake of a food additive. The main assumption in the budget-method is that the maximum daily consumption for an adult is 1.5 kg of foods and 6 L of beverages and water. It is also assumed that only half the foods are industrially processed and thus contain food additives. As far as the liquid intake is concerned the assumption is made that only 25 per cent of beverages contain food additives. The ADI can be divided between solid and liquid foods according to technological needs. If the required level is too high compared to the ADI available the additive may be limited to either solid or liquid foods or to certain groups of foods.

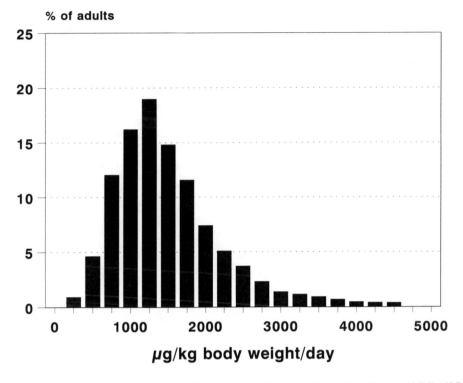

% of adults

µg/kg body weight/day

Figure 7. Maximum benzoic acid/benzoates intake, Danes 15–80 yrs (ADI: 625 µg/kg body weight/day)

The calculations show that each of these assumptions is reasonable for 90 per cent of the adult population. The type of calculations illustrated in Figures 6 and 7 confirm that the budget-method is a reliable tool in the administration of food additives.

■ Conclusion

The Danish Food Monitoring System has proven to be a valuable tool for identifying nutritional or toxicological areas where action has to be taken, as well as actions in the area of food administration and regulation. Systematic monitoring of foods is necessary, also in the future, to ensure the supply of healthy foods to the Danish population. As dietary habits are constantly changing, it is important to adjust the monitoring system on a continuing basis so that areas without problems are monitored less often, while newly detected problems are taken up for inclusion in the system.

■ References

(1) National Food Agency (1984) *Establishment of a Food Monitoring System,* Statens Levnedsmiddelinstitut, Søborg

(2) National Food Agency (1990) *Food Monitoring in Denmark: Nutrients and Contaminants 1983-1987,* National Food Agency of Denmark, Søborg

(3) Haraldsdottir, J., Heidemann, F. & Leth, T. (1982) *Establishment of a Monitoring System for Nutrients in Foods,* Statens Levnedsmiddelinstitut, Søborg

(4) Haraldsdottir, J., Holm, L., Jensen, J.H. & Møller, A. (1986) *Dietary*

Habits in Denmark 1985, 1. Main Results, Publication No. 136, Levnedsmiddelstyrelsen, Søborg

(5) Haraldsdottir, J., Holm, L., Jensen, J.H., & Møller, A. (1987) *Dietary Habits in Denmark 1985, 2. Who Eats What?,* Publication No. 154, Levnedsmiddelstyrelsen, Søborg

(6) FAO/WHO (1972) *Sixteenth Report of the Joint FAO/WHO Expert Committee on Food Additives,* WHO Technical Report Series No. 505, Geneva

(7) FAO/WHO (1989) *Thirty-third report of the Joint FAO/WHO Expert Committee on Food Additives,* WHO Technical Report Series No. 776, Geneva

(8) National Food Agency (1988) *Fortegnelse Over Godkente Tils'tningsstoffertil Levnedsmidler,* Levnedsmiddelstyrelsen, Søborg, Publication No. 171

(9) Hansen, S.C. (1979) *J. Food Protect.* **5**, 429-434

Food Composition Data Requirements for Nutritional Epidemiology of Cancer and Chronic Diseases

Nadia Slimani, Elio Riboli

Programme of Nutrition and Cancer,
WHO International Agency for Research on Cancer, Lyon, France

Heather Greenfield

Department of Food Science and Technology,
University of New South Wales, Kensington NSW 2033, Australia

Nutritional epidemiology is concerned with, among other things, establishing the association of diet and disease. The principles of nutritional epidemiology drive the requirements for nutrient databases for valid measurement of dietary exposure. The potential impact of random and systematic errors in food composition data on computation of nutrient intakes in prospective multi-center studies is discussed and the needs for modeling studies and time-related databases highlighted.

Nutritional epidemiology is concerned with, among other things, establishing the association between diet, health and disease. Establishing a relationship relies on measurement of exposure to a dietary factor and estimating the absolute (incidence) or relative risk (odds ratio) of having a given disease associated with a given level of exposure. The categorization in quantiles of a population distribution represent one type of classification of subjects that can be used usually with three to five classes of exposure from lowest to highest. The establishment of a statistical association relies on the absence of bias in all of the observations including the dietary observations. Systematic errors (bias) have to be excluded as they could affect classification of disease cases and control subjects unequally. Random errors, which have an equal chance of occurring in affected and unaffected individuals, thus affect the classification process equally for all groups. Nevertheless even random errors can affect the validity of a study's findings by distorting the estimation of relative risk towards the null value of 1 and increasing the variance of observations, thus blurring true relationships. Procedures exist for minimizing bias, controlling measurement errors, and preventing misclassification. These procedures rely to an important degree on collecting data according to clearly defined, rigorous, standardized protocols for all aspects of the scientific observations (1).

Epidemiological investigations of the role of diet in cancer and other chronic diseases to date have revealed in many cases a weak association (2), but even such a weak association is potentially of great biological significance due to the large numbers of people likely to experience high or low exposures to dietary factors since everyone eats. There is a strong case, therefore, for continuing work to establish the dietary links.

The major method of measuring dietary exposure has been the collection of data on food intakes and converting these data to nutrient intakes by means of food composition databases. While there has been progress in understanding the errors which can arise in measurement of food intake, the role of errors in conversion of these intakes to nutrient intakes is not so well investigated. In fact, much published literature about food composition databases in epidemiological studies is descriptive rather than analytical (3,4,5,) and Willett (3) noted that no formal analysis had been done of the impact of variability (systematic) in nutrient content of food in nutritional epidemiology. The only analytical study appears to be that of Beaton (6) who investigated the impact of *biological* variability in the

composition of foods (a source of random error) on nutrient intakes calculated from two different one-day intakes (sample diets) by use of the US nutrient composition tables for which measures of dispersion are given (7). Some caution is needed in interpreting these findings given the nature of food table compilation which rejects statistical outliers and may also include some subjective judgement in acceptance of the individual values from which the mean and standard deviations of values are computed. However, Beaton's analyses give valuable indications of the *low* impact of random biological errors on computed nutrient intakes especially in diets composed of large numbers of foods. It would be useful if such analyses could be extended to investigations of systematic bias in food composition values, a topic which is of great concern in epidemiology.

◾ Nutrient Databases for Nutritional Epidemiology

In examining nutrient database options for any study in nutritional epidemiology, it is important to consider the aims and

Table I. Ideal versus usual approach to planning a diet study

Ideal Approach	Usual Approach
Identify nutrients of interest	Select data collection method based on cost and ease of administration
Determine level of specificity of food descriptions required to assess the nutrients of interest	Collect dietary data prior to selecting an appropriate database for nutrient analysis
Select a data collection method that will accommodate the desired level of specificity	
Develop or modify an existing database to:	Select an existing nutrient nutrient database without evaluating:
■ accommodate the desired level of specificity	■ the level of specificity of foods included in the database
■ provide complete, accurate, specific, and updated values for the nutrients of interest	■ the completeness, the accuracy, the specificity or the currency of the nutrient database

Adapted from Buzzard et al. (8)

methods of the discipline particularly in order to avoid the ad hoc selection of a database portrayed as the "usual approach" in the model described by Buzzard and co-workers (Table I) (8). The first step is the definition of the nutritional hypothesis which is to be tested in the study. The several different possible approaches in descriptive and analytical nutritional epidemiology require separate and lengthier consideration both in terms of the nutrient composition database and the dietary methodology. However, this discussion will be restricted to the concerns associated with a prospective multicenter study which it is hoped will shed considerable light on the relationship of diet to cancer and other chronic diseases.

■ Database Requirements for Prospective Studies

The EPIC study (European Prospective Investigation into Cancer and Nutrition) has the advantages of a large study population living in several geographical areas with different dietary patterns and cancer incidences (northern and southern Europe), with an appropriate age and socioeconomic distribution, which has the power to establish valid relationships between diet and even relatively rare cancers (2).

A multi-country prospective study requires within-cohort and between-cohort analyses, and further has implications for the period over which data will be collected (changes in environment and observers) as well as the volume of data to be gathered. The between-cohort analysis is particularly important to determining the impact of large variations of diet on disease incidence since many within-cohort studies are of national populations with relatively homogeneous dietary intakes.

Any prospective epidemiological study planning to analyze and compare dietary information for several countries will need to take into account several considerations for the food composition database used to analyze the food intake data. These are discussed below.

Need for a Tailored Database

Nutritional epidemiology requires the database to be specifically tailored to the actual foods reported consumed, and according to the dietary method used, to increase the accuracy of nutrient intakes computed; thus the concept is of a user database which may need to draw on several reference databases in its compilation. The important distinction must be drawn between this approach and other applications in which it is acceptable to tailor the dietary intake obtained to the database (i.e. matching a food with the most similar food in the database). In epidemiology it is the reverse, a point not always understood in the field. For example, a comparative study of two databases (9) found a new national database deficient since it did not have values for lean meat unlike the foreign database used previously. This was despite the availability of the published "lean only" data for the local meats in the literature which the authors cited (10) and which could have been used to tailor the local database in order to avoid over-estimation of the fat intakes of study populations to which the database was subsequently applied.

Needs for Local Data for Local Foods

Nutrient composition data for the local foods as consumed in the specific countries will be necessary for a multi-country prospective study of nutrition. To use non-indigenous data, particularly for staple foods, could suppress the effects of an important potential source of dietary variability. For example, fat from meat is often of interest in surveys of diet and degenerative disease. However, meat is a food which is known to vary dramatically in its fat content over time and between countries. When new compositional data for meat became available in one particular country and was found to be up to 50 per cent leaner than the previous data set (data origins obscure) (10), the total fat available from the food supply daily per capita dropped from 145 g to 119 g (i.e. 19 per cent), the total fat available daily per capita from meats fell by 27 g (from 52 g to 25 g) and the total fat available daily per capita expressed as per cent energy available fell from 37 per cent to 33 per cent, in other words, it fell below the (then) dietary target (11). The ratio of vegetable to animal fat increased from 0.55:1 to 0.74:1. Hence it can be expected

that use of meat fat data which are "too high" for one country, and "too low" for another country (in relation to the "true" values) could either obscure a true difference in fat intakes between the two countries or artificially create a difference where there is none.

Some simple tests using pilot dietary data from two countries participating in the EPIC study varying the fat content of meat showed some effect on the difference between national samples (as expected). In fact, a 10 per cent increase in fat content of two food groups combined (meats, milk and their products) in country A and a 10 per cent decrease in country B produced a 50 per cent decrease in the difference in total fat intake between countries.

So far as within cohort analyses are concerned, when the fat content of meat was varied by up to 50 per cent in a mathematical simulation by computer there was no effect on classification of subjects (as expected), but also no effect on classification when the content of fat in milk and milk products was lowered by 30 per cent at the same time that the fat content of meat was increased by 30 per cent. This result was unexpected and was not affected by any correlation between meat consumption and consumption of milk and milk products. However, different results can be expected in populations with different dietary habits.

Further simulations on other nutrients and other food groups could act to improve estimates of error in nutrient intakes obtained using databases. It could be hypothesized that other foods may be less heterogeneous between countries (particularly some fruits and vegetables) and therefore local data would not be needed but the final answer cannot be known until some analytical data for such foods are available and the hypothesis tested.

Nutritional Epidemiology Needs Time-Related Data

Foods change in composition over time, particularly when there are changes in breeding of plants and animals, changes in feeding regimes, and changes in preparation of foods for retail sale (e.g. butchering). Changes in regulations affecting foods (e.g. the introduction of mandatory fortification with a nutrient such as thiamin) also have the potential to alter their composition over time. Food tables and databases, on the other hand, tend to be up to a decade out of date, given the delays experienced between collecting and analyzing the food, the delays in publishing the data and the delays in compiling data into databases. There is potential therefore for any database to be out of phase with the dietary intake data to which the database is applied (12). This point is of importance for studies of trends over time within a country.

A recent study (13) examined the sodium and potassium intakes of a group of 27 females using urinary excretion and several dietary methods. One part of the study involved computing the dietary intake of sodium and potassium by means of analyzing sets of 24 hour food intake data against three subsequent versions of the Australian nutrient database *NUTTAB* (*NUTTAB89* vs *NUTTAB90* vs *NUTTAB91/92*) (14, 15, 16). Note that the food intake data sets were constants. The values for sodium and potassium in foods had changed over this period, but since some foods increased in sodium or potassium by 10–100 per cent, while others decreased by 10–100 per cent, the net effect was of no change in group means for total intake from foods of these two minerals; the changes in food composition canceled each other out.

Needs for Analytical Data for Foods

The lack of compositional data for indigenous foods consumed in some of the southern European countries is a soluble problem for EPIC. Many useful data are being produced in local laboratories, and once they have been assessed and scrutinized can be used to update and amend the databases used to analyze the food intake data. Re-analyses done in the future will refine the estimates of nutrient intakes calculated (rather than alter them completely). The analyses undertaken can of course be expanded once data for important but often missing components such as carotenoids, vitamers E and other bioactive compounds become available. This kind of laboratory work and food intake re-analyses could be expected to shed additional light on dietary relationships with the cancers and other diseases which emerge during the 10–15 year course of the observations of the prospective study. Such re-analyses of biological samples such as blood have already been provided for in the EPIC study (2).

Needs for a Complete Database

The nutrient database will need to be complete (i.e. include all relevant foods for a given nutrient) if nutrient intakes are not to be underestimated; this is a point which has been well-accepted (9) and some data have been provided, e.g., by Stockley (17) who reviewed studies of error associated with missing values in databases, citing underestimates of B vitamin intake ranging from 1.5 per cent to 14.3 per cent, and recoveries of only 69 per cent of total polyunsaturated fatty acids analyzed in duplicate diets as opposed to computed nutrient intakes, improving to 89 per cent when the missing fatty acid values were inserted. Also mentioned were the new starch values for UK potatoes ranging from 11 g/100 g to 23.0 g/100 g, according to cultivar, with the average value (weighted by tonnage) being 17.0 g/100 g compared to the value of 20.3 g/100 g given in the food tables then current. Starch intake from potatoes may therefore be only 60 per cent of that computed from the tables. It should be relatively easy to design simulations to investigate the effects of missing data using pilot studies of dietary intake carried out for the EPIC investigation.

Nutrient values should be, as far as possible, analytical values representative of the foods consumed by the study population. It might be expected that this approach would minimize bias. The food composition analyses, ideally, should reflect any potential regional differences in foods which are key sources of nutrients. The extent of regional variation in foods and nutrients is not well established and the potential biases which may occur by the use of non-representative data are a potential source of misclassification of subjects, as well as obscuring between-cohort effects.

Data Imputation

Data imputation, which may be necessary for tailoring the database is, by definition, a biased procedure and is likely to affect classification of subjects. Bias will be minimized by basing imputations on analytical data wherever possible from the country concerned. There is some misunderstanding about imputed data, and whether they are better than analytical data or not. The point is that an imputation, by definition, is done against a previous set of analytical data, and the assertion of validity cannot be tested without new analyses, creating a circular situation. For epidemiological studies a trade-off between missing data and imputed data has to be made. Again a series of simulation tasks could possibly identify the priorities for chemical analysis and indicate where compromises could be made.

Quality Control

On the practical side, the problems for a food composition database are relatively simple to understand. Prospective studies have to address (among other problems) the implications of personnel and methods of measurement being subject to change during the study. As the database has to be maintained over an extended period, quality control will demand extensive computerized data documentation, including dating of food analyses (12).

Mode of Data Expression

To compare countries, even where indigenous data sets are available for each country, conversions to the same basis of data expression will be needed for nutrients and foods. Specific software is needed to meet all of the requirements identified and initial requirements for such software have been described (18). These requirements for a comprehensive, multi-country user database differ considerably from a national reference database and will have to be specifically incorporated in purpose-built software.

Documentation of Nutrient Database

The nature of epidemiological work makes difficult the question of replication of a study as a method of validation. An indispensable part therefore of the reporting of any epidemiological research is a requirement to document the nutrient database used in sufficient detail to enable detailed scrutiny when under review or when comparisons are made with other studies. This point has recently been re-emphasized (17).

∎ Conclusion

A major barrier to achieving the "ideal approach" is the difficulties the majority of users experience in expressing their needs in a way which permits a custom database to be compiled.

There are two powerful tools potentially applicable to the problems posed by large-scale multi-country studies. First, so long as great attention is paid to the collection of the dietary intake and other data, these data could be re-analyzed against date-stamped sets of food composition data in the future enabling a clarification of the nutrient exposure. Second, further studies involving computer modeling which examine the potential impact of defined systematic errors in food composition data on dietary intake data, particularly by using sample populations with a wide variety of food habits, and with intakes corrected to energy intake, would undoubtedly be useful in validating differences in dietary exposure.

Finally, future prospective studies could consider the option of collecting "food archives" in which sample diets from study populations are collected and stored at low temperatures for future (and replicated) analysis in much the same way in which plasma or urinary samples for biochemical markers are currently collected and stored (2).

∎ References

(1) Hennekens, C.H., & Buring, J.E. (1987) *Epidemiology In Medicine*, Little, Brown and Company, Boston, MA

(2) Riboli, E. (1992) *Ann. Oncol.* **3**: 783-91

(3) Willett, W. (1990) *Nutritional Epidemiology*, Oxford University Press, Oxford

(4) West, C.E., & van Staveren, W.A. (1991) in *Design Concepts in Nutritional Epidemiology*, B.M. Margetts & M. Nelson, (Eds.), Oxford University Press, Oxford, pp. 101-119

(5) Paul, A.A., & Southgate, D.A.T. (1988) in *Manual on Methodology for Food Consumption Studies*, M.E. Cameron & W.A. van Staveren, (Eds.), Oxford University Press, Oxford, pp. 121-144

(6) Beaton, G.H. (1987) in *Food Composition Data: a User's Perspective*, W.M. Rand, C.T. Windham, B.W. Wyse, & V.R. Young, (Eds.), UNU Press, Tokyo, pp. 194-205

(7) US Department of Agriculture (1976–) *Composition of Foods: Raw, Processed, Prepared*, Agric. Handbook No. 8 series, USDA, Washington, DC

(8) Buzzard, I. M., Price, K.S., & Feskanich, D. (1991) in *The Diet History Method*, L. Kohlmeier (Ed.), Smith-Gordon and Company Ltd, London, pp. 39-51

(9) Magarey, A., & Boulton, T.J.C. (1991) *Aust. J. Nutr. Diet.* **48**, 128-31

(10) Greenfield, H. (Ed.) (1987) *Food Technol. Aust.* **39**, 181-140

(11) Cashel, K.M., & Greenfield, H. (1995) *J. Food Comp. Anal.* (in press)

(12) Buzzard, I.M. (1991) in *Proceedings of the 16th U.S. National Nutrient Databank Conference*, The CBORD Group Inc, Ithaca, pp. 73-77

(13) Jia, Y. (1992) MSc thesis, University of New South Wales, Sydney

(14) Commonwealth Department of Health and Community Services (1989) *NUTTAB89*, diskette, AGPS, Canberra

(15) Commonwealth Department of Health and Community Services (1990) *NUTTAB90*, diskette, AGPS, Canberra

(16) Commonwealth Department of Health, Housing and Community Services (1991) *NUTTAB91/92*, diskette, AGPS, Canberra

(17) Stockley, L. (1988) *J. Hum. Nutr. Diet.* **1**, 187-195

(18) Greenfield, H., Hémon, B., Slimani, N., & Riboli, E. (1991) NUBEL/EURONIMS Meeting, Antwerp

(19) Murphy, S.P. (1993) *Aust. J. Nutr. Diet.* **50**, 176

Food Composition Data and Population Studies

Developing a Food Composition Database for Studies in the Pacific Islands

Jean H. Hankin, Loïc Le Marchand, Laurence N. Kolonel

Epidemiology Program, Cancer Research Center of Hawaii, Honolulu, HI 96813, USA

Brian E. Henderson

Salk Institute, La Jolla, CA 92037, USA

Gary Beecher

Nutrient Composition Laboratory, U.S. Department of Agriculture, Beltsville, MD 20705, USA

As part of collaborative surveys of lifestyle risk factors for cancer and other chronic diseases in several Pacific Islands, diet studies were conducted among samples of semi-urban 45-65 year old men and women living in each island. Local nutritionists, dietitians, and other health workers identified the food items usually consumed, along with the seasonal fruits and vegetables that were major sources of carotenoids. The food composition table used to calculate nutrient intakes was developed during and following the survey, using a variety of procedures, including recipe calculations, laboratory analyses for carotenoids, and sourcing data from national and international food composition tables. The original carotenoid data for the Pacific Islands fruits and vegetables are presented in this paper.

D eveloping a food composition database for emerging and some-what isolated nations, such as the South Pacific Islands, presents an interesting challenge for nutrition researchers. There are problems in identifying the various traditional and imported foods, determining the usual food preparation methods, and assigning appropriate nutrient values to rare items not found in published food composition tables. We had an opportunity to meet this challenge in our recent study of diet and other lifestyle risk factors for cancer in several South Pacific Islands. For the dietary component of the study, the objectives were to obtain representative data on the usual diets of the islanders and to characterize the dietary intakes according to particular nutrients and other dietary components, as well as selected food items and food groups. This paper will review the background of the study and the procedures followed for identifying the foods usually eaten, developing the diet history questionnaire, determining the composition of the local foods, and creating the database for each island. In addition, we will discuss some of the problems that may occur in developing a database for an emerging country and offer a few suggestions that may be helpful.

∎ Background of the Study

Since 1980, the South Pacific Commission (SPC), with the assistance of the University of Southern California Comprehensive Cancer Center (USCCCC) and the Cancer Research Center of Hawaii (CRCH), has been recording all reported cases of cancer in the South Pacific region. Analysis of the incidence data revealed marked variation in the rates of several site-specific cancers among the different ethnic and island populations (1,2). For example, the Polynesians in Hawaii, French Polynesia, Cook Islands, and New Zealand, tend to have high rates of several cancers which most likely are related to diet. For instance, stomach cancer rates are generally higher among Polynesians as compared to the other islanders. Lung cancer rates are high among all Pacific Islanders except among the Melanesians and Indians in Fiji. Breast cancer and prostate cancer are also relatively high among the Polynesians. However, the rates of colon cancer among

Polynesians living in Hawaii and New Zealand are low in comparison to the Caucasians living in these respective countries. Among the Melanesians, New Caledonians have considerably higher rates of lung cancer than the Fijians, as well as the Indians in Fiji. This is of particular interest because the Fijians have high lifetime rates of smoking.

The variation of incidence rates within and among the ethnic groups suggested that environmental, and in particular lifestyle factors, may be associated with these variable cancer patterns. To identify particular risk factors, the SPC, CRCH, USCCCC and the Ministry of Health of each island conducted cross-sectional surveys in the Cook Islands, Fiji, French Polynesia, and New Caledonia between 1988 and 1992. The objectives were to collect data on the prevalence of lifestyle factors (such as smoking, drinking, diet, reproductive history, physical activity and obesity) among representative samples of semi-rural adults and to correlate these data with the observed cancer incidence patterns. These island communities are undergoing rapid economic, technological and social change, which is having an impact on their eating patterns, especially in urban areas. For instance, the use of imported foods has resulted in a modification of their traditional food practices. We hoped that the study findings would lead to greater knowledge about the causes of cancer in the South Pacific Region and would be utilized by the Ministries of Health for planning public health interventions to control cancer and other chronic diseases.

Methods

The same methodology was followed in each country to obtain comparable results. The surveys were conducted in the same season (June through August) of the year. Random samples of approximately 250 semi-rural males and females, 50 to 65 years of age, from each main ethnic group living on the island were included in each of the surveys. The questionnaires included a diet history, information on cigarette smoking, alcoholic consumption, physical activity, and medical and reproductive histories. Additional components included anthropometric data (weight, height, triceps and skinfold measurements); plasma and serum samples which were subsequently analyzed for carotenoids and tocopherols; and urine samples which were analyzed for sodium and cotinine (an indicator of smoking history).

Identifying the Food Items for the Dietary Assessment

To assess the role of diet in the etiology of diseases, such as cancer and heart disease, investigators seek information on the usual dietary intake of individuals. Generally, a diet history method which provides an estimate of the frequencies and amounts consumed during a specified period of time is recommended (3-5). To estimate the usual diet of the islanders, we utilized a diet history that included those food items that were likely to be consumed during a one-month period. This time interval seemed appropriate because of the similarity in the dietary patterns of the villagers from month to month. In addition, seasonal fruits that were major sources of carotenoids and ascorbic acid were included in the questionnaire.

The selection of the particular food items for the diet history began several months before the survey. The nutritionists, dietitians and epidemiologists from the Ministry of Health in each country identified the foods usually consumed at least once a month, along with the seasonal items. They reviewed recent dietary surveys, conferred with other nutrition, health and agricultural personnel, and prepared a list of food items for the diet history questionnaire. The items included both western and traditional foods that covered several food groups, such as starches, breads and spreads, meat, poultry and fish, vegetables, fruits, snacks, beverages, etc. Information on the usual methods of food preparation, including the use of particular fats and oils and coconut cream in food preparation, was also identified.

Developing the Diet History Questionnaire

The diet history listed each item individually. The local names of each food were included in the questionnaire, which was administered by trained nutrition and health education personnel. The format included columns for recording weekly or monthly frequencies and usual serving sizes. To assist participants in nominating the quantities consumed, the island's nutritionists or dietitians developed appropriate visual aids, such as root vegetables preserved with a shellac coating, Polaroid photographs of medium and large servings of vegetables, plastic meat models, and different sizes of familiar bowls and cups.

As another measure of dietary intake, we collected a 24-hour recall of foods consumed the day before the interview.

This was done before the diet history, so that participants would become familiar with recalling what they ate and how to use the visual aids for estimating amounts consumed.

Determining the Composition of Foods Consumed in Each Island

On arrival in each island, we visited the various produce markets and village stores to observe firsthand the available food supply. Unfamiliar foods were purchased and identified, and the contents of commercially prepared items were separated and weighed to develop estimated quantities of the ingredients. Recipes of various mixed or traditional dishes were also obtained. In addition, procedures were designed for collecting and preparing the fruits and vegetables for carotenoid analysis. The labels of cereals, rice, flour, breads, crackers, and similar items were scrutinized to identify the ingredients and to determine if the products were enriched or fortified. It was also necessary to investigate the available meat, poultry and fish. Beef was generally frozen and imported, and it was difficult to identify the particular cut and its fat content in the frozen state. The chief nutritionist of each island suggested the probable cut of meat, percentage of fat, and usual method of preparation. Lamb from New Zealand was utilized in the Cook Islands and Fiji. Food composition data on New Zealand lamb were available from the U.S. Department of Agriculture (USDA) (6), whereas data on mutton flaps, consumed by the Cook Islanders, were found in a report by Platt (7). The Fijians consumed both fresh and canned goat. Values for fresh roasted goat were found in USDA (6), but no data were available for canned goat. We compared the taste and appearance of the two products, and based on their similarity, decided to use the same values for both items. Chicken was similar to the stewing chickens of Hawaii, and we estimated the cooked items as about 20 per cent fat (6).

All of the islanders consumed a large variety of reef and ocean fish and shellfish. In general, people described them by their size (small, medium or large) or by their traditional names. The nutritionists recommended that fish be classified according to their estimated fat content. Fresh fish of high fat content, such as salmon, were rarely available. The names of the local fish were then classified according to low or medium fat and were used by the interviewers for coding the reported fish items.

One of our major objectives was to obtain estimates of the carotenoid values of the vegetables and fruits grown on each island. One of us (GB) performed the laboratory analyses of these items. In each area, 15 to 20 highly consumed foods were selected from local markets or home gardens. All foods were prepared as normally consumed within each population. A representative sample of each food was packaged, frozen, and shipped on dry ice to Beltsville, MD, for subsequent analysis. Carotenoids in extracts from each food were separated and quantified by a combination of high performance liquid chromatography and UV-visible spectroscopy (8). The items included dark leafy greens, other green, yellow and red vegetables, and a few yellow and orange fruits. The green vegetables, in particular, included some unfamiliar items, such as hibiscus leaves, amaranthus, wild fern, and drumstick leaves. We located some of these items in various food composition tables (6,9,10). If nutrient data were not available, we compared the items to similar vegetables of the same color and shape and imputed the food composition values. Although these procedures are not error-free, they are acceptable for comparing the diets of various groups of islanders.

Each group of islanders consumed some items unique to their own setting. For example, in French Polynesia, two "Chinese" plate lunches were popular and were listed in the diet history. The first was a mixture of pork, dried white beans, macaroni, green beans, rice and soy sauce, and the second contained chicken, cabbage, noodles, sausage, carrots and soy sauce. The soy sauce was obviously the Oriental component! We purchased the lunches, separated and weighed the ingredients, estimated the amount of soy sauce, and developed approximate "recipes" for the database. Similarly, canned products imported from France, such as "cassoulet", were purchased, and the kind and amount of each ingredient weighed to develop a "recipe". This procedure was followed for estimating the contents of various mixed dishes or sandwiches that were eaten frequently. In addition, the diet histories in each area included a number of traditional main dishes, desserts and snacks. The nutritionists, other staff, and family members contributed information, which was used to develop a formula for the composition for each of these mixed dishes.

Creating the Database

Because there were no comprehensive food composition data for the Pacific Islands, we utilized reliable sources of published data whenever possible. Our most frequent resources were the USDA *Nutrient Database for Standard Reference* (6), *McCance and Widdowson's Composition of Foods* (10), *Food Composition Table for Use in East Asia* (9), and an article by Mangels et al. (11). In addition to energy and macro- and micronutrients, the data set includes values for dietary fiber, starch, nonstarch polysaccharides, carotenoids and tocopherols. All values represent foods as commonly consumed including recipes which were calculated from the data for cooked ingredients. No further adjustments were made for potential losses after food preparation. Energy and carbohydrate values were not adjusted when data from different sources were combined.

Some of the items included in the data set may be of interest. The root vegetables presented little problem, because the various sweet potatoes, taro, and breadfruit are also popular among the Polynesians in Hawaii. Assuming that the values of the same tuber would be comparable among the Pacific Islands, we utilized the USDA values (6) for each area. A few "new" root vegetables were consumed, for example, "wild yams" in Fiji. We used the same values as regular yams, but assigned different code numbers so the items could be identified. We also used the same values for plantains and green bananas which are most likely comparable in composition. They differ, of course, in their size, but not in the way they are consumed. We decided to use the values of barracuda (2.6 per cent fat) and Spanish mackerel (6.5 per cent fat) (6) for the low fat and medium fat categories of fish, respectively. With a few exceptions, values for shellfish were generally available. A "new" item was "bêche-de-mer" or sea slugs, and we were fortunate to locate it in the East Asia tables (9). To insure that our values for canned fish were appropriate, we purchased samples to determine the percentage of oil and solids and modified the USDA nutrient data, if warranted.

A few rather exceptional food items were consumed by some of the islanders, such as "roussettes" or flying foxes in New Caledonia. The proximate values were obtained from Cecily Dignan of SPC (personal communication), However, we could not find values for raw and grilled worms ("vers de bancoule"), which were occasionally consumed by Melanesians in New Caledonia. This was one of the very few items not included in the dietary analysis.

The carotenoid values of the analyzed vegetables and fruits were added to the data set. If analytical data were not available for a particular vegetable or fruit, we averaged the laboratory values for the same item from the other islands and utilized the imputed data. Published values from Mangels et al. (11) were selected for fruits and vegetables that were not analyzed. It is of interest to note the variability of the carotenoid contents of the same items from the different islands. Table I shows the variation of carotenoids

Table I. Carotenoid content of selected green vegetables from Pacific Islands (mg/100 g edible portion) [a,b]

Food	α-carotene	β-carotene	Lutein
Chinese cabbage[c]			
Cook Islands	0	2900	1270
Fiji	0	4570	7470
French Polynesia	0	1111	1470
Taro leaves[d]			
Cook Islands	62	4580	3630
Fiji	0	4210	8660
French Polynesia	0	7400	9640
Leaf lettuce, raw			
Cook Islands	0	1810	903
Fiji	0	2150	2040
French Polynesia	0	1230	1560
Hibiscus leaves[e]			
Cook Islands	187	5660	4300
Fiji	280	5700	8890

[a] Nutrient Composition Laboratory, USDA, Beltsville, MD
[b] Green vegetables from New Caledonia were not analyzed (see text for method of imputing the values)
[c] Chinese cabbage (bok choy) was steamed 3-5 minutes and drained
[d] Taro leaves were boiled 40 minutes and drained
[e] Hibiscus leaves were steamed 10 minutes and drained

in Chinese cabbage, taro leaves, leaf lettuce, and hibiscus leaves in three of the islands, whereas Table II presents the difference of carotenoids in pumpkin, tomatoes, and papayas in the four geographic areas. The variations among the islands are probably due to sampling, geographic location, light and soil, and other factors. For the other dietary components of fruits and vegetables, we assigned the same values used for the comparable foods in the Hawaii database (unpublished data). Analysis of the association of dietary risk factors and cancer incidence in the South Pacific Islands is in progress and will be reported within the near future.

∎ Problems and Suggestions

Based on our experience in developing a food composition database for the Pacific Islands, we are aware of the potential problems that may occur in analyzing dietary data from isolated populations. First, it is important to know the local names used for various foods. For example, in Fiji, each item had a Melanesian name and a Hindi name, whereas in French Polynesia, most adults used the Tahitian name rather than the French. Second, although foods may have the same name in different countries, they may differ in food composition. For instance, Chinese cabbage ("bok choy") was dark green in one island, medium green with white stems in a second, and light green with yellow flowers in a third.

Table II. Carotenoid content of selected yellow and red vegetables and fruits from Pacific Islands (μg/100 g edible portion) [a]

Food	α-carotene	β-carotene	Lycopene	Lutein	β-cryptoxanthin
Pumpkin, peeled[b]					
Cook Islands	236	951	2240	131	0
Fiji	1760	3040	1900	2210	0
New Caledonia	1290	4000	0	560	0
Tomato, raw, whole					
Cook Islands	0	515	1620	0	0
Fiji	0	160	2550	130	0
French Polynesia	0	620	4730	210	0
New Caledonia	0	570	7540	110	0
Papaya, yellow, raw, flesh only					
Fiji	0	100	0	0	560
French Polynesia	0	260	0	140	2470
New Caledonia	0	60	0	70	760
Papaya, red, raw, flesh only					
Cook Islands	0	137	1940	0	6180
French Polynesia	0	260	3040	90	960
New Caledonia	0	100	3960	50	620

[a] Nutrient Composition Laboratory, USDA, Beltsville, MD
[b] Pumpkin was peeled, boiled 30 minutes, and drained

These differences probably explain the variation in their carotenoid values. Similarly, in some areas, we observed a difference in the color of a vegetable that was locally grown as compared to the same vegetable that was imported. These items were treated as separate foods according to the local or ethnic names. It may be helpful to photograph unfamiliar vegetables and to match their colors with a set of colored markers. This information, along with laboratory analysis of various antioxidants and appropriate botanical data, may permit reasonable imputations of values for the food composition database.

Third, processed foods are likely to be imported from various countries. For example, canned, frozen and packaged products from New Zealand, Australia and France were available in different islands. The labels may suggest that the items are similar to those found in the investigator's native country. However, this cannot be assumed. Items, such as baked beans, canned or frozen mixed vegetables, sausages, etc., need to be checked to identify their approximate contents before selecting published values. Fourth, most islanders used the term "juice" (or the local name) loosely. For instance, concentrated syrups were often diluted with water and called "juice"; if real juice was used, it generally was sweetened with considerable sugar and diluted with water. Observing the preparation of "juice" is recommended, so that the appropriate nutrient values can be assigned.

Fifth, recipes are needed for traditional and ethnic mixed dishes, desserts and snacks. Although island recipes may be printed in tourist publications, it is preferable to ask several local people for their recipes and use this information to develop prototype recipes for the food composition database. Finally, knowledgeable nutritionists and dietitians familiar with the eating patterns of the population are the keys to achieving a realistic database that is area-specific and meaningful for analyzing the dietary intakes of the population.

■ Acknowledgments

We are grateful to the following nutritionists for their generous assistance in our surveys: Taiora Matenga Smith, Ministry of Health, Rarotonga, Cook Islands; Mona J. Chand, Ministry of Health, Suva, Fiji; Maeva Barral, Ministry of Health, Papeete, Tahiti; and Dominique Daly, Noumea, New Caledonia. We also thank Cecily Dignan, Nutritionist, South Pacific Commission, for her generous support.

■ References

(1) Henderson, B.E., Kolonel, L.N., & Foster F. (1982) *Nat. Cancer Inst. Monog.* **62,** 73-78

(2) Henderson, B.E., Kolonel, L.N., & Dworsky, R. (1986) *Nat. Cancer Inst. Monog.* **69,** 73-81

(3) Willett, W. (1990) *Nutritional Epidemiology*, Oxford University Press, Oxford

(4) Hankin, J.H. (1991) in *Research: Successful Approaches*, E.R. Monsen (Ed.), American Dietetic Association, Chicago, IL, pp. 173-194

(5) Block, G., & Hartman, A.M. (1989) in *Nutrition and Cancer Prevention. Investigating the Role of Micronutrients*, T.E. Moon & M.S. Micozzi (Eds.), M. Dekker, New York, NY, pp. 159-180

(6) US Department of Agriculture (1993) *Nutrient Database for Standard Reference*, Release 10, USDA, Washington, DC

(7) Platt, B.S. (1980) *Tables of Representative Values of Foods Commonly Used in Tropical Countries*, Special Report Series No. 302, Medical Research Council, London

(8) Khachik, F., Beecher, G.R., Goli, M.B., & Lusby, W.R. (1991) *Pure Appl. Chem.* **63,** 71-80

(9) Leung, W.T.W., Butrum, R.R., & Chang F.H. (1972) *Food Composition Table for Use in East Asia*. Nat. Inst. of Arthritis, Metabolism and Digestive Diseases, Bethesda, MD

(10) Holland, B., Welch, A.A., Unwin, I.D., Buss. D.H., Paul, A.A., & Southgate, D.A.T. (1991) *McCance and Widdowson's The Composition of Foods*, 5th Ed., Royal Society of Chemistry, Cambridge

(11) Mangels, A.R., Holden, J.M., Beecher, G.R., Forman, M.R., & Lanza, E. (1993) *J. Am. Diet. Assoc.* **93,** 284-296

The Effects of Australian, US and UK Food Composition Tables on Estimates of Food and Nutrient Availability in Australia

Karen M. Cashel

School of Human and Biomedical Sciences, University of Canberra,
P.O. Box 1, Belconnen, ACT 2616, Australia

Heather Greenfield

Department of Food Science and Technology,
The University of New South Wales, Sydney, NSW 2052, Australia

Until the late 1980s, Australia used national food composition tables that were compiled in the late 1960s, predominantly from overseas sources, or foreign tables, particularly those of the UK or the USA. New tables, The Composition of Foods, Australia (COFA), based on an ongoing national analytical program, have been progressively released from 1989. The quantity and adequacy of the foods and nutrients available for consumption in Australia, 1990–91, calculated on the basis of the new Australian tables are compared here with those obtained using the US or UK tables. There are marked differences in the edible weights of foods and the amounts of nutrients available for consumption when the different databases are used. The most marked effect is on the quantity, type and sources of fat in the food supply, assessed as at least 60 per cent higher from meats, and 15-22 per cent higher in total using the data from the US or UK. Iron and zinc are all higher and retinol activity, vitamin C and magnesium lower using the foreign data. Calcium is 35 per cent higher when UK data are used and thiamin 59 per cent higher when US data are used.

Food composition databases are essential components of nutritional monitoring and surveillance, and of much health-related research, yet many countries have traditionally relied on the United States of America (US) or United Kingdom (UK) tables rather than develop their own national tables. Many individual users also rely on non-local data as their source of information. Inappropriate food composition data have the potential to undermine or misdirect the research or nutrition effort, but few studies have been done to provide quantitative evidence of this.

Until the late 1980s, Australia, like many other countries, relied on a national food composition database which incorporated data from a variety of sources, including from overseas tables, scientific publications and food industry information (1). By the late 1970s, the inadequacies of the information provided in the range of food items and nutrients, had many major users, particularly researchers, turning to other sources of data. In Australia, in the main, users were either developing their own databases by supplementing the Australian tables with data from overseas tables, the food industry and journal publications, or using overseas computer-based packages as their principal source. This approach was exacerbated by the growing availability of overseas databases, including in software packages, well in advance of their Australian print only counterpart. The most widely introduced and used overseas food composition data in Australia were those from UK (2), or the US (3), available in print or on computer tape and/or incorporated into software packages. The use of US or UK data in Australia was usually justified by arguments that the health problems and food patterns were similar, and the Australian tables were too limited in their coverage of foods and nutrients.

In 1989, revised food composition data for Australia (4), began to be released. These data were based entirely on an ongoing national food analysis program initiated at the beginning of the 1980s (5). The previous national tables (TCAF) (6,7) included fewer than 650 food items, and just 16 nutrients, while in 1993, the new tables (COFA) (4,8-12) include some 1400 food items and a greatly expanded range of nutrients, including data on fatty acids, sugars, amino acids and organic acids. This database continues to grow on an annual basis.

The new analytical data on Australian foods provide a unique opportunity to compare the gross and nutrient composition data of local foods with data from overseas sources for apparently similar foods, and to assess the effect of using local data on the determination of foods and nutrients consumed rather than overseas data. In this paper, the foods available for consumption per capita (13) are used to demonstrate and compare the US, UK and Australian tables.

Data on the per capita food supply have provided the only consistent measure of trends in foods and nutrients consumed in Australia. The food supply data are used to monitor the nutritional adequacy of the food supply, and, in the absence of more specific consumption data at household or individual level, have provided the basis for developing a range of public health nutrition policy and programs, including the nutrition component of the National Health Goals and Targets (14,15).

The food supply data represent foods as available, rather than as prepared and consumed (i.e. in cooked and/or mixed form). This level of definition of "food consumed" allows ready identification of the scope and source of any differences found specific using alternate sources food composition data. Some of these differences may be difficult to identify, or may be overlooked in foods as consumed due to the effects of different methods of food preparation and combination.

In this paper, the effects of using US or UK rather than Australian national food composition databases are assessed. Specifically, factors influencing the quantity and adequacy of the foods and nutrients available for consumption in Australia will be determined and compared.

■ Methods

Food Composition Data

The data used are the food composition tables, or series of tables developed for national use in Australia, the US and the UK. These are, in Australia, *Composition of Foods, Australia* (4,8-12); for the US, the USDA series *Composition of Foods* (3); and from the UK the 1978 HMSO edition of *McCance and Widdowson's The Composition of Foods* and the subsequent supplements released in the 1980s (2,16,17).

The official printed data sources rather than commercial packages were used. As many of the commercial computer-based packages have modified or extended databases, this approach was to ensure that only the official data were used. Further, the printed versions include detailed information and explanatory notes and appendices to assist the user to interpret and apply the data.

■ Food Consumption Data

The quantity and type of foods available for consumption per capita (AC) in 1990-91 (13) in Australia are used (AC). The edible weight of foods and associated nutrients available are calculated using the

most appropriate data selected from the three data sources. For example, the edible portion factors (EPF) for carcase meats should allow for losses at the level of both the butcher (carcase to retail meats) and the consumer (retail to raw edible meat) (18).

To assess the adequacy of the food supply to meet the nutrient requirements of the population, the calculated nutrients available per capita are compared with the weighted population recommended dietary intakes (WPRDI). Prior to this comparison, thiamin and vitamin C are adjusted to make some allowance for losses during food processing and cooking and niacin equivalents are calculated (13). The WPRDI is derived by calculating the sum of nutrients needed to provide the RDIs (19) for the proportion of the population in each age and sex group, and the WPRDI is then expressed per capita.

Analyses undertaken

Quantity of Food. The effect of differences in edible portion factors (EPF) was assessed using fruit, vegetable and meat data from the three sources. These factors reflect the proportion of the food that is edible and usually eaten by the population. For example, for a fruit such as the raw orange, the COFA EPF of 0.74 indicates that 74 per cent of the food item is considered edible flesh, the other 26 per cent (in this instance, skin, seeds, pith) is usually discarded.

Nutrients Available — Effect of Differences in EPF. Meats and vegetables were used as the basis for this assessment. The EPF of each of the three data sources were used to calculate the nutrients available from the determined edible weights of meats and vegetables using COFA nutrient composition data.

Nutrients Available — Effect of Differences in Nutrient Composition. For this example, the COFA EPF were used as the basis for determining the edible weight of meats and vegetables. Nutrients available in the food supply from these

Table I. Effect of different edible portion factors from different food composition tables on the weight of fruits, vegetables and meats available for consumption (kg per capita per year)

Foods	Quantity FEW[a] kg	COFA EPF[b]	COFA EW[c] kg	UK EPF	UK EW kg	US EPF	US EW kg
Fruits							
Oranges	30.0	0.74	22.2	0.75	22.5	0.73	21.9
Apples	16.7	0.92	15.4	0.77	12.9	0.85	14.2
Bananas	12.7	0.64	8.1	0.59	7.5	0.65	8.3
Grapes[d]	9.7	0.98	9.5	0.88	8.5	0.96	9.3
Pineapples	9.1	0.67	6.1	0.53	4.8	0.52	4.7
Melons	7.5	0.60	4.5	0.56	4.2	0.50	3.8
Other citrus	6.3	0.70	4.4	0.51	3.2	0.52	3.3
Pears	6.0	0.90	5.4	0.72	4.3	0.92	5.2
Peaches	3.1	0.90	2.8	0.87	2.7	0.76	2.4
Other[e]	6.9	0.86[g]	5.9	0.87[g]	6.0	0.86[g]	5.9
Total[f]	**108.0**		**84.3**		**76.6**		**79.2**
Percent COFA EW[c]	NA		NA		90.9%		94.0%
Weighted EPF		0.78		0.71		0.73	
Vegetables							
Potato	63.5	0.82	52.1	0.86	54.6	0.75	47.6
Tomato	25.8	0.99	25.5	1.00	25.8	0.91	23.5
Onions	10.3	0.88	9.1	0.97	10.0	0.90	9.3
Carrots	8.2	0.90	7.4	0.96	7.9	0.89	7.3
Peas	6.7	0.36	2.4	0.37	2.5	0.38	2.5
Lettuce	5.9	0.87	5.1	0.70	4.1	0.95	5.6
Pumpkin	5.7	0.80	4.6	0.81	4.6	0.70	4.0
Cabbage & other green leafy	5.4	0.77	4.2	0.78	4.2	0.73	3.9
Cauliflower	4.8	0.57	2.7	0.62	3.0	0.39	1.9
Sweet corn	3.9	0.52	2.0	0.66	2.6	0.36	1.4
Celery	3.4	0.79	2.7	0.73	2.5	0.89	3.0
Other[h]	12.6	0.86[g]	10.8	0.73[g]	9.2	0.83[g]	10.4
Total[f]	**156.2**		**128.6**		**131.0**		**120.8**
Percent COFA EW[c]			NA		101.9%		93.9%
Weighted EPF		0.82		0.84		0.77	
Meats							
Beef	39.2	0.66	25.9	0.83	32.6	0.80	31.4
Veal[j]	1.5	0.59	0.9	(0.83)	(1.2)	(0.69)[k]	(1.0)
Lamb	21.8	0.63	13.7	0.84	18.3	0.84	(18.3)
Pigmeat	18.0	0.65	11.7	0.74	13.3	0.82	14.8
Offal[l]	3.8	0.98	3.7	0.96	3.6	0.98	3.7
Poultry	25.4	0.62	15.7	0.64	16.3	0.69	17.5
Total[f]	**109.7**		**71.7**		**85.3**		**85.2**
Percent COFA EW[c]			NA		119.1%		118.9%
Weighted EPF		0.65		0.78		0.78	

a = fresh equivalent weight
b = edible portion factor
c = edible weight
d = includes FEW of grapes to be dried
e = apricots, figs, plums, berries, figs, cherries, custard apples, mangoes, pawpaws, strawberries, olives
f = rounded from more detailed individual data items
g = total edible weight/total FEW
h = beetroot, beans, cucumber, eggplant, marrows, mushrooms, sweet potato etc
j = data in brackets derived using EP factors for beef
k = data in brackets derived using EP factors for composite boneless meat

foods were then calculated using each of the three nutrient composition data sources.

Nutrients Available — Effect of Differences in EPF and Nutrient Composition. The effects of differences in edible portion *and* nutrient composition data in each of the three data sources were assessed for all food groups, including the meat and vegetable groups. The relative contributions of the macronutrients to total energy were calculated.

Nutrient Adequacy. The total nutrients available in the food supply were then assessed for adequacy against the WPRDI. The proportion of energy contributed by the macronutrients was also determined. The range of nutrients included was selected on the basis of consistency across all data sources, and on the basis of those for which there are RDIs for use in Australia (19).

▮ Results

In this paper, the COFA data are used as the basis for all comparisons made.

Quantity of Food Consumed

Each of the three food composition tables provides EPF for foods such as fruits, vegetables and meats. Table I shows the EPF for a range of raw fruits, vegetables and carcase meats from each of the three data sources. On a weight basis, the fruit and vegetable items comprise 93 per cent of all fruits, and 92 per cent of all vegetables available for consumption in Australia. The remaining items from these food groups are included in the "other" category. For both fruits and vegetables there are marked differences in the EPF for individual foods reported in each source.

Despite differences in the EPF of up to plus 27 per cent or minus 32 per cent of the edible weight (EW) of the individual fruits and vegetables, the impact on *the total* edible weight of these commodities available for consumption is much smaller (minus 10 per cent to plus 2 per cent). The use of the UK and US data

gives a total EW of vegetables 101.9 per cent and 93.9 per cent of that obtained using COFA. The effect on total EW of fruits is greater, with results 90.9 per cent and 94.0 per cent using UK and US data compared to COFA.

The other major food group on which EPFs have a marked effect is the meats. Table I shows that for beef, lamb and pigmeat there is a consistently higher EPF for carcase meats in the UK and US databases than in COFA. The effect of using these EPFs to calculate the raw EW of meat available for consumption is an EW of meats and poultry of 119.1 per cent and 118.9 per cent when UK or US factors are used, respectively, compared to COFA. The basis for the revised EPF for Australian carcass meats is reported elsewhere (18).

Nutrients Available for Consumption

Effect of Differences in EPF. Using COFA nutrient data as a constant in all calculations, Table II indicates the effect of the different EPF from each of the three sources on the nutrients calculated as available for consumption from vegetables and meat. The effects are generally consistent with the differences in total EW shown in Table I. The exception to this is retinol activity contributed by the meats. The EPF for meats (beef, veal, lamb, pigmeat) are low in COFA compared to all other sources, but the EPF for offal are similar. While small amounts of retinol are contributed by muscle meats, as shown in brackets in Table II, offal is the major determinant of the quantity of retinol contributed by meat. This is responsible for the similar retinol contributed by all three sources.

Effect of Differences in Nutrient Composition per 100 g Edible Portion. Table III shows the impact of the differing nutrient data from the three data sources on the contribution of vegetables and meats to the nutrients available in the food supply. The quantities of EW of food are calculated using the COFA EPF.

Table II. Effect of differences in source of EPF on nutrient contribution from vegetables and meats, quantity per capita per day. COFA used as nutrient composition source

Source	Protein	Fat	Carbo-hydrate	Energy	Ca	Fe	Mg	Zn	Retinol activity	Thiamin	Ribo-flavin	Niacin	Vitamin C
	g	g	g	kJ	mg	mg	mg	mg	µg	mg	mg	mg	mg
Vegetables													
COFA	6.8	0.5	26.0	583	45	2.0	51	1.1	477	0.25	0.16	3.3	73
UK	7.0	0.5	27.3	611	45	2.0	52	1.2	499	0.25	0.15	3.4	74
US	6.3	0.5	23.8	538	43	1.9	47	1.1	460	0.23	0.15	3.1	67
Meats													
COFA	37.4	32.6	0.2	1850	15	3.5	36	5.0	1839 (21)[a]	0.31	0.64	7.8	2
UK	44.3	39.0	0.2	2198	17	4.0	43	6.2	1813 (24)	0.36	0.69	9.2	2
US	44.3	39.0	0.2	2198	17	4.0	43	6.0	1838 (25)	0.37	0.69	9.2	2

[a] = values in parentheses are for retinol activity from non-offal meats

This table shows that the fat contribution from meats was 147 per cent and 133 per cent of that of COFA using the UK and US data, respectively. Combined with the associated variations in protein levels, this results in the energy contributed from meats also being 124 per cent and 121 per cent, respectively, compared to COFA. Using fat-trimmed composite data for boneless meats when available in the US databases reduces this to 115 per cent of the COFA fat contribution. The energy contributed by vegetables using UK and US nutrient data are similarly higher compared to COFA due mainly to the considerably higher carbohydrate levels. Calcium, riboflavin and thiamin contributed by vegetables are higher when US and UK data are used. Magnesium and retinol activity levels from vegetables are also higher than COFA when the US or UK data are used, as is niacin from meats. These results reflect the generally higher levels of these nutrients reported in these data sources. Retinol activity, however, is lower from meats when data sources other than COFA are used. Differences in the composition of offal are primarily

responsible for the variation obtained. While offal is the main source of retinol activity contributed by the meats group, the use of US data suggest a considerably greater contribution from other meats, particularly poultry, and a considerably lower contribution when the UK data are used.

Effect of Differences in EPF and Nutrient Composition Data. Table IV provides a similar comparison for all food groups, except that the different source data EPF factors have also been applied. For vegetables, for example, Table I showed that while the EPF from the different data sources varied considerably for any particular vegetable, the differences were small for the total weight of vegetables. The combination of differences in EPFs and nutrient data at the individual vegetable level, however, result in very different estimates of the nutrients available for consumption from vegetables. The carbohydrate contribution from vegetables compared to COFA is higher using the UK (154 per cent) and US (138 per cent) data. The minerals all show variation with data source. Calcium

Table III. Effect of differences of nutrient composition on nutrients available from vegetables and meats, quantity per capita per day. COFA used as an EPF source

Source	Protein	Fat	Carbo-hydrate	Energy	Ca	Fe	Mg	Zn	Retinol activity	Thiamin	Ribo-flavin	Niacin	Vitamin C
	g	g	g	kJ	mg	mg	mg	mg	µg	mg	mg	mg	mg
Vegetables													
COFA	6.8	0.5	26.0	583	45	2.0	51	1.1	477	0.25	0.16	3.3	73
UK	5.9	0.4	38.1	729	69	2.0	63	1.0	591	0.29	0.20	3.1	66
US	5.9	0.7	38.8	726	52	2.4	62	1.0	736	0.28	0.18	3.5	70
Meats													
COFA	37.4	32.6	0.2	1850	15	3.5	36	5.0	1839 (23)[a]	0.31	0.64	7.8	2
UK	31.0	47.9	0.1	2303	16	3.3	35	4.9	1430 (6)	0.32	0.63	9.4	1
US	33.4	43.4	0.3	2237	18	3.4	35	5.5	683 (100)	0.36	0.68	10.5	2

[a] = values in parentheses are for retinol activity from non-offal meats

and magnesium levels are higher when the UK and US food composition tables are used, being up to 156 per cent that of COFA for calcium from vegetables when UK data are used. Zinc contributed by vegetables using US data, is nearly twice that obtained using COFA. The use of UK or US data also suggest a considerably higher total retinol activity from vegetables compared to COFA: 129 per cent and 151 per cent, respectively. This is also seen with thiamin and riboflavin (120 per cent and 125 per cent, respectively, that of COFA when UK data are used). In contrast, vitamin C is around 90 per cent that of COFA when UK or US data are used.

For meats, the differences in both EPF and nutrient composition in the three data sources further exacerbate the trends observed in Tables II and III. Fat, energy, and the minerals calcium, iron and zinc are all higher when data other than COFA are used. The fat contribution from meats is 178 per cent and 161 per cent of that of COFA when UK or US data are used, while energy levels are 150 per cent and 145 per cent, respectively. The retinol activity levels are all lower using data

sources other than COFA; being 77 per cent (UK) and 38 per cent (US) of the level obtained using COFA.

When the nutrients available for consumption from all foods, with thiamin, niacin and vitamin C adjusted as described in the methods section, levels are higher when data other than COFA are used. The exceptions are magnesium, retinol activity and vitamin C for both UK and US data, and thiamin, riboflavin and niacin equivalents when the UK data are used. The higher contribution of meat fat to total available fat suggested by the use of UK and US data has the effect of reducing the relative importance of the added fats and oils as a source of fat in the national diet. Using COFA data, added fats contribute 60 per cent more fat in the national diet than the meats; using the other data sources suggests that the contributions of meats and added fats are about equivalent. Consequently, the ratio of animal fats to vegetable fats obtained using UK and US data is also higher.

Alcohol content varies with the data source, being lower when UK data are used (93 per cent) and slightly higher when US data are used (102 per cent). The

Table IV. Effect of different sources of EPF and nutrient composition on nutrients available for consumption per capita per day

Source	Protein	Fat	Carbo-hydrate	Alcohol	Energy	Ca	Fe	Mg	Zn	Retinol activity	Thiamin	Ribo-flavin	Niacin	Vitamin C
	g	g	g	g	kJ	mg	mg	mg	mg	µg	mg	mg	mg	mg
COFA														
Meats	37.4	32.6	0.2	0	1850	15	3.5	36	5.0	1839	0.31	0.64	7.8	2
Seafood	5.1	1.3	0	0	138	23	0.3	8	1.0	6	0.01	0.03	1.0	0
Milk & milk products	19.4	21.4	19.8	0	1442	659	0.6	52	2.5	215	0.20	0.76	0.4	5
Fruits	1.9	0.2	26.2	0	480	39	0.8	22	0.4	42	0.12	0.07	0.6	53
Vege-tables	6.8	0.5	26.0	0	583	45	2.0	51	1.1	477	0.25	0.16	3.3	73
Grains	26.8	3.7	183.0	0	3700	49	5.3	113	1.6	0	0.85	0.71	9.6	0
Eggs	2.2	1.7	0.1	0	101	7	0.3	2	0.2	27	0.01	0.07	0	0
Nuts	1.9	4.6	0.6	0	210	15	0.3	36	0.5	0	0.04	0.08	0.7	0
Oils & fats	0.2	52.6	0.2	0	1952	4	0	0	0	294	0	0.01	0.1	0
Sugars	0	0	122.5	0	1958	4	0.1	0	0.1	0	0	0	0	0
Alcohol	1.0	0	6.9	17.5	648	15	0.1	21	0	0	0	0	1.3	7
UK														
Meats	36.6	58.1	0.1	0	2775	18	3.9	41	6.0	1410	0.37	0.70	10.9	2
Seafood	4.9	1.8	0	0	150	18	0.3	9	1.1	8	0.03	0.04	1.3	0
Milk & milk products	19.9	21.4	20.1	0	1452	668	0.3	53	2.2	293	0.14	0.81	0.4	5
Fruits	1.4	0.2	23.5	0	408	42	0.8	29	0.3	53	0.12	0.06	0.6	48
Vege-tables	6.1	0.5	40.1	0	763	70	2.0	65	1.0	614	0.30	0.20	3.2	66
Grains	23.9	4.2	195.6	0	3687	300	5.5	85	2.3	0	0.75	0.07	5.0	0
Eggs	2.2	1.9	0	0	105	10	0.3	2	0.2	33	0.02	0.08	0	0
Nuts	1.8	4.1	1.5	0	177	12	0.2	17	0.2	0	0.03	0.04	0.6	0
Oils & fats	0.1	52.9	0	0	1961	2	0.1	0	0	281	0	0	0	0
Sugars	0	0	128.1	0	2051	54	0.1	0	0.9	0	0	0	0	0
Alcohol	0.9	0	8.0	16.2	613	38	0.6	30	0	0	0	0.12	1.3	0

Table IV. Effect of different sources of EPF and nutrient composition on nutrients available for consumption per capita per day-*Continued*

Source	Protein	Fat	Carbo-hydrate	Alcohol	Energy	Ca	Fe	Mg	Zn	Retinol activity	Thiamin	Ribo-flavin	Niacin	Vitamin C
	g	g	g	g	kJ	mg	mg	mg	mg	µg	mg	mg	mg	mg
US														
Meats	39.5	52.5	0.2	0	2691	21	3.9	33	6.5	693	0.42	0.75	12.2	2
Seafood	5.2	0.6	0.1	0	119	13	0.4	8	0.5	5	0.01	0.05	0.7	0
Milk & milk products	20.0	19.8	20.7	0	1416	679	0.4	59	2.4	189	0.16	0.76	0.4	4
Fruits	1.6	0.6	31.5	0	515	39	0.5	22	0.2	55	0.11	0.09	0.68	49
Vegetables	5.5	0.6	35.8	0	672	51	2.2	57	2.0	720	0.26	0.18	3.3	64
Grains	26.0	2.8	194.1	0	3853	46	11.3	106	2.5	2	1.82	1.10	14.2	0
Eggs	2.1	1.9	0.2	0	112	10	0.4	2	0.2	27	0.02	0.05	0	0
Nuts	1.8	4.1	1.5	0	196	15	0.3	19	0.2	0	0.03	0.04	0.6	0
Oils & fats	0.3	52.6	0.1	0	1953	7	0	1	0	240	0	0.01	0	0
Sugars	0	0	122.5	0	1958	4	0.1	0	0.9	0	0	0	0	0
Alcohol	0.9	0	10.9	17.9	719	19	0.3	22	0.1	0	0.02	0.09	1.4	0
Summary totals (adjusted)[a]														
COFA	103	119	385	17.5	13060	873	13.3	342	12.5	2901	1.52	2.51	42.6[b]	102
UK[c]	98	145	416	16.2	14140	1181	14.1	331	14.2	2693	1.50	2.12	39.5[b]	85
US[d]	103	136	418	17.9	14205	904	19.8	329	15.5	1931	2.42	3.10	50.6[b]	86

a = rounded from more detailed individual data items.
   Thiamin and vitamin C adjusted for losses with processing and cooking. Niacin equivalents calculated
b = niacin equivalents
c = without fortification of flour, total calcium = 926 mg; iron = 13.1 mg; thiamin = 1.14 mg and niacin
   equivalent = 37.5 mg; without fortification of skim milk powder, retinol activity = 2672 mg
d = without fortification of flour and rice, iron = 12.1 mg; thiamin = 1.20 mg, riboflavin = 2.18 mg and
   niacin equivalent = 40.5 mg

Table V. Macronutrient contribution to total energy[a] (per cent)

Data source	Protein	Fat	Carbohydrate	Alcohol
COFA	13.6	34.3	48.1	4.0
UK	11.7	37.9	47.1	3.3
US	12.5	36.0	48.0	3.5

[a] adjusted to ignore minor contributions to total energy from minor sources such as organic acids

retinol activity data vary from 67 per cent (US) to 93 per cent (UK) of those of COFA. Vitamin C is also 16 per cent lower using data sources other than COFA.

The use of the UK data indicates that grain products are a major source of calcium, providing 25 per cent of the total, as compared with only 5 per cent obtained using the other food composition sources, while the use of the US data suggests that grains contribute twice as much iron and thiamin and nearly 50 per cent more niacin and riboflavin. Both results are due to fortification of wheat flour, with calcium in the UK, and wheat flour and rice with iron, thiamin, niacin and riboflavin in the US. The fortification of wheat flour with iron, thiamin and niacin in the UK is not as apparent in these results.

Table V presents the macronutrient data using the three data sources, as per cent contribution to total energy. Data sources other than COFA result in a higher contribution from fat and a consequent lower contribution from carbohydrate, alcohol and protein.

Nutritional Adequacy of the Food Supply

Table VI shows that the use of the three data sources give values for protein, retinol activity (even with contribution of offal discounted), thiamin, riboflavin, niacin equivalents, and vitamin C that are at least 50 per cent in excess of recommended intakes. For calcium, COFA and the US data suggest that there is little excess available in the food supply relative to the requirements of the population, while the use of the UK data suggests

there is a comfortable excess of 41 per cent of this nutrient. With the exception of COFA, the available level of zinc is at least 29 per cent in excess of requirements. The use of COFA data also gives lower levels of iron in excess of the WPRDI than the other data sources. The adjustment of the US and UK databases used to "remove" the fortifying nutrients from wheat flour or rice reduces these differences, with the excess of WPRDI for iron, thiamin and niacin equivalents then being lower (compared to COFA) when US or UK data are used.

▪ Discussion

Quantity of Food Consumed

EPFs are highly variable and have the potential to markedly affect the estimates of nutrient intakes. There are many possible reasons for the variation reported in the different databases. It may be cultivar related, or due to local preference for a particular unit size or stage of maturity; or it may reflect the degree of pre-market trimming of inedible or unattractive components. For example, mature carrots used to be marketed in Australia with their green leaves. These are now removed prior to sale. Alternatively, differences in EPF may reflect differences in the parts of the food that are considered edible in the local community. For example, in some food cultures, spinach stalks are discarded, in others they are consumed. Further, in Australia, in response to the demand for lower fat meats, there have been changes in developing animals with different characteristics, in pre-

Table VI. Effect of differences in source of EPF and nutrient composition on the assessment of the nutritional adequacy of the food supply (per cent in excess of WPRDI[a])

Source	Protein	Energy	Ca	Fe	Mg	Zn	Retinol activity[b]	Thiamin	Ribo-flavin	Niacin equivts.	Vitamin C
	g	kJ	mg	mg	mg	mg	µg	mg	mg	mg	mg
WPRDI	45.8	9283	838	9.2	261	11	685	0.89	1.36	15.2	34
COFA	125	41	4	45	31	14	324 (58)	70	85	180	200
UK[c]	114	52	41 (11)	53 (42)	27	29	293 (87)	69 (28)	56	160 (147)	150
US[c]	125	53	8	115 (32)	26	41	182 (97)	172 (35)	128 (60)	233 (166)	153

a = WPRDI (ABS, 1993); Mg & Zn calculated for this paper
b = values in parentheses are for comparisons without contribution from offal meats
c = values in parentheses for calcium, thiamin, riboflavin and niacin equivalents are for comparisons without fortification of wheat flour or rice.

slaughter feeding and handling practices, in butchering techniques and in retail fat trimming practices (20). These affect both EPF and nutrient composition.

Nutrients Available for Consumption

Users have a number of sources of food composition databases available to them. This is particularly apparent in countries such as Australia where a national food analysis program is only of recent origin. Local food availability, food regulations, food preferences and preparation practices all influence the actual gross and nutrient composition of foods. The food composition database selected for use, unless specific to the local food supply, can have a marked effect on the outcome of a study, both on nutrients, and on foods as sources of nutrients.

These and other factors influence the actual composition of a food, and the relevance of the food composition database used. There are, however, other factors that influence the interpretation of food composition data, and the comparability of data from different sources. For example, the analytical methods used to determine nutrient levels and the mode of

expression of these nutrient data may vary between food composition tables.

Methods of Analysis. These can have a large effect on the reported value of a nutrient in a food. This effect can be so striking that data from two different tables cannot necessarily be combined and be expected to provide a meaningful assessment of the dietary intake for that nutrient.

The most obvious example is carbohydrate. The carbohydrate data in COFA and the UK tables represent a direct analysis of the sugars and starch content of foods. The carbohydrate data in the US do not represent direct measures, but rather are calculated "by difference", a method which includes dietary fibre in the carbohydrate data. The US tables add to the confusion by reporting other measures of fibre components, namely crude fibre and pectin.

The method of determining carbohydrate in foods also affects the associated energy calculations. When carbohydrate is determined "by difference", the carbohydrate energy conversions factors used are food type specific, and allow for the potential fibre component. This is not the case when carbohydrate is determined by analysis.

Other common examples of the effect of different methods of analysis are vitamin C, vitamin A and dietary fibre. The analytical methods used in the COFA and UK tables for vitamin C, for example, include ascorbic acid and dehydroascorbic acid. The US data are measures of reduced ascorbic acid only. Data for total ascorbic acid including the dehydroascorbic acid form is given in footnotes where available.

Modes of Expression. Nutrients may be expressed differently in different tables. The term dietary fibre may include different components dependent upon the method used. Carbohydrate components (starch, sugars and dietary fibre) are expressed as monosaccharide equivalents in the UK tables (2), but as the direct measure in the Australian tables (4,8-12). Vitamin A is expressed as retinol and β-carotene equivalents in the UK; retinol equivalents, retinol and β-carotene equivalents in COFA and the measures are direct weights, but in the US tables the term used is vitamin A, and the values expressed as retinol equivalents or International Units. Energy may be expressed as kilojoules or kilocalories, and the factors used to calculate energy vary as described above. Total energy may include other energy-contributing components such as organic acids, as in COFA.

Missing Data. In the printed version of the UK tables (2), for example, the fact that there are no measures of zinc for a variety of foods, particularly fish, is clearly indicated. In computer based tables, zeros may be inserted with obvious problems for the user who is unaware that "0" may represent either no nutrient detected at the level of delectability of the analytical method used or, no data available on the level of this nutrient in this food. This can result in an incorrect perception of a food such as fish as a food source of zinc, an inappropriately low value for the total dietary intake of this nutrient, and an incorrect interpretation of

the results obtained. This is an obvious example of the value of checking the data on the computer version against the official published copy. A related problem for users of computer databases is that of national differences in nutrient fortification regulations and practices. The impact of this on study outcomes and appropriate interpretation of data is clearly shown in this paper. Specific information is needed to both identify and adjust for these effects and even then the effects may be masked by variable voluntary nutrient additions (e.g. in breakfast cereals).

Nutritional Adequacy of the Food Supply

Assessment of the amounts of a nutrient available per capita against the WPRDI is the basis for monitoring the trends in the nutritional adequacy of the Australian food supply. The level of nutrient in excess of the WPRDI, is used as an indication of the "safety margin" for that nutrient. In recent years, the National Health and Medical Research Council has expressed concern about several nutrients in the Australian food supply — thiamin, calcium and iron (21,22).

Thiamin. The data in Table VI data indicate thiamin at 70 per cent in excess of the WPRDI using COFA, whereas if the standard US data were the basis of the assessment, the 172 per cent excess would be grounds for complacency. Grains are the major source of thiamin when all three data sources are used, the absolute level of thiamin contributed by grains when US data are used is much greater compared to the other two sources. This reflects the level of thiamin fortification of wheat flour in the US. Conversely, "removing" this added thiamin from the US or UK wheat flour suggests that there is a lower excess of 35 per cent of WPRDI compared to COFA at 70 per cent. The reasons for this are the naturally higher level of thiamin in Australian flour due to higher extraction rates, and, at that time, a segment of the flour supply contained voluntarily added thiamin.

Iron. The use of COFA shows that iron levels are 45 per cent in excess of WPRDI (considerably lower than obtained using the previous Australian food tables at 93 per cent of the WPRDI (25). This information coupled with a national survey of schoolchildren in 1985 indicating that 9 per cent of 15 year old girls had compromised iron status based on biochemical assessment (23) led directly to a recommendation to "increase the consumption of iron containing foods" in the national dietary guidelines (21). By contrast, the use of the UK or US food composition tables would not have caused such a degree of concern, at 53 per cent and 115 per cent in excess of WPRDI, respectively, the US results reflecting the iron fortification of wheat flour and rice. Differences in breakfast cereal fortification with iron also have an effect, but varies with product as well as country.

Calcium. Calcium intakes are of considerable concern in Australia due to the prevalence of osteoporosis and data indicating a decrease in consumption of milk and milk products in adolescence (24). In 1992 a recommendation "to increase the intake of calcium containing foods" was added to the revised dietary guidelines for Australians (21). The use of COFA or US data to assess the adequacy of this nutrient in the food supply, indicate only a small safety margin. The level of calcium suggested by the standard UK data, however, would not raise the same degree of concern because of the calcium fortification of flours in the UK.

Country Specific Food Composition data

All the data sources are derived from national food composition databases developed to best represent the local food supply. COFA is based primarily on a national food analysis program. The UK database is underpinned by a national analytical program, however, the US database is primarily compiled from analytical data produced by independent, mainly US based researchers.

From the results in this paper, the use of UK and US food tables gives nutrient estimates that are closer to those obtained using TCAF, the "old" Australian tables, than using COFA (25) probably reflecting the previous reliance on the data from these two sources in the compilation of the "Australian" food composition tables. Even with access to the more recent US and UK data used in this paper, the Australian food analysis program has shown that there are real differences in the composition of locally produced and consumed foods.

∎ Conclusion

The analysis in recent years of foods currently available and consumed in Australia has provided the first opportunity to assess the effect of using data from other countries on perceptions of foods and nutrients available in Australia.

The data presented in this paper show that using overseas data sources to estimate nutrient availability can produce significant errors in the assessment of the nutrient adequacy of the food supply, and of the relative significance of foods as sources of nutrients. The implications for the development of nutrition programs, goals and targets are obvious.

This paper makes a strong case for ongoing support for the local food composition program, and for the use of the Australian food composition database in all Australian nutrition programs and research studies.

While the value of good food composition data which are relevant to the local food supply has been demonstrated in this study, high standards in use of the data will not occur unless users are adequately trained. Such education should include the need to know about local food determinants, as well as how to use and interpret information such as different analytical methods, modes of data expression, and the rates for sampling, method choice and analytical quality assurance (26,27).

■ Acknowledgments

The Australian Bureau of Statistics kindly made available unpublished details of the estimates of foods available for consumption. We thank Michael de Looper, Australian Institute of Health and Welfare, for assistance with the WPRDI calculations.

■ References

(1)   English, R. (1981) *Food Tech. Aust.* **33**, 103-106.

(2)   Paul, A.A., & Southgate, D.A.T. (1978) *The Composition of Foods*, HMSO, London

(3)   US Department of Agriculture (1976–) *Composition of Foods: Raw, Processed, Prepared*, Agric. Handbook No. 8 series, USDA, Washington, DC

(4)   Cashel, K., English, R., & Lewis, J. (1989) *Composition of Foods, Australia*, Australian Government Publishing Service, Canberra

(5)   English, R. (1986) *Trans. Menzies Found.* **11**, 25-34

(6)   Thomas, S. & Corden, M. (1970) *Tables of Composition of Australian Foods*, Australian Government Printer, Canberra

(7)   Thomas, S., & Corden, M. (1977) *Metric Tables of Composition of Australian Foods*, Australian Government Printer, Canberra

(8)   English, R., Lewis, J., & Cashel, K. (1990) *Composition of Foods, Australia, Volume 2, Cereals and Cereal Products*, Australian Government Publishing Service, Canberra

(9)   Lewis, J., & English, R. (1990) *Composition of Foods, Australia, Volume 3, Dairy Products, Eggs and Fish*, Australian Government Publishing Service, Canberra

(10) English, R., & Lewis, J. (1990) *Composition of Foods, Australia,*

(11) Lewis, J. & English, R. (1990) *Composition of Foods, Australia, Volume 5, Nuts and Legumes, Beverages and Miscellaneous Foods*, Australian Government Publishing Service, Canberra

(12) Lewis, J., Holt, R., & English, R. (1992) *Composition of Foods Australia, Volume 6, Infant Foods*, Australian Government Publishing Service, Canberra

(13) Australian Bureau of Statistics (1993) *Apparent Consumption of Foodstuffs and Nutrients, Australia, 1990–91*, ABS, Canberra

(14) English, R. (1987) *Towards Better Nutrition for Australians*, Australian Government Publishing Service, Canberra

(15) Health Targets and Implementation Committee (HTIC) (1988) *Health for All Australians*, Australian Government Publishing Service, Canberra

(16) Holland, B., Unwin, I.D., & Buss, D. (1988) *Third Supplement to McCance and Widdowson's The Composition of Foods, 4th edition: Cereals and Cereal Products*, Royal Society of Chemistry, Nottingham

(17) Holland, B., Unwin, I.D., & Buss, D. (1988) *Fourth Supplement to McCance and Widdowson's The Composition of Foods, 4th edition: Milk Products and Eggs*, Royal Society of Chemistry, Nottingham

(18) Cashel, K., & Greenfield, H. (1994) *Br. J. Nutr.* **71**, 753-773.

(19) National Health and Medical Research Council (1992) *Recommended Dietary Intakes For Use in Australia*, Australian Government Publishing Service, Canberra

(20) Warren, B., & Channon, H. (c1990) *Lamb Cutting Notes 1. More Fat Means Less Saleable*

Volume 4, Fats and Oils, Processed Meats, Processed Fruit and Vegetables, Australian Government Publishing Service, Canberra

Meat, Rutherglen Research Institute, Victoria

(21) National Health and Medical Research Council (1992) *Dietary Guidelines For Australians,* Australian Government Publishing Service, Canberra

(22) National Health and Medical Research Council (1989) *Report of the 108th Session of the Council,* Australian Government Publishing Service, Canberra.

(23) English, R., & Bennett (1990) *Med. J. Aust.* **152,** 582-586.

(24) English, R., Cashel, K., Lewis, J., Bennett, S., Berzins, J., Waters, A., & Magnus, P. (1988) *National Dietary Survey of Schoolchildren Aged 10–15 Years, No. 1, Foods Consumed,* Australian Government Publishing Service, Canberra

(25) Cashel, K., & Greenfield, H. (1995) *J. Food Comp. Anal.* (in press)

(26) Greenfield, H. (1990) *Food Aust.* **42,** S1-S44

(27) Greenfield, H., & Southgate, D.A.T, *Food Composition Data: Production, Management and Use,* Elsevier Applied Science, London

Quality Control in the Use of Food and Nutrient Databases for Epidemiologic Studies

I. Marilyn Buzzard, Sally F. Schakel, Janet Ditter-Johnson

Nutrition Coordinating Center, Division of Epidemiology, School of Public Health, University of Minnesota, 1300 South Second Street, Minneapolis, MN 55454-1015, USA

This paper describes procedures used by the Nutrition Coordinating Center (NCC) at the University of Minnesota for maintaining food and nutrient databases. NCC's databases are designed to support an automated system for dietary data collection and nutrient calculation for clinical trials and other nutrition research and large population-based studies. The three major databases include the Nutrient Database, the Food Database, and the Brand Database. The Nutrient Database consists primarily of food composition data for "core" (non-recipe) foods. The Food Database drives the system's interactive prompting for detailed food descriptions and specification of amounts consumed. This database also contains all of the non-nutrient data required to link food descriptions with one or more entries in the Nutrient Database and convert amounts consumed to gram weights for nutrient calculation. The Brand Database, which contains food and nutrient information for commercial products, is used to update the other two databases. Each of these databases and the quality control procedures used for maintaining them are described. Because many of the studies using NCC databases are long term projects, time-related database maintenance and quality control procedures are required. These procedures permit routine updating to reflect the changing marketplace and the availability of new or improved data, while also ensuring comparability of dietary data collected at any point in time.

The Nutrition Coordinating Center (NCC) at the University of Minnesota maintains food and nutrient databases to support a system for the collection and nutrient calculation of dietary data. The system is designed primarily for clinical trials and other medical research and epidemiologic studies investigating relationships between diet and health (1-3). The Minnesota nutrition data system has been used for hundreds of research studies over the past two decades. The majority of these studies have been funded by the US National Institutes of Health. A brief overview of the requirements for the system will provide a basis for understanding the functionality of the databases that drive the system.

■ Overview of the Minnesota Nutrition Data System

The Minnesota nutrition data system was designed to meet the needs of its users—primarily large, population-based nutrition research studies. These needs include the following: standardized procedures for collecting food intake data, especially for multi-centered studies collecting data at many different centers by many different individuals; a high level of specificity for describing foods, including methods of food preparation and brand identification; food and nutrient databases that are frequently updated and which contain no missing values of nutritional significance; a food composition database that continues to expand to include the nutrients of current research interest; rapid data processing; and database maintenance procedures that permit accurate

comparison of food and nutrient intakes over time.

To avoid the need to maintain different versions of the system for different users, the most stringent requirement demanded by any one user is provided to all users. For example, if only a few studies need specificity for sodium, this level of specificity is provided to everyone; those who are not interested in sodium intake may opt not to ask questions about salt use in food preparation, and the system will automatically assign the default amounts. If one study needs foods added to the database for a special study population, these foods become available to all users.

The three major components of the current version of the Minnesota nutrition data system are shown schematically in Figure 1. They include interactive data collection, automated coding, and nutrient calculation. Over the years the system

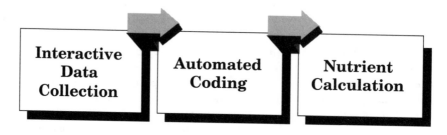

Figure 1. Major components of the Minnesota nutrition data system

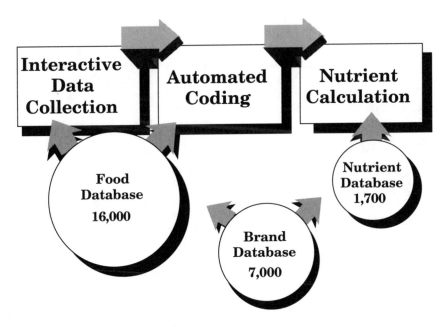

Figure 2. The three databases that drive the Minnesota nutrition data system

has evolved to take advantage of techno-logical advances and more accurate and efficient procedures for collecting and processing the data (4). When the system was first developed about 20 years ago, the first two steps were not automated (1,2). Food intake data were collected on paper, and the quality of the data de-pended largely on the skills of the inter-viewer or on how well subjects were trained to keep food records. The data collection process has now been auto-mated so that the computer provides all of the prompts required to describe foods at the appropriate level of detail (5).

Similarly, coding was initially done on paper by trained food coders, and the coded data were then entered into the computer by data entry operators. Despite the use of duplicate data entry and sub-sequent computerized edit checks, there was potential for transcription and other errors. About ten years ago, an on-line coding system was developed which al-lowed coders to enter the data directly into the computer (6). Edit checks could then be invoked at the point of data entry,

which greatly enhanced the accuracy and efficiency of the coding process.

The final step of completely auto-mating the coding process was not possi-ble until we had completed the development of the interactive data col-lection component. Only when all of the detail required for coding is captured by the computer can the coding be totally automated. This enhancement, which was implemented about five years ago, re-sulted in substantial improvements in ac-curacy and standardization, as well as savings in time and effort, since coding has traditionally been the most labor in-tensive part of processing dietary data.

The three major components of the automated system have now been incor-porated into a software package that is currently being used at approximately 150 research institutions in the US and Canada (5,7). A customized version of the system was developed for collecting 24-hour dietary recalls for the Third Na-tional Health and Nutrition Examination Survey (NHANES III) which is now in its fifth year of data collection (8).

The three databases required to maintain the automated nutrition data system are shown schematically in Figure 2. They include the Nutrient Database, the Food Database, and the Brand Database. Each of these databases will be described in greater detail below.

■ The Nutrient Database

The NCC Nutrient Database is the smallest of the three databases. It consists of the following data fields:

- food codes for approximately 1700 "core" (i.e., non-recipe) foods

- food descriptions for each food code

- amounts per 100 g for each of 94 food components for each food

- reference codes for each nutrient value

- serving sizes designated by the US Food and Drug Administration and the US Department of Agriculture (USDA) for labeling purposes

- food group designations for several different food grouping classification schemes.

Our philosophy is to keep the number of foods in the Nutrient Database as small as possible to minimize maintenance efforts and facilitate rapid updating (6). Foods are included only in their "as eaten" state; for example, foods that are never eaten raw are not included in this database. The majority of the foods in the Nutrient Database are single ingredient foods, but there are also a number of commonly consumed multi-ingredient processed foods such as cheese, bread, and sausage. Each food entry is described in detail in a text field; the Latin or scientific name is also included if applicable.

The 94 food components in the current NCC Nutrient Database include: energy; the proximate nutrients (protein, fat, carbohydrate, and alcohol, plus water and ash); animal and vegetable protein plus 18 amino acids; 23 individual fatty acids; cholesterol; starch; six simple sugars; total dietary fiber and three fiber fractions;

nine minerals; 17 vitamins, including two vitamin A fractions and four fractions of vitamin E; plus caffeine, aspartame, and saccharin. Every nutrient value in the database is associated with a reference code documenting the source of the data and/or the method used to impute the data, if applicable (9). The database also includes fields for three different food grouping schemes to facilitate analysis by food groups and to accommodate different research objectives.

Sources of data for the NCC Nutrient Database are described in detail elsewhere (9). The primary sources are USDA data tapes and publications, information from manufacturers of brand name products, and the scientific literature. The USDA Nutrient Data Base for Standard Reference is the major USDA data set used by NCC (10). The USDA Survey Database (11) provides many imputed values that are not included in the Data Base for Standard Reference. USDA Handbook No. 8 (12) provides additional information not included in the Standard Reference data sets such as specific factors for calculating energy values, standards for enrichment of grain products, and values for the amounts of separable lean and fat of retail beef cuts. Other USDA data sets used by NCC include various provisional tables and bulletins (9).

Nutrient data for brand name products are becoming increasingly important as the consumption of processed foods continues to increase in the US. Values for commercial products are obtained from the NCC Brand Database (described below). The scientific literature is another important source of nutrient data, especially for those nutrients included in the NCC database that are not currently provided by USDA. Food composition tables from other countries are occasionally used to obtain values for foreign foods not included in the USDA data sets.

■ The Food Database

The NCC Food Database exceeds the size of the Nutrient Database by approximately ten-fold. It includes the hierarchy of food descriptions that drives the interactive prompting for detailed food identification (5,7). The hierarchy consists of about 17,000 food descriptions for foods consumed in North America. This includes brand name descriptions as well as generic descriptions, in addition to a large number of ethnic and regional foods, dietary supplements, and medications containing caffeine and sodium. The hierarchy is organized in a manner that reflects the way people think about foods, rather than according to any scientific classification. The hierarchical organization facilitates the prompting for food description detail by presenting a series of menu selections that become progressively more detailed until the food is adequately described.

For each food in the hierarchy of food descriptions, the Food Database provides all of the data required to link the food with one or more entries in the Nutrient Database and to convert amounts expressed in various common units to gram weights for nutrient calculation (5,7). Examples of other data fields in the Food Database include codes that designate the type of food preparation method; ingredient listings and amounts for recipes and formulations; designation of ingredients that require further description (such as the type of fat used in a recipe); default assignments, based on nationally representative market research or food consumption data, which designate the most common of the available options when a subject cannot provide the level of detail requested; any geometric shapes (e.g., cube, sphere, wedge, or cylinder) in which the food might be described; one or more density conversion factors, depending on the various forms in which a food can be measured (e.g., solid, chopped or grated); and other amount conversion factors, such as the weights of food-specific portions (e.g., small, me-

dium, or large piece; slice; or package), raw to cooked yields, and edible portion conversions. Also included is a maximum serving size for each food in the database to serve as a quality control check for unusually large amounts.

Sources of data for the Food Database are documented by reference codes. The primary sources are the coding manual section of the USDA survey database (11) and information from manufacturers. Several other USDA publications related to food weights, yields, and portion sizes are also used for the Food Database. These publications are referenced by Schakel et al. (9).

NCC currently maintains two separate versions of the Food Database. Food descriptions in the one version are linked to the NCC Nutrient Database, whereas in the other version, the foods are linked to the USDA Survey Database (11). The latter version, which has been customized for collecting 24-hour dietary recalls for NHANES III (8), includes some additional modifications to enhance comparability of nutrient calculations with calculations from the USDA surveys.

■ The Brand Database

The NCC Brand Database contains food and nutrient information for selected categories of commercial products. This database continues to grow as the food marketplace expands and changes. In the US there are approximately 1000 new products introduced every month (13). So trying to keep up with even the most popular foods is a never ending process. We currently maintain data for about 7000 products in the Brand Database. Information from this database is used routinely to update both the Nutrient Database and the Food Database.

Brand name information is used for several different purposes. In some cases it is needed to adequately identify the food that is consumed. For example, subjects may describe a food by its brand name, such as "Coke," rather than by a more generic description, such as "car-

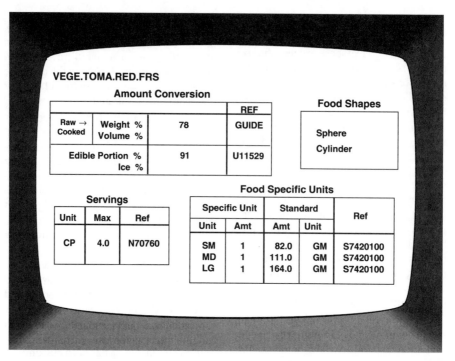

Figure 3. Example of a screen from the Food Database Maintenance System used for the NHANES III survey

bonated cola beverage." Brand name data may also be needed to differentiate between similar products that differ significantly in composition. For example, if different brands of carbonated cola beverages differ with respect to caffeine content, knowing the brand facilitates identification of the appropriate caffeine level. Another very important use of brand information is to help determine the amount of the food consumed. For example, a subject may report consuming a small container of low fat yogurt. Since low fat yogurt is available in several different "small" sizes, knowledge of the brand will often permit accurate determination of the amount consumed.

Although our goal is to update each food category at least annually, changes in the marketplace often determine priorities for updating. For example, we might update frozen entrees and ready-to-eat cereal several times during the year due to the influx of many new products and product reformulations in these catego-ries, whereas other categories that are not changing so rapidly might not be completely updated for several years, other than obtaining manufacturers' information on a few new products that appear on food intake records obtained from research subjects.

Not all brand name food categories are included in the Brand Database. If there are no significant differences among brands within a food category with respect to nutrient content or serving amount, that category is not included in the database. For example, brand name canned vegetables are not included in the database. The current version of the Brand Database includes 25 food categories.

Examples of the types of data fields in the Brand Database include: the product code, an arbitrary number assigned by NCC; the product name; a detailed description of the product; the name of the manufacturer and the product's Universal Product Code (UPC); the product cate-

Table I. A partial list of NCC edit limits for entering nutrient values

Nutrient	Food groups	Limit/100 g
Alcohol	Alcoholic beverages	16 g
	Other	0 g
β-carotene equivalents	Fruits/vegetables	7000 µg
	Margarine	1100 µg
	Other	800 µg
Calcium	Cheeses	1000 mg
	Other dairy, soups, sauces, candy	300 mg
	Cold cuts, seafood	120 mg
	Other	100mg
Cholesterol	Eggs	1700 mg
	Cold cuts, organ meats, shellfish	500 mg
	Animal fat, shortening	230 mg
	Dairy products	140 mg
	Meat, poultry, fish	100 mg
	Salad dressing, gravy	80 mg
	Bread, crackers	75 mg
	Other	20 mg

gory designation; density information, if available; package size; serving size; servings per package; ingredient listing; and preparation instructions. Nutrient values provided by the manufacturer, including label data as well as analytical or calculated data, are included in the database. Although analytical data are preferred for nutrient calculation, studies sometimes prefer label values for developing educational materials. Nutrient values obtained from other sources, such as from the literature, are also included. Sources of all information are indicated by reference codes, and the dates of receipt of the data at NCC are noted.

∎ Quality Control Procedures

Quality control procedures are critical for maintaining food and nutrient databases because the potential for error in dealing with hundreds of thousands of data ele-

ments is very great. Quality control procedures are designed both to reduce the potential for error and to increase the likelihood of identifying errors that occur inadvertently. The quality control procedures used by NCC for database maintenance are similar for the three databases described above. These procedures include the following: data evaluation based on established criteria; automated data entry whenever possible; comparison of new with pre-existing data; well-organized data entry screens; edit checks at the point of data entry; review of all manually entered data; checks for consistency among related data fields; and review of data fields within food groups for consistency with expected ranges of values.

When data are available from multiple sources, criteria are used to select the most appropriate values (9). Analytical data are generally preferred over calculated data; however, the quality of the analytic procedures used, the extent to which the data represent nationwide sampling and eating habits, and the currency of the data are also important considerations. USDA data are generally preferred over other data sources, and refereed publications are preferred to other publications, such as meeting proceedings or text books. If no published data are available, we occasionally use unpublished data, such as those provided by a reputable laboratory. Because missing nutrient values are calculated as zeros, they can result in significant underestimations of nutrient intakes (14,15). Therefore, when values are not available from any sources, we calculate or impute them using established procedures (3,15-17). A great deal of nutritionist effort is involved in imputing data to ensure that there are no missing values of nutritional significance in the database. Imputed values are replaced with analytical data when they become available.

Whenever possible, data entry is automated to enhance efficiency and reduce the potential for data entry errors. Most USDA data are now available in electronic form, and we are able to link many of our Nutrient Database entries with USDA food descriptions via the reference codes. We hope that manufacturers will eventually provide product information electronically, which would greatly reduce the potential for error. When database changes are required for an entire classification of foods, rather than for a single food item, a computer program is written to implement these global changes. For example, when the default for "margarine, regular stick, brand unknown" was changed to reflect more recent market research data, the new default code number was globally inserted into all recipes that included the default margarine.

Well-designed data entry screens can reduce the potential for error. Such screens may be formatted in a manner that simulates the format of the input documents, thus decreasing the amount of eye movement required by the data entry operator. An example of a well designed data entry screen is shown in Figure 3. Note that the different types of data are separated by labeled boxes, so specific data are easy to locate. The screen is not too crowded, which makes it easy to view.

To further reduce the potential for error, data are entered into the database in the format in which they are received. For example, nutrient values provided by the manufacturer may be entered into the Brand Database as amount per serving, amount per Reference Daily Intake (RDI), or amount per 100 g. Edit checks at the point of data entry permit immediate correction of keying errors. These checks flag data that are out of a given range or do not conform to other field specific restrictions. A partial list of edit limits used for entering nutrient values is presented in Table I. Since nutrient composition may vary substantially among food groups, the limits are usually food group specific. Another type of edit check is the flagging of incomplete data sets; for example, some data fields require that the reference codes be designated before the computer will accept the data.

All data entered manually into the database are cross-checked by a second database nutritionist. Data that are manually entered into the Nutrient Database are stored in a temporary file. Each database nutritionist is assigned a color that identifies the values entered by that individual; if changes are recommended by the second nutritionist, these changes must be verified by the nutritionist who originally entered the data. Only after verification of any changes are the new data accepted for posting to the permanent data file.

Reports are routinely generated comparing new data with previous data. For example, when a new version of the USDA Nutrient Database for Standard Reference is installed, a report of differences between the new and the pre-existing values is generated. Any unusually large differences are verified through

Table II. Examples of relational edits for the Nutrient Database

Compare:	With:	Acceptable difference:
Sum of proximates[a]	100 g	±5 g
4(pro) + 4(carbo) + 9(fat) + 7(alc)[b]	Total energy	±12%
Sum of amino acids	Total protein	−20%
Sum of fatty acids	Total fat	−5 to −20%[c]
Soluble fiber + insoluble fiber	Total dietary fiber	±10%

[a] proximates include protein, carbohydrate, fat, alcohol, water and ash
[b] pro=protein; carbo=carbohydrate; alc=alcohol
[c] acceptable difference depends on type of food

communication with USDA staff. Similarly, reports are generated to compare new data from manufacturers with any pre-existing data for the same product. If differences are noted, the manufacturer is contacted to determine if the differences are due to a reformulation of the product or to improved composition data. This information allows us to determine whether a new entry needs to be created or an existing entry updated. For this reason, we routinely request information for *all* food products marketed by a manufacturer, not just for the new products.

New versions of the Food and Nutrient Databases are generally released concurrently. During the four-week period prior to the release of the new versions, all modifications to the databases cease while the efforts of the database nutritionists are devoted to the various quality control procedures. Three types of quality control reports are generated prior to the release of the new versions. One type, the relational edits, are reports that examine consistency among different fields in the database (3). For example, appropriate relationships among nutrients in the Nutrient Database are verified by comparison of calculated values with expected values. The calculated values must fall within an acceptable range of the expected result. Table II lists a few examples of the 28 relational edits currently generated for verification of the Nutrient Database. Examples of relational edits for the Food Database include verification of rules such as: every recipe ingredient re-

ported by volume must have a density; and every food that can be described in terms of a geometric shape must have a solid density. There are currently 26 of these relational edits for the Food Database. Although many of these edits are invoked at the point of data entry, others must be verified before a new version of the Food Database is released.

Another type of quality control check conducted before the release of a new version of one of the databases is a review of computer listings of selected fields by food category. For example, vitamin A values for all processed cheeses in the Brand Database are scanned for any outliers which must then be verified from the original data source. This type of review is conducted for all nutrients in the Nutrient Database that are not included in the relational edit type of consistency checks shown in Table II. Many of the non-nutrient data fields are also subjected to this type of review. For example, the options for various food shapes in the Food Database are compared within food groups, and any differences must be justified.

A final quality control report that is generated before the release of a new version of the Food and Nutrient Databases is the calculation of nutrients for a test set of menus specifically designed to include a wide variety of foods, as well as all of the functionalities of the calculation software. These calculations are compared with calculations from the previous versions of the databases; any differences must be verified as the result of intended modifications to the databases or to the calculation software.

The three NCC databases are currently maintained separately, but a project is underway to integrate them into a single database management system. This will enhance our quality control by permitting us to automate more of the data entry than is now possible. For example, selected information from the Brand Database will be able to be automatically transferred to the Food Database rather than having to be manually entered.

■ Time-Related Database Maintenance and Quality Control Procedures

The need for comparability of dietary data over time requires use of time-related procedures for maintaining the Food and Nutrient Databases (18). Time-related database maintenance procedures permit recalculation of previously collected food intake data at any subsequent time to take advantage of new or improved data, including updates to both the Food Database and the Nutrient Database. Use of these procedures ensures comparability within long-term studies and among studies by eliminating the confounding due to using different databases and coding practices at different time periods.

Database changes that reflect real changes in the foods people are eating or in food preparation methods, must be differentiated from those changes that represent new or improved data for foods that have not changed. Time-related changes include most marketplace changes, such as new products, new serving sizes of existing products, product reformulations, and discontinued products. Changes in food preparation methods, such as increased trimming of fat from

meats or use of less salt and fat in recipes, may also represent time-related changes. Non-time-related database changes include such changes as new or improved analytic data, or better data for calculation of nutrient retentions in cooked or processed foods.

Procedures for time-related database maintenance require quality controls to ensure consistency among subsequent database versions. For every change made to the Food Database, the nutritionist must indicate whether or not the change is retroactive to previous versions of the database. The computer will not accept a change unless this information is entered. For example, improved data, such as more accurate values for raw to cooked conversion factors, are always retroactive to all previous versions of the Food Database. Edit checks at the point of data entry prevent making changes that would compromise consistency with previous versions of the database. For example, deletion of a food in the Food Database cannot be retroactive to previous versions because studies must be able to edit food intake records collected on previous versions.

New versions of the Food and Nutrient Databases are released approximately every six months. Time-related changes are handled differently for maintaining the Food Database, which is used for data collection and coding, than they are for maintaining the Nutrient Database, which is used for nutrient calculation. The current version of the Food Database must always reflect the current marketplace. Products no longer on the market must be deleted from the database to make sure that they are not selected when they are no longer available. For the Nutrient Database, however, foods must never be deleted, since a new version of this database may be used for calculating nutrients for dietary data collected at any time in the past. Discontinued foods continue to be updated to reflect improved nutrient data and the addition of new nutrients to the database.

Thus, for a long term study, many versions of the Food Database must be used for collecting and coding the data, whereas a single version of the Nutrient Database is used for calculating nutrients for the entire study. Whenever a new version of the Nutrient Database is released, dietary intake data for the entire study may be recalculated on that version. This will ensure that the most current data are used for nutrient calculations and that the calculations are comparable throughout the study.

To facilitate ongoing editing of dietary data for long-term studies, NCC has developed a Multi-Version Food Database that collapses all existing versions of the Food Database into a single database. Each subsequent release of the Multi-Version Food Database incorporates only those data which have changed since the previous release of the database. This eliminates the redundancy that exists among individual versions of the database. Use of the Multi-Version Food Database permits the editing of food intake data collected at any point in time. For example, NHANES III will have used 12 different versions of the Food Database for collecting and coding dietary data over the six years of the survey. Because all editing of dietary recalls must be done using the version on which the data were collected, the editing would be very cumbersome without the functionality of the Multi-Version Food Database.

All of the quality control procedures previously mentioned have been incorporated into the maintenance software for the Multi-Version Food Database. Careful adherence to time-related procedures for maintaining databases allows investigators to recalculate their dietary data automatically at any future time to take advantage not only of new nutrients and other food components that have been added to the Nutrient Database, but also of improved nutrient and non-nutrient data that have become available. These procedures make it possible to monitor trends in food and nutrient intakes over time, which is especially important for meeting the objectives of ongoing dietary surveys and long term research studies.

■ Acknowledgments

Funding to support this work has come primarily from the National Heart, Lung, and Blood Institute and the National Cancer Institute of the National Institutes of Health, Bethesda, MD, and from the National Center for Health Statistics, Centers for Disease Control and Prevention, Hyattsville, MD. Specific grants and contracts include the following: NIH/N01-HV-12903, NIH/RO1-HL-42165, NIH/R01-CA-36522, and CDC/200-89-7014.

■ References

(1) Dennis, B., Ernst, N., Hjortland, M., Tillotson, J., & Grambsch, V. (1980) *J. Am. Diet. Assoc.* **77,** 641-647

(2) Tillotson, J.L., Gorder, D.D., & Kassim, N. (1981) *J. Am. Diet. Assoc.* **78,** 235-240

(3) Sievert, Y.A., Schakel, S.F., & Buzzard, I.M. (1989) *Contr. Clin. Trials* **10,** 416-425

(4) Buzzard, I.M., Price, K.S., & Feskanich, D. (1991) in *The Diet History Method*, L. Kohlmeier (Ed.), Smith-Gordon and Company, London, pp. 39-51

(5) Feskanich, D., Buzzard, I.M., Welch, B.T., Asp, E.H., Dieleman, L.C., Chon, K.R., & Bartsch, G.E. (1988) *J. Am. Diet. Assoc.* **88,** 1263-1267

(6) Buzzard, I.M. (1989) in *Nutritional Status Assessment of the Individual*, The Food and Nutrition Press, Inc., Trumbell, pp. 87-98

(7) Feskanich, D., Sielaff, B.H., Chon, K., & Buzzard, I.M. (1989) *Comp. Meth. Prog. Biomed.* **30,** 47-57

(8) McDowell, M., Briefel, R.R., Warren, R.A., Buzzard, I.M., Feskanich, D., & Gardner, S.H. (1990) in *Proceedings of the 14th National Nutrient Databank Con-*

ference, The CBORD Group, Inc., Ithaca, NY, pp. 125-131

(9) Schakel, S.F., Sievert, Y.A., & Buzzard, I. M. (1988) *J. Am. Diet. Assoc.* **88,** 1268-1271.

(10) US Department of Agriculture (1993) *Nutrient Database for Standard Reference,* Release 10, USDA, Washington, DC

(11) US Department of Agriculture (1993) *Nutrient Data Base for Individual Food Intake Surveys*, Release 6, National Technical Information Service, Springfield, VA

(12) US Department of Agriculture (1976–) *Composition of Foods: Raw, Processed, Prepared*, USDA Agric. Handbook No. 8 series, USDA, Washington, DC

(13) Gorman, B. (1990) *Prep. Foods New Prod. Ann.* **159,** 16-18, 47-52

(14) Buzzard, I.M., Price, K.S., & Warren, R.A. (1991) *Am. J. Clin. Nutr.* **54,** 7-9

(15) Posati, L. (1985) in *Proceedings of the Tenth National Nutrient Databank Conference,* National Technical Information Services, Springfield, VA, pp. 124-133

(16) Schakel, S.F., Warren, R.A., & Buzzard, I.M. (1990) in *Proceedings of the 14th National Nutrient Databank Conference,* The CBORD Group, Inc., Ithaca, NY, pp. 155-165

(17) Westrich, B.J., Buzzard, I.M., Schakel, S.F., & McGovern, P.G. (1993) in *Proceedings of 18th National Nutrient Databank Conference*, Washington, ILSI Press, p.276

(18) Buzzard, I.M. (1991) in *Proceedings of the 16th National Nutrient Databank Conference,* The CBORD Group, Inc., Ithaca, NY, pp. 73-77

Construction of a Database of Inherent Bioactive Compounds in Food Plants

Andrew D. Walker, Roger Preece

Institute of Food Research, Computing Group,
Norwich Research Park, Colney Lane, Norwich, NR4 7UA, UK

Jenny A. Plumb, Roger Fenwick, Bob K. Heaney

Institute of Food Research,
Food and Molecular Biochemistry Department,
Norwich Research Park, Colney Lane, Norwich, NR4 7UA, UK

Numerous incidences have been recorded where naturally-occurring dietary components have contributed to chronic and acute illness and occasionally to human fatalities. The causative agents, termed "natural (or inherent) toxicants", are commonly present in food plants in order to provide protection against fungal, insect and herbivore attack. Perhaps the best known example of the effects of such a toxicant is the severe gastrointestinal and neurological disturbances observed following consumption of damaged, green or sprouted potatoes containing high levels of glycoalkaloids. Other classes of compounds with well-defined physiological effects include glucosinolates (in brassica vegetables and condiments), lectins (in legumes), isoflavones (in soya), cyanogenic glycosides (in cassava and legumes) and psoralens (in parsnip and celery).

In order to study the varying biological effects of these natural toxicants (or of naturally occurring non-nutritional compounds offering protection against heart disease or cancers), it is essential that the available information on the content of these bioactive compounds in foods is readily accessible to workers in the plant science, food science, nutrition and clinical areas. Although databases exist which contain data on the nutrient compositions of foods, readily accessible/critically evaluated data on the occurrence and levels of inherent biologically active compounds in foods is not yet available. Researchers at the Institute of Food Research (IFR) have designed and are currently compiling a database to include information on occurrence, levels and factors affecting levels of natural toxicants, anti-nutrients and protective factors in foods.

The database, constructed using the *ORACLE* Relational Database Management System (RDBMS) (1), provides information on the levels of specific compounds in food plants, on the country of origin, the plant part analyzed, any preparation methods used; information on varieties and sample numbers is included together with full citations for all references used. The relational data model used can be used to construct the database using other RDBMS. The system was originally developed on a DEC VAX minicomputer and has been successfully installed on an IBM PC 486 compatible.

Primary literature searches on specific natural toxicant occurrence and factors affecting levels have been carried out using CD ROM databases (e.g. *Agricola* and *Food Science and Technology Abstracts*) and are routinely updated using *Current Contents* on disk. Collected references are read and any relevant references cited therein are additionally obtained for use as a secondary source of data. Reprints describing occurrence data for a number of naturally-occurring toxicants are critically assessed for data quality according to defined criteria. These criteria, developed at IFR after wide consultation, contain guidelines on acceptability of analytical method, in sampling, unequivocally-identified plant species, etc. Only data which satisfy these criteria are entered into the database.

Currently, eight compound classes (covering 65 compounds) including glycoalkaloids, glucosinolates, psoralens (furocoumarins), alkenylbenzenes, saponins and hydrazines have been entered. One hundred and twenty foods have been coded giving a total number of records of about 1100.

Together with the records from individual references, further fields have been entered including a thesaurus of alternative compound names, a thesaurus of food names, and a textual "comments" screen containing information on the way in which levels may change as a result of processing, storage, cooking, agronomic and environmental conditions etc. All references relevant to this field have been entered. Output screens have been developed linking food name, food part, preparation method and compound name. The mean levels of each compound together with maximum and minimum levels are calculated from all the data in the database assigned a satisfactory quality code, and are presented with supporting information on the number of records and references used to obtain these data.

Planned developments include expansion of the number of foods and compounds within the database, inclusion of data relating to toxicological effects, and the setting up of a European database on non-nutrient composition of foods.

▮ Acknowledgment

This project has been funded by the Ministry of Agriculture, Fisheries and Food.

▮ Reference

(1)   *ORACLE 6* The ORACLE Corporation UK Ltd, Bracknell, UK

Copyright, Food Industry and Food Safety Considerations

This last Session of the Conference was chaired by Professor Geoff M. Wilson of the University of New South Wales, and commenced with a keynote address entitled *International and Australian Copyright Considerations in Data and Data Compilations* by S. Ricketson. This was followed by papers on *Non-nutrient Databases for Foods* by K. Louekari (presented by V. Piironen), *Food Composition Databases in the Food Industry* by O. de Rham, *The Databases of the Australian National Food Authority*, by J. Lewis and S. Brooke-Taylor, *Data Considerations for Nutritional Labeling in the United States*, by J. Tanner, and *Functional Foods for Specific Health Use - the Needs for Compositional Data*, by K. Shinohara. These papers are all published in this Section.

International and Australian Copyright Considerations in Data and Data Compilations

Sam Ricketson

Faculty of Law, Monash University, Wellington Road, Clayton,
Vic 3168, Australia

Copyright protection of data and data compilations both in Australia and internationally is both qualified and incomplete. The paper reviews the basic principles of copyright, and then considers their specific application to data, tables and compilations. The principal domestic law examined is the Copyright Act 1968 (Cth) and the case law arising under this Act and in jurisdictions with similar common law backgrounds, such as the USA and UK. The principal international instrument considered is the Berne Convention for the Protection of Literary and Artistic Works which is currently in the process of revision. The paper examines the scope of protection for data and tables and compilations of data, with particular reference to the requirements for protection, the exclusive rights obtained and the question of entitlements. Brief consideration is also given to non-copyright protection which may be available.

U nlike other statutory intellectual property rights, such as patents, designs and trade marks, Australian copyright law, which is contained in the *Copyright Act* 1968, is not dependent upon a system of registration or compliance with any other kind of formality, such as the giving of notice or the deposit of copies. Protection arises once a work is "made", that is, once it is reduced to some kind of "material form". This form may be visible or invisible (1). Apart from this, all that needs to be established is that the author of the work is qualified for protection in Australia by reason of her nationality or residence status (2) as extended by the international conventions to which Australia is party (3), or by reason of first publication in Australia (4) or in another country which is party to the same international conventions as Australia (5). Protection is available to a wider range of productions under the general classifications of "works" and "subject matter other than works". The first covers "literary, dramatic, musical and artistic works", which in turn embrace a disparate collection of subcategories such as books, plays, paintings, tables and compilations, computer programs, photographs, buildings, choreographic works and sculptures (6). These are protected so long as they are "original" (7) (see further below). The second covers material of a more "industrial" character, namely sound recordings, films, broadcasts and published editions of works (8). Copyright protection confers quite extensive "exclusive" rights on the copyright owner. Of these, the most important are the reproduction, adaptation, public performance and broadcasting rights (2). Duration of protection is also extensive, the basic rule being that, in the case of works, it applies for the life of the author of the work plus 50 years (9). In the case of subject matter other than works, the basic term is shorter (50 years from first publication or making).

Copyright in Relation to Databases

In essence, databases are simply a particular species of the broader genus of tables and compilations which have long been the subject of protection under Anglo-Australian copyright law. Thus, the definition of "literary work" in subsection 10 (1) of the *Copyright Act* 1968 includes

> "... (a) a table, or compilation, expressed in words, figures or symbols (whether or not in a visible form); ..."

The words in brackets seem to be an express legislative indication that tables and compilations expressed in electronic form are comprehended within the meaning of literary work and this is confirmed in the Explanatory Memorandum to the *Copyright Amendment Bill* 1984 which states that it was intended to include computerized data banks which might not be expressed in any visible form of notation (10).

However, it is not the case that all tables and compilations (however expressed) are automatically protected under the *Copyright Act* 1968. As with all other works, it is still necessary that the table or compilation in question be an "original" literary work in order to qualify for protection (11). Anglo-Australian copyright law has never placed a particularly high premium on the requirement of originality in comparison with other jurisdictions where some level of personal intellectual creation is often required (12). There is no requirement of novelty or inventiveness, such as are necessary in patent or design law. All that is required is that the alleged author has contributed skill, time and effort to the creation of the alleged work and that the latter is not the result of copying from elsewhere (13). This approach has a liberating effect in many instances, in so far as it frees courts from the invidious task of comparative aesthetic judgment in considering the eligibility for protection of works such as the pulp novel, the hackneyed dramatic script and the amateur painter's daub. It has also provided protection to a vast array of subject- matter that would otherwise have little claim to be "literary" or "artistic" but which nonetheless embody the results of the application of high levels of intellectual and/or physical effort on the part of their creators. Early instances of this included railway timetables (14), anthologies of poetry (15), catalogues of merchandise (16) and betting coupons (17); more recently, protection has been accorded to subject-matter as diverse as the forms of a card index accounting system (18), a table of scores and winning symbols for a poker machine (19), computer programs in source code (20) and engineering and design drawings (21). Some of the above would properly be classified as tables or com- pilations and, while the protection accorded to them as "original literary works" can be readily seen as an appropriate safeguard against third parties who would "reap where they have not sown", such protection nonetheless can lead to difficulties.

The essence of a table or compilation is that it comprises a mass of raw data or information, on which the tabulator or compiler has then imposed a particular order or arrangement. So far as the individual items of data are concerned, if these enjoy copyright protection this is entirely separate from the protection which may subsist in the table or compilation (see further below): what is protected in the case of the table or compilation is simply the element of arrangement, selection or ordering that has gone into its construction. This is certainly an extension of the everyday meaning of "authorship" and, for this reason, the courts have not been prepared to confer protection on all tables or compilations. Even if the unfair competition rationale of copyright protection is admitted, the courts have still required that a particular level of skill in compilation,

selection and arrangement be displayed (22).

Where the skill of selection and arrangement requires considerable literary knowledge and taste, as in the case of an anthology of poetry, the judgment that the resultant compilation is an original literary work is not a difficult one to make. Nonetheless, it is clear that the element of compilation must be clearly identifiable, if not substantial, for protection to be accorded under this heading. Thus, Anglo-Australian courts have often been reluctant to extend protection to "mere lists", where the skill applied has been simply that of gathering and presenting items of information in a fairly mechanical way. For instance, in the famous High Court decision of *Victoria Park Racing & Recreation Grounds Co Ltd v Taylor* (23), it was held that copyright did not subsist in information posted by proprietors of a race course inside the course as to the names and numbers of the starting horses, the horses scratched, the numbers of the winners and so on. In the words of Latham CJ, the reason for this was that:

> "The law of copyright does not operate to give any person an exclusive right to state or describe particular facts" (24).

In other words, the element of selection and compilation involved in this case was so small that to grant protection would have been equivalent to protecting the raw data itself. There are a number of other Australian and English decisions to similar effect (25), although this is an area where there is room for judicial disagreement (26), and there are a number of decisions to be found in common law jurisdictions where only minimal quantities of selection and arrangement have been held capable of attracting copyright protection (27). In this regard, it is worth noting that the courts have generally been reluctant to separate the mental skill and effort involved in ascertaining or calculating a particular item of information, such as a wager on the outcome of a football match, from the skill and effort which is applied to the actual presentation and ordering of that item in the final table or compilation for which protection is sought — chronological list of football fixtures (28); weekly fixed-odds betting coupon (29); score table used on poker machine (30). The effect of this is to protect the mental and physical effort involved in collecting data just as much as the effort devoted to ordering and presenting it. Thus, if a party wishes to use that information for his own purposes, he must gather it himself, rather than take advantage of the plaintiff's efforts in compiling it. In the colorful words of a nineteenth century judge speaking in relation to a roads directory, the defendant must "count the milestones" himself (31). On the other hand, it should be stressed that this protection of the data in a plaintiff's table or compilation is parasitic, in the sense that there must still be some element of tabulation or compilation which has been imposed upon that data by the plaintiff: there can be no protection just for raw unprocessed data and the effort that has gone into their collection.

In this regard, there may be now be a distinction between US and Anglo-Australian copyright law. In a recent decision, the US Supreme Court has made it clear that it will not give protection to "simple" compilations of data, where the elements of compilation lack the necessary degree of "personal intellectual creation" on the part of the compiler. On this basis, an alphabetical list of telephone subscribers was held incapable of attracting copyright protection (32).

By contrast, Australian and English courts still appear satisfied by a lower level of intellectual input by the compiler (33).

Copyright as Applied to Food Databases

How are these principles to be applied to food databases or compilations? The immediate, and simple, answer is that the above principles apply to these kinds of compilations in exactly the same way as they apply to compilations in general. Thus, it will be necessary to show that (a)

effort has gone into the collection of the food data contained in the table or compilation, and (b) that some identifiable skill and effort has been applied to the organization and presentation of that data, that is, that it is not simply an undigested mass of "raw information". Given the general character of food data compilations and tables, this necessary element of arrangement will usually be present. In this regard, and subject to one qualification noted below, it should not matter that the database is in electronic form, as required for computer use and storage, or whether it is in the form of "hard copy", whether printed or in microfiche or microfilm. So long as the data are presented with some minimum degree of tabulation, ordering or collation, Australian copyright law should protect the particular format in which the database compiler has chosen to present the data. While the minimum of skill required may not be high, it should nonetheless be remembered that the "authorial" quality that is protected is that of tabulation or compilation and the protection thereby given to the data is to the data so tabulated or compiled, not to the data themselves.

The qualification referred to above concerns data compilations and tables stored in electronic form in, or for use in, a computer or computer network. It is a requirement of the *Copyright Act* 1968 that each protected work should have an "author" and, further, that this author should be a human being (34). This is by contrast with other subject matter protected under the Act (sound recordings, cinematographic films, broadcasts and published editions) where protection is given to the maker, broadcaster or publisher (as the case may be) and where these persons may be bodies corporate (35).

The requirement of human authorship for compilations may lead to difficulty in the case of those stored in electronic form. It is possible, perhaps probable, that in such cases the necessary element of tabulation or compilation will not have been supplied by a human operator, but by a separate computer program that has classified and organized the data in accordance with the directions of the human operator. While the computer program itself may have a clearly identifiable human author, it may be more difficult in such a case to identify the necessary element of human authorship in the compilation which has been constructed with the use of that program. In the recent British *Copyright, Designs and Patents Act* 1988, this potential difficulty has been overcome by a specific provision dealing with "computer-generated" works:

"In the case of a literary, dramatic, musical or artistic work which is computer-generated, the author shall be taken to be the person by whom the arrangements necessary for the creation of the work are undertaken"(36).

While this provision is of general application to all works created by computer, for example, computer-aided design drawings, in the case of an electronic database it would mean that the person who made the arrangements for the collection of the data, their storage in the computer and the use of any compilatory program for the organization of the data would be regarded as the author (and therefore first owner of copyright).

In the absence of such a provision, the Australian copyright law is not so certain, but I would suggest that a similar result would probably be reached by an Australian court faced with the question. Thus, it can be argued that there will still be the need for considerable human input into the construction of an electronic database, even where a computer program is used for this purpose. Decisions as to the kind of data to be stored, the method of organization to be adopted and the mode of retrieval will still need to be made by a human operator and the appropriate instructions given to the computer to achieve these results. By way of rough analogy, the use of the program can be seen as a tool or aid in this process, in much the same way as a typewriter, word processor or camera can be seen as aids in the creation of other kinds of literary and artistic works (37).

Greater difficulties, however, may arise where there are a number of persons involved in the creation of the compilation. Rarely will it ever be just one or two persons who have contributed to the making of a database: there will usually be a team of many persons who have participated in the project. While Australian copyright law readily recognizes the concept of joint authorship (38), there may simply be too many persons to make this workable, particularly when questions of ownership and duration of protection arise (39). Furthermore, many databases are continuing productions that are added to on a regular basis, for example, by updating or revising entries, incorporating new data, and providing different kinds of methods of presenting and analyzing those data. These additions to the database may come from one source, or may come from many, for example, where the database is networked and may be added to from any station on the network. In these circumstances, the copyright status of a person who makes one or two of these ongoing entries into the database is far from clear. Problems of this kind indicate that the protection of electronic databases as original literary works does not sit easily with the traditional concepts of authorship and originality that apply under the present Copyright Act. A provision of the kind contained in the British Act given above would therefore assist in assigning authorship ownership to one party alone, namely the person who makes the arrangements for the construction of the database.

Ownership Issues. The determination of authorship questions in relation to a database is of crucial significance in determining the important issue of who owns the copyright in the database. Not only is there a requirement of human authorship for the subsistence of copyright under the Australian Act, but there is a general rule that the author is also the first owner of that copyright. This situation is modified in the case of employee authors, where the ownership vests in the employer if the database has been made in the course of their employment (40). In other cases, it will be necessary for the would-be copyright owner to receive an assignment (or transfer) in writing of that copyright from the author or authors (41). This will be of vital significance where the compilation is prepared by a third party under some contractual arrangement. If the data are provided by A, and B then prepares the compilation, in the absence of an express assignment B will own the copyright in the resultant compilation. Where there are multiple authors who are not A's employees, it will be necessary to have separate assignments from each so far as their contributions to the compilation are concerned.

Protection of Data Used in Data Compilations

The above discussion has been concerned only with the question of copyright protection for the data compilation itself. What of the data that are used in the compilation? The answer to this depends on the nature and quality of the data in question. However, the following general propositions can be stated.

- There can be no copyright protection for "simple" facts on their own, for example, a statistic, chemical formula, short verbal description, or the like. It is possible that data in any of these forms could form part of a food database. However, copyright law has always refused to protect facts or items of an insubstantial nature. Thus, there is a series of old English cases in which it was held that copyright did not subsist in the titles of books (42) and, in one celebrated later case, the Privy Council denied protection to the title of a song, "The Man who Broke the Bank at Monte Cristo" (43). More recently, a New Zealand court has held that there was no copyright in the words "Opportunity Knocks" as the title of a television program (44) and a British court refused protection for the word "Exxon" (45). The unspoken reason for these decisions seems to be an application of the de minimis principle, namely that such items are too insubstantial to be protected as literary works in their own right (46). An alternative view is that they are lacking in the necessary degree of originality (47), although this may be another way of saying the same thing. On the other hand, originality, in the sense of skill and research, was not lacking in the choice of the word "Exxon" in the Exxon case, and the reason given by the English Court of Appeal for denying it protection as a literary work was that, in itself, it conveyed neither "information and instruction, [n]or pleasure, in the form of literary enjoyment" (48). Accordingly, the storing of a title or name in a database will not generally raise any copyright issue, and the same would be true with respect to single items of data in relation to food and food composition.

- While single items of data may not constitute original literary works in their own right, it is possible that a combination or assembly of data relating to a particular matter could attract protection as a table or compilation on the same principles discussed above. An example might be a table which analyzes the nutritional content of a particular food (49). If this were so, it would be necessary for the compiler of a database who wished to include that table within his own compilation to seek permission from its authors. From some of the examples I have seen, it is possible that this has not happened in many situations involving the compilation of food composition databases, and strictly this would involve an infringement of the copyright in any separate tables or compilations of data that were used without permission (50).

- It is also possible that some individual items of data will be capable of attracting protection in their own right if they are more "substantial" in size than those referred to in the first paragraph. It is impossible to indicate what the quantum required here will be, but, on occasion, the courts have been prepared to protect works such as short poems, newspaper summaries, a series of numbers, and abridgments or abstracts of longer works, on the basis that they displayed sufficient original effort on the part of the alleged author. It is not clear how relevant this head of protection might be to the compilers of food databases, but possibilities would include written analyses and summaries of the nutritional components and value of particular foods, abstracts of longer papers or reports, items of explanatory material, and so on. Once these works have reached a certain length and go beyond the simple factual items referred to in the first paragraph, the possibility of protection will arise and the permission of the owner of that copyright will need to be sought in respect of any use made of it in a database.

The Scope of Copyright Protection in Relation to Data and Data Compilations

As noted above, the exclusive rights conferred on owners of copyright in literary works under the *Copyright Act* 1968 are quite extensive. It is worth saying something further about the more important of these rights.

Reproduction. This is the most basic right of the copyright owner, and essentially gives protection against copying or derivation. The latter need not be literal or "word-for-word": it is sufficient if the copy is substantially similar or only "colorably" different from the original. It is also unnecessary for the copy to be in the same medium as the original: a printed work may be copied in any "material" form (51), and this would include storage in the hard disk of a computer, on a CD ROM, on film or microfiche, or magnetic tape. Nor is it necessary for the whole of the protected work to be taken: under

subsection 14(1) of the *Copyright Act 1968*, it is enough if a "substantial" part is appropriated. "Substantiality" in this context is not simply a reference to quantity: Anglo-Australian courts have always stressed that the quality of what is taken is just as important in determining whether a substantial part of a work has been taken (52). Thus, courts will look at the significance or importance of the part taken in relation to the work as a whole, and it may not matter that a relatively short section is taken.

In the case of databases, the requirement of substantiality can give rise to problems. As noted above, the protected aspect of such works is the element of selection and arrangement that has gone into their construction, and does not extend to the individual items that make up the compilation. The latter may enjoy copyright protection in their own right, or not at all, as the case may be, but this is beside the point. If the allegation is that X has reproduced part of the database of Y, this claim will only be good if that act has been done in relation to a substantial part of that database. Taking individual items of data, or even a number of items, will usually not be enough: liability will only arise where a substantial part of the arrangement or compilation of data is taken. This may provide a severe limitation on the exploitation of their rights by the owners of copyright in databases, as is well illustrated by the English case of *Warwick Films v Eisinger* (53) . The compilation here comprised edited transcripts of the trials of Oscar Wilde, but, although the defendant had taken considerable extracts from the transcripts (in which the plaintiff had no rights), these portions did not contain any of the plaintiff's editorial changes or accompanying commentary. Accordingly, as they now lacked the element of selection and arrangement which the plaintiff had supplied in his compilation, they did not constitute a substantial part of it (54). The same point was also made in *Ladbroke (Football) Ltd v William Hill (Football) Ltd* (55), a case involving a claim for copyright in the layout of a football coupon. On the question of whether the appellants had reproduced a substantial part thereof, Lord Pearce said:

"Whether a part is substantial must be decided by its quality rather than its quantity. The reproduction of a part which by itself has no originality will not normally be a substantial part of the copyright and therefore will not be protected. For that which would not attract copyright except by reason of its collocation will, when robbed of that collocation, not be a substantial part of the copyright and therefore the courts will not hold its reproduction to be an infringement" (56).

In crude terms, the principle here can be expressed as follows with respect to databases: it will only be the taking of the "processed" data that will attract copyright liability, in the absence of any other copyright that might subsist separately in the data itself. Nevertheless, this principle may require modification in certain circumstances. As noted above, an important part of a compilation may lie in the skill and judgment exercised by the maker of the compilation in deciding what to include. If this is the case, then the taking of several items that would not otherwise form a substantial part of the compilation may well constitute an infringement of the compilation as extended to this element of initial selection (57). In such a case, the defendant has helped himself to the efforts and skill of the plaintiff, rather than going back to the data himself and making his own selection. In this respect, however, the technical and storage capabilities of computer databases may be a disadvantage so far as the availability of protection is concerned. It is now possible for these to be comprehensive within their particular field and this, indeed, may be the essence of their commercial appeal. Thus, if a database contains every item of information relevant to a particular field, there can be no element of selection that is infringed by the taking of any number of these items. It will only be if the arrangement or collocation of these items within the database is also taken that any question of the taking of a substantial part of the overall compilation will arise. In the case of food data, unless the individual items are capable of copyright protection, there may be no infringing act on the part of a person who simply takes the data and stores it in her own database where it is used with that person's data management system.

Adaptation. A further exclusive right of a copyright owner is the right to adapt the work. "Adaptation" in this context covers a wide range of transformations of a work, such as dramatizations of non-dramatic works, fictionalizations of dramatic works, arrangements of musical works and translations from one language to another (58). Following amendments made in 1984, "adaptation" now includes a different version of a computer program (whether or not in the language, code or notation in which the program was originally expressed). None of these transformations seem apt to cover what might be done with data or a database by a third party, for example, where the latter takes one or both and then puts them in his own database where they are organized and used in accordance with an entirely different data management program. Although it is possible that the items of data and/or the database may constitute original literary works in their own right (see above), the adaptation right is simply not relevant in the present context unless one or the other of these works can also be regarded as a computer program. On the other hand, the reproduction right may still be relevant here, and the initial act of storage may constitute an infringing act, irrespective of what is done after this with the data or data compilation.

Public Performance, Broadcasting, Cable Diffusion. The exclusive rights of the copyright owner also extend to authorizing the public performance or display of the work, broadcasting it, and, in limited circumstances, transmitting it to subscribers to a diffusion or wire service (59). All these acts, together with the reproduction right discussed above, are relevant to the way in which data may be retrieved and distributed. In this regard, there is a marked contrast between electronic and "traditional" or hard copy databases, where the common means of retrieval is for the user to turn the pages or shuffle the cards — acts that clearly do not involve an infringement of the copyright owner's rights. With an electronic database or data stored in electronic form, however, the processes of transmitting or communicating data to the user may in themselves involve infringements of copyright, while the actual retrieval of this data by the user may involve other kinds of infringing acts.

Distribution of Data to Users

There are three basic ways in which this can occur in the case of electronic databases: through the supply of external storage devices to the user, such as CD-ROMs; transmission by television signals; and transmission over wire, such as cable or telephone lines. The first of these, sometimes referred to as "off-line distribution", clearly involves the making and distribution of "copies" of the database and of any works stored in the database. This is on the basis that the storage devices can be regarded as "reproductions in a material form" of any protected works that are stored in this fashion.

As to the second, television transmission as a means of disseminating information in computer databases is apparently not common, although "teletext" or "videotext" systems using television signals have clear potential for expansion. From a copyright point of view, however, communication of data in this way will clearly be an infringement of the exclusive broadcasting rights in any protected works comprised in the transmission (60).

To date, the third method of transmission by wire or cable remains the most common means of "on-line" distribution of data stored in computer systems. In so far as this involves the dissemination of protected works, the provisions of the *Copyright Act* are reasonably clear. One of the exclusive rights of copyright owners of original works is the right to transmit those works to "subscribers to a diffusion service" (61). This is a distinct activity to that of broadcasting, which means transmission by means of wireless telegraphy (62). By contrast, transmission to subscribers to a diffusion service entails the distribution of "broadcast or other matter (whether provided by the person operating the service or other persons) over wires, or over other paths provided by a material substance, to the premises of subscribers to the service" (63). The latter definition appears apt to cover the circumstances under which the information from many computer databases is distributed to users. The latter may well be "subscribers to a service" within the terms of the legislation, namely through a service agreement with the owner of the database, and will be receiving the data via visual display units or printers in their own premises. This would probably not extend to networks within particular institutions or networks provided on some kind of co-operative basis.

Retrieval of Data by Users

Irrespective of whether data are transmitted to users by off-line or on-line communication, the question still arises as to whether the retrieval and use of those data by the user constitute an infringing act in relation to any copyright work embodied in that material. Basically, there are two ways in which retrieval may occur: through the display of data on a visual display unit or through the production of printed or other "hard" copies.

Visual Display. There are two ways in which this activity may be analyzed under the *Copyright Act* 1968. The first is that the visual display is a public performance of the work displayed (64). The second is that this is a reproduction in a material form of that work (65). The two are by no means mutually exclusive.

*Public Performance.*This does not require performance by a human actor or performer. Under subsection 27(1), a reference to "performance" includes "any mode of visual or aural presentation, whether the presentation is by the operation of wireless telegraphy apparatus, by the exhibition of a cinematographic film, by the use of a record or by any other means; ..." It is further provided that:

> "Where visual images or sounds are displayed or emitted by any receiving apparatus to which they are conveyed by the transmission of electromagnetic signals (whether over paths provided by a material substance or not), the operation of any apparatus by which the signals are transmitted, directly or indirectly to the receiving apparatus shall be deemed not to constitute performance ... but, in so far as the display or emission of images or sounds constitutes a performance, ... the performance ... shall be deemed to be effected by the operation of the receiving apparatus" (66).

It therefore seems reasonable to regard the display of protected works on the visual display unit of a computer terminal as the "performance" of those works by means of a receiving apparatus (where the work is communicated by cable or some other material path) or "by any other means" (where the work is retrieved off-line).

The next question is whether the act of visual display occurs "in public". No definition of this term is to be found in the Act (save for section 28 which excludes performances given exclusively in the course of educational instruction and section 46 which provides an exclusion for the visual display of broadcast data where this is done in premises where persons reside or sleep), and it therefore remains a matter for judicial interpretation. Essentially, the courts have adopted a restrictive approach, confining non-public performances to those in the domestic or quasi-domestic sphere (for an extreme interpretation of "quasi-domestic" in the case of nurses and doctors living within the confines of Guy's Hospital, see *Duck v Bates* (67). Thus, the fact that the "audience" is limited in some way, for example, to those who pay an admission fee or who are members of a club or association,

will normally be irrelevant (68). The prime consideration in determining whether a particular performance is "in public" is the character of the audience: whether this is the type of audience which can be described as the copyright owner's audience in the sense that the owner would look to deriving financial benefit from authorizing a performance of his work before it. In the present context, it is relevant to note a significant New South Wales decision in which this principle has been applied to the case of free in-house movies that were offered as part of the services to guests at a motel (69). There was clearly a market there for the display of such films and the persons who viewed them were members of the copyright owners' public, even if they viewed the films in the privacy of their individual rooms. Another decision of the Federal Court of Australia has held that there was a public performance where video films were played to a small group in a bank as part of an in-house training program (70). By the same token, where users of a computer database retrieve information on a visual display unit, they are displaying or performing in public any protected work which appears on the screen and it should not matter whether the unit is situated in a publicly accessible place such as a library or in the office of an individual user.

Reproduction in a Material Form. The other alternative is that visual display is a reproduction in material form of the work displayed. However, it is more difficult to reach a firm conclusion here. There can be no doubt that, unlike storage of a work in a computer hard disk or CD-ROM, in this instance the work is perfectly visible and comprehensible to the human eye. Furthermore, it is often in a page format that is similar to that of any printed version of the work. On the other hand, the form of fixation is transitory and only lasts so long as the human user desires to have the work displayed on the screen. In this regard, reference can be made to the use of the word "storage" in the definition of "material form" in subsection 10(1) of the *Copyright Act* 1968.

"Storage" implies some degree of permanency and it seems a misuse of language to describe the transitory display of a work on a visual display unit as a form of storage. On the other hand, the definition of "material form" is inclusive only and it is therefore arguable that "material form" can embrace other less permanent forms of fixation. Thus, in an early case under the *Copyright Act* 1911, it was held that a tableau vivant representing a cartoon from Punch Magazine was a reproduction in a material form of the cartoon (71).

There is no reason under the present Act why visual display should not simultaneously constitute both the act of performance in public and the act of reproduction in a material form. As a matter of principle, however, it is obviously undesirable that the one act should give rise to two distinct grounds of liability and it would therefore be advantageous for the Act to indicate which one should apply to the exclusion of the other. In this regard, it is of interest to note the recent recommendation of the Commonwealth Copyright Law Reform Committee that the Act should be amended to make it clear that screen displays do not constitute *either* a reproduction in material form or a public performance of works stored in computer memory (72)

Other Forms of Storage. This expression is used simply by way of contrast to visual display and is intended to cover all other forms in which data may be retrieved, including hard-copy printout, facsimile reproduction or by way of transfer into other devices for internal or external storage. The relevant right here is the reproduction right, and as a general proposition it would appear that any acts of this kind will involve an infringement of this right. However, a question remaining to be resolved in each instance will be whether a substantial part of the data or database has been reproduced, and the matters that are relevant to this have already been discussed above.

Some Practical Issues. In the light of the above, it will be clear that many uses of the data contained in a protected database will be controlled by the owner of the copyright in that database and that permission will therefore need to be sought for the use or uses that is sought to be made of this data. As there is no registration system for copyright in Australia, it may not always be easy to identify the copyright owner for the purposes of obtaining permission. Nonetheless, this does not excuse the intending user from seeking out the copyright owner, and it will be dangerous to proceed in the absence of permission. As the use of data in protected databases is not covered by any compulsory license scheme under the *Copyright Act* 1968, there is no clearly established benchmark for the level of fees or royalties that will be payable for the intended use. This will be a matter for negotiation between the copyright owner and user, although in practice there may be clearly accepted levels of royalty that exist in particular fields. In each instance, it will be necessary to comply with any other conditions that are laid down by the copyright owner, for example, limitations on the amount that may be used, the need for acknowledgment of source, and the like.

At the same time, it should be noted that some database copyright owners do not object to appropriate use being made of their data where this is clearly in the public interest. This would seem to be the case under the *Australian Food Standards Code*, Section A, Clause 13, where the reproduction or adaptation of Australian food composition data from the government database is expressly permitted for certain purposes, such as for display on food labels for advertising and information purposes. From the copyright perspective, this kind of permitted use should give rise to no problems, so long as any specified limitations or conditions on the use are observed (In the event that they are not, this will be a breach of the license given and therefore an infringement of copyright).

International Aspects of Copyright Protection

Several matters need to be noted here: first, the protection of Australian data and databases abroad; secondly, the protection of foreign data and databases in Australia; and thirdly, some brief comparative treatment of developments that are occurring in other countries with respect to increased protection of these kinds of subject matter.

Protection Abroad and in Australia

Australia is a party to the *Berne Convention for the Protection of Literary and Artistic Works* which now binds over 105 countries. These include almost all of the important developed countries and a great majority of developing and former socialist states (the separate states of the Commonwealth of Independent Nations are significant exceptions, but are probably still bound to a lesser extent through their membership of another international convention, the *Universal Copyright Convention*).

The effect of the *Berne Convention* is to accord protection to Australian works in all other countries which are members of the Convention, and to extend similar protection here to works that originate from those countries. So far as Australia is concerned, this is done through regulations made under the *Copyright Act* 1968, the effect of which is to extend protection in Australia to works with authors who are nationals of these other countries or to works which have been first published in one of those countries (73). In broad terms, this means that a British or French database will be entitled to protection in Australia, in the same way as an Australian database, and this will also be the case for individual items of data that are capable of being treated as separate copyright works (see above). A similar position will also apply so far as the protection of Australian data and databases in these other countries is concerned. This occurs without the need for any formalities, such as registration, although in the USA registration will provide the foreign copyright owner with certain procedural advantages that may make it easier for her to enforce her rights in that country. Some differences in treatment may arise from country to country, depending on the level of originality or intellectual creation that is required for protection, but, in any event, it is a fundamental requirement of the Convention that foreign and local works are to be treated in exactly the same way (the principle of "national treatment": *Berne Convention*, article 5(1)). In other words, if German law, for example, requires a higher level of personal intellectual creation for an item of data or a database, the same standard will apply to the foreign claimant for protection as to the local claimant.

International Comparisons with Respect to Databases

It is only possible here to make brief reference to the substantive level of protection for databases both internationally and in other jurisdictions. As a general matter, compilations are protected elsewhere on a similar basis to that under Australian law, but with some variation as to the levels of originality or intellectual creation required. Relatively little attention, however, has been paid to the particular problems that may be raised by electronic databases. Thus, article 2(5) of the *Berne Convention* provides that:

> "Collections of literary or artistic works such as encyclopedias and anthologies which, by reason of the selection and arrangement of their contents, constitute intellectual creations shall be protected as such, without prejudice to the copyright in each of the works forming part of such collections."

This provision refers only to collections of copyright works, but as its emphasis is upon the elements of selection and arrangement this does not seem to restrict member countries extending protection to collections of non-copyright material that display the same qualities (74). This is, for example, the position in the Federal Republic of Germany, where "collections of works or of other contributions" are protected as works where, "by virtue of the selection or arrangement thereof, [they] constitute personal intellectual creations" (75). Likewise, the US *Copyright Act* 1976 protects "compilations" of data as works, defining "compilation" as:

> "... a work formed by the collection and assembling of pre-existing materials or of data that are selected, co-ordinated or arranged in such a way that the resulting work as a whole constitutes an original work of authorship."(76)

Similar provisions apply in Japan (77), where an amendment made in 1986 now makes specific reference to "data base works". "Data base" is defined as "an aggregate of information such as articles, numerals or diagrams, which is systematically constructed so that such information can be searched for with the aid of a computer." (78) It is then provided that these are protected as independent works, "where, by reason of the selection or systematic construction of information contained therein, [they] constitute intellectual creations" (79).

In general, it seems that many national copyright laws provide protection for databases, irrespective of whether they contain protected works or not (80). However, it also appears that, as in Australia, these laws will generally require the database to possess some minimum level of originality or intellectual creation by reason of its selection and arrangement. These levels may differ between countries, and the result is to produce uncertainty for database producers who wish to obtain copyright protection on as broad a basis as possible. (For example, in the USA the number of protected databases may now be considerably less following the decision of the Supreme Court in *Feist Publications Inc v Rural Tele-*

phone Service Co Inc (81). It may also be the case that a number of databases that would otherwise qualify for protection in that country will be in the public domain because they are "works of the United States Government" (82). This uncertainty has led to international proposals that databases lacking the necessary quantum of originality should nevertheless be entitled to special protection so as to safeguard the considerable investment that is represented therein. Such protection would be analogous to that granted to subject-matter such as sound recordings and broadcasters under neighboring rights legislation in many countries or under Part IV of the Australian Act, but would not be to the prejudice of any fuller copyright protection that might be available for truly original databases. A precedent for this form of protection already exists in some countries in respect of compilations lacking the necessary degree of originality. Thus, in the Nordic countries, there is a common provision that provides as follows:

> "Catalogs, tables and similar productions in which a great number of items of information have been compiled, as well as programs, may not be reproduced without the consent of the producer until 10 years have elapsed from the year in which the production was published" (83).

A proposal for a similar kind of protection for electronic databases was discussed at a WIPO/UNESCO Committee of Governmental Experts on the Printed Word in Geneva in late 1987. It was submitted that this special protection should comprise the following: the exclusive right of database producers to authorize the reproduction, in any manner or form, of their databases; similar limitations to this right as are applicable in respect of literary and artistic works included the database; and a minimum term of protection of 10 years from the end of the year in which the database is made available to the public (84). These proposals were embodied in a series of draft principles. A final principle (85) provided that:

"The specific protection granted to data base producers according to Principles PW17 to PW19 should leave intact and should in no way affect the protection of copyright in literary and artistic works included in electronic data bases."

This received varying degrees of support from the 31 nations represented on the Committee. Some delegations expressed their reservations concerning sui generis protection of databases, on the ground that this would fall outside the scope of the international copyright conventions and the principle of national treatment (as occurs in the case of the Nordic countries). It was also argued that such protection would serve to dilute copyright protection where it might otherwise be applicable and, on the other hand, might result in the protection of "fairly meager collections which were not worthy of protection" (86). Reservations were also expressed concerning the shortness of the proposed period of protection and the difficulty that any requirement of publication might pose in particular countries. Nonetheless, although there was no clear consensus among delegates as to the details of protection, it does seem that there was a general recognition that some protection was appropriate to safeguard the efforts and investment involved in the compilation of electronic databases (87). In a Green Paper on Copyright published in 1989, the Commission of the European Communities proposed that there should be a separate sui generis form of protection for those databases ineligible for copyright protection (88). A subsequent Draft Directive (1991) prepared by the Commission and still under discussion creates a new right of "unfair extraction" in both non-original databases and those protected by copyright.

At the broader international level, the World Intellectual Property Organization (1992) has proposed modest amendments to the *Berne Convention*, but these would not represent any advance on the current Australian law and do not go as far as the EC proposals. Finally, so far as Australia is concerned, the Copyright Law Review Committee has taken the view that, with some minor exceptions, there is no need for changes in our domestic law in relation to databases (89). It is clear, therefore, that it will be some time before there is international agreement on whether special treatment for databases is warranted.

■ Other Forms of Protection

While the bulk of this paper has been concerned with the copyright status of food data and databases, brief reference should be made, for the sake of completeness, to two other forms of protection that may be highly relevant. These are: (a) the equitable action of breach of confidence, and (b) contractual restrictions.

Breach of Confidence

This is a purely judge-made form of protection that safeguards information that has been prepared and utilized in circumstances of confidence (90). If this information is communicated in confidence to another party and the latter misuses or discloses the information to another without permission, the law will often grant a remedy (either an injunction restraining the activity or some form of monetary award) against the offending party. This is a completely informal form of protection that will depend very much upon the plaintiff establishing the confidentiality or secrecy of his information and some kind of improper misuse of that information by the person to whom it has been confided. It can even extend to third parties who come into possession of the information. The action of breach of confidence is of great importance in the commercial and industrial area where it is used to protect trade secrets, confidential data and know-how. It therefore has obvious implications so far as the compilers of databases are concerned, particularly where these involve information that is out of the public domain.

Contractual Restrictions

As a practical matter, these may be the most effective form of protection as between data providers and users. This will not affect third parties, that is, persons who are not parties to the contract, but it can be very effective as between the contracting parties. Thus, they could agree on the precise terms of use of data, the question of ownership of copyright in data that are created by one or the other, the level of remuneration for use, e.g. display, retrieval, recompilation, and so on. Obviously, much more could be said on this topic, but, as a general matter, the courts will seek to enforce what the parties agree and, in specific cases, this may be more effective than relying upon such heads of protection as copyright and breach of confidence.

■ References

(1)   *Copyright Act* 1968, Section 10(1)
(2)   *Copyright Act* 1968, Section 31(1)
(3)   *Copyright (International Protection) Regulations* 1969
(4)   *Copyright Act*, Section 31(2)
(5)   *Copyright (International Protection) Regulations* 1969
(6)   *Copyright Act* 1968, Part III
(7)   *Copyright Act*, Section 31(1)(2)
(8)   *Copyright Act*, Part IV
(9)   *Copyright Act*, Section 34(2)
(10) Lahore, J.C. (1977) *Intellectual Property Law in Australia: Copyright*, 1st Ed., Butterworths, Sydney, pp. 280-282
(11) *Copyright Act* 1968, Subsections 32(1) for unpublished works and (2) for other works
(12) West German *Copyright Act of 1965 (Act Dealing with Copyright and Related Rights of 9 September 1965)*, Article 2(2); Italian *Law for the Protection of Copyright and Other Rights Connected with the Exercise Thereof (No 633 of 22 April 1941, as amended)*, Article 1
(13) *Water v Lane* [1900] *AC* 539, *MacMillan & Co Ltd v K & J Cooper* (1925) 93 *LJPC* 113; *Sands & McDougall Pty Ltd v Robinson* (1917) 23 *CLR* 49; *Ladbroke (Football) Ltd v William Hill (Football) Ltd* [1964] 1 *All ER* 465
(14) *H Blacklock & Co Ltd v C Arthur Pearson Ltd* [1915] *ILRC* 2 *Ch* 376
(15) *MacMillan v Suresh Chunder Deb* (1890) 17 *ILRC* 951
(16) *Purefoy Engineering Co Ltd v Sykes Boxall & Co Ltd* (1955) 72 *RPC* 89
(17) *Ladbroke v William Hill* (Ref 13)
(18) *Kalamazoo (Australia) Pty Ltd v Compact Business Systems Pty Ltd* (1985) 5 *IPR* 213
(19) *Ainsworth Nominees Pty Ltd and Ainsworth Holdings Pty Ltd v Anclar Pty Ltd* (1989) 12 *IPR* 551
(20) *Computer Edge Pty Ltd v Apple Computer Inc* (1986) 60 *ALJR* 313
(21) *S W Hart & Co Pty Ltd v Edwards Hot Systems* (1985) 159 *CLR* 466
(22) *MacMillan & Co Ltd v K & J Cooper* (1924) 93 *LJPC* 113, 118
(23) (1937) 58 *CLR* 479
(24) *Ibid*, 498
(25) *Chilton v Progress Printing and Publishing Co* [1895] 2 *Ch* 28; *Odham's Press Ltd v London and Provincial Sporting News Agency* [1935] *Ch* 672; *Smith's Newspapers Ltd v The Labour Daily* (1925) 25 *SR (NSW)* 593
(26) *G A Cramp & Sons Ltd v Smythson Ltd* [1944] *AC* 329; *ITP Pty Ltd v United Capital Pty Ltd* (1985) 5 *IPR* 315
(27) *Canterbury Park Race Course Ltd v Hopkins* (1932) 49 *WN (NSW)* 27; *John Fairfax & Sons v Australian Consolidated Press* [1960] *SR (NSW)* 413.
(28) *Football League Ltd v Littlewoods Pools Ltd* [1959] 1 *Ch* 637
(29) *Ladbroke (Football) Ltd v William Hill (Football) Ltd* [1964] 1 *All ER* 465
(30) *Ainsworth Nominees Pty Ltd and Ainsworth Holdings Pty Ltd v Anclor Pty Ltd* (1989) 12 *IPR* 551
(31) *Kelly v Morris* (1866) 1 *LR Eq* 697

(32) *Feist Publications Inc v Rural Telephone Service Co Inc* (1991) 22 *IPR* 129

(33) *Waterlow Publishers Ltd v Rose* (1990) 17 *IPR* 493; *Kalamazoo (Australia) Pty Ltd v Compact Business Systems Pty Ltd* (1985) 5 *IPR* 215

(34) *Copyright Act* 1968, Section 32 (author must be a "qualified person", meaning an Australian citizen, an Australian protected person or a person resident in Australia)

(35) *Copyright Act* 1968, Section 84

(36) *Copyright, Designs and Patents Act* 1988, Section 9(3)

(37) *Roland Corporation v Lorenzo and Sons Pty Ltd* (1992) 22 *IPR* 245, 252-253, per Pincus J

(38) *Copyright Act* 1968, Subsection 10(1) (definition of "work of joint authorship") and Division 9 Part III

(39) *Copyright Act* 1968, Section 80

(40) *Copyright Act* 1968, Subsection 35(6)

(41) *Copyright Act* 1968, Subsection 197(1).

(42) *Maxwell v Hogg* (1867) 2 *Ch App* 307; *Kelly v Hutton* (1868) 3 *Ch App* 203; *Mack v Peter* (1872) *LR* 114 *Eq* 431; *Schove v Schminke* (1886) 33 *Ch D* 546; *Licensed Victuallers' Newspapers Co v Bingham* (1888) 38 *Ch D* 139

(43) *Francis, Day & Hunter Ltd v Twentieth Century Fox Corporation* [1940] *AC* 112.

(44) *Green v Broadcasting Corporation of New Zealand* (1983) 2 *IPR* 19

(45) *Exxon Corporation v Exxon Insurance Consultants International Ltd* [1982] *RPC* 69.

(46) *Kalamazoo (Australia) Pty Ltd v Compact Business Systems Pty Ltd* (1985) 5 *IPR* 213 at 232, per Thomas J

(47) *Francis Day & Hunter Ltd v 20th Century Fox Corporation Ltd* [1940] *AC* 112, 123, per Lord Wright for the Privy Council

(48) *Ibid*, 88 per Stephenson LJ quoting the observations of Davey LJ in *Hollinrake v Truswell* (1894) 3 *Ch D* 420

(49) *Kalamazoo (Australia) Pty Ltd v Compact Business Systems Pty Ltd* (1985) 5 *IPR* 213

(50) Brown, R.L. (1985) *Rutgers Comp. Technol. Law J.* **11**, 17-49

(51) *Copyright Act* 1968, Subsections 10(1) and 22(1)

(52) *Hawkes & Sons (London) Ltd v Paramount Film Productions Ltd* [1934] *Ch* 593; *LB (Plastics) Ltd v Swish Products Ltd* [1979] *FSR* 145

(53) [1969] *Ch* 508

(54) *Ibid*, 385

(55) [1964] 1 All *ER* 465

(56) *Ibid*, 481

(57) *Jarrold v Houlston* (1859) 3 *K & J* 708, 69 *ER* 1294; *Harman Pictures NV v Osborne* [1967] 2 *All ER* 324; *Elanco Products Ltd v Mandops (Agrochemical Specialists) Ltd* [1979] *FSR* 46

(58) *Copyright Act* 1968, Subsection 10(1)

(59) *Copyright Act*, Section 31(1)

(60) *Copyright Act* 1968, Sections 31(1)(a)(iv) (literary, dramatic and musical works) and 31(1)(b)(iii) (artistic works)

(61) *Copyright Act* 1968, subparagraphs 31(1)(a)(iv) (literary, dramatic and musical works) and 31(1)(b)(iii) (artistic works); para 86(d) (cinematograph films); there is no diffusion right in the case of sound recordings).

(62) *Copyright Act* 1968, Subsection 10(1))

(63) *Copyright Act* 1968, Subsection 26(1))

(64) *Copyright Act* 1968, subpara 31(1)(a)(iii) (literary, dramatic and musical works), paras 85(b) (sound recordings) and 86(b) (cinematograph films); there is no performance right in respect of artistic works

(65) *Copyright Act* 1968, subpara 31(1)(a)(i) (literary, dramatic and musical works); subpara

31(1)(b)(i) (artistic works); para 85(a) (sound recordings); para 86(a) (cinematograph films)

(66) *Copyright Act 1968*, Subsection 27(4)

(67) (1884) 13 *QBD* 843

(68) See, for example, *Jennings v Stephens* [1936] *Ch* 469; *Ernest Turner Electrical Instruments Ltd v Performing Right Society Ltd* [1943] *Ch* 167; *Australian Performing Right Association v Canterbury-Bankstown Leagues Club Ltd* [1964-1965] *NSWLR* 138; *Performing Right Society Ltd v Rangers Football Club Supporters Club* [1975] *RPC* 626.

(69) *Rank Film Productions Ltd v Dodds* (1983) 2 *IPR* 113

(70) *Australasian Performing Right Association Ltd v Commonwealth Bank of Australia* (1993) 25 *IPR* 157

(71) *Bradbury Agnew & Co v Day* (1916) 32 *TLR* 349

(72) Copyright Law Review Committee, *Draft Report on Computer Software Protection*, June 1993, p. 17

(73) *Copyright (International Protection) Regulations* 1969, Reg 4

(74) WIPO Preparatory Document for the meeting on "The Printed Word", 7-11 December 1987, Geneva, in [1988] *Copyright* 42 at 81 Ricketson, S. (1987) *The Berne Convention for the Protection of Literary and Artistic Works: 1886-1986,* Centre for Commercial Law Studies, London, p. 298

(75) Copyright Law of 9 September 1965, article 4. Also Dietz, A. in M. Nimmer and P. Geller (Eds.), *International Copyright Law and Prac-tice*, Matthew Bender, New York, FRG-22

(76) US *Copyright Act* 1976, Section 101

(77) *Copyright Act 1970 (Law No 48 of 1970,* article 12

(78) See now article 2(1)$^{\text{(xter)}}$

(79) *Ibid*, article 12bis(1)

(80) See WIPO Preparatory Document, Ref. 74, 81

(81) (1991) 22 *IPR* 129

(82) *Copyright Act* 1976, Section 105

(83) *Swedish Law No 729 of 30 December 1960 on Copyright in Literary and Artistic Works*, Article 49; *Danish Act No 158 on Copyright in Literary and Artistic Works*, of 31 May 1961, Article 49; *Norwegian Act relating to Property Rights in Literary, Scientific or Artistic Works*, No 2 of 12 May 1961, Article 43; *Finnish Law No 404 relating to Copyright in Literary and Artistic Works of 8 July 1961*, Article 49

(84) (1988) *Copyright* 42 at 82 (Principles PW 17(2), 18 and 19))

(85) *Ibid,* Principle PW20

(86) *Ibid*, 83

(87) *Ibid*, 84

(88) Commission of the European Communities, (1988) *Green Paper on Copyright and the Challenge of Technology — Copyright Issues requiring Immediate Action*, Communication from the Commission, Brussels, p. 216

(89) *Draft Report on Computer Software Protection*, June 1993, pp. 16-17

(90) Ricketson, S. (1984) *The Law of Intellectual Property*, Law Book Co., Sydney, Ch. 42-46

Non-Nutrient Databases for Foods

Kimmo Louekari

Institute of Occupational Health,
Topeliuksenkatu 41 a A, SF-0250 Helsinki, Finland

Non-nutrient databases for foods contain analytical data on toxic elements, pesticides, additives, mycotoxins, allergens or natural components which have no nutritional function. Non-nutrient databases can be used to monitor the trend of potentially harmful components in food; to estimate dietary intakes, provided that another file containing food consumption data can be linked with non-nutrient concentrations in foods; to clarify possible interactions between nutrients and non-nutrients; and to assess and measure exposure and risk in population groups. Examples of non-nutrient databases are discussed.

The reason for including a certain food component in a non-nutrient database is (i) that it can cause allergic or other adverse reaction; (ii) that it is potentially toxic to the consumer in excessive amounts or in long-term exposure (e.g. heavy metals or pesticide residues); or (iii) that it may interact with nutrients (e.g. decrease of calcium absorption caused by phytates) (Table I). In practice, it seems reasonable to establish and maintain a non-nutrient database only, when the necessary research capacity for updating the database contents is available and when there is the scientific and/or regulatory interest to use the data. Some categories of non-nutrients presented in Table I are not necessary included in any existing non-nutrient database (e.g. natural toxic substances and pyrolysis products), since data on their concentrations in the relevant food items are not yet available.

Table I. Categories of non-nutrients in foods

Category (Examples)	Nutritional or harmful effects	User needs
Toxic elements and contaminants (Pb, Cd, Hg, Al, PCBs, dioxins)	Accumulation in the body, chronic effects	Intake monitoring, survey of trends
Pesticides (organochlorine and organophosphate pesticides)	As above	As above
Food additives (nitrates, nitrites, BHA, BHT, colours)	Toxic effects, hypersensitivity reactions	Diet planning and the above needs
Allergens	Intolerance reactions, allergies	Labeling, usage restrictions, consumer information
Nutrient inhibitors (phytates, tannins)	Decreased bioavailability of nutrients	Analysis of interactions and effects on nutrient status
Naturally occurring toxicants (patulin, aflatoxin, flavonoids)	Acute and chronic toxicity	Risk and intake assessment
Pyrolysis products (quinoline and indole compounds)	Suspected carcinogenicity	Exposure estimation, process optimisation, consumer information

A non-nutrient database should contain average concentrations, ranges and tolerances to enable the calculation of dietary intakes and comparison with regulations. The range of the observed non-nutrient concentration is useful when estimating maximum intakes. Data on preparation of the sample are also necessary, since different types of handling and preparation (washing, peeling, cooking, canning, frying etc.) can decrease concentration of non-nutrients, especially those attached to the surface of vegetables and fruits (toxic metals and pesticides) and those which are decomposed by heat (mycotoxins). Description of the food sampling should be included to allow evaluation of how well the results represent different products, agricultural areas and seasons. Analytical method, year of analysis, and quality control of the analysis should also be presented in non-nutrient databases to enable the assessment of reliability and comparability of data. The detection limit of the analytical method may be much higher in older studies and this affects the comparability of old and recent concentrations and estimated intakes. The code of the food item can be useful when a non-nutrient database is combined with other databases on food

constituents of food consumption. The relation code links a record in the calculation database (enabling numerical analysis) to the reference database which is necessary as a documentation of data sources and evaluation of data. Often one record in the reference database can be linked with several records in the calculation database, which is convenient in terms of database maintenance (Table II).

Unlike nutrients, local conditions, especially sources of food contaminants, often cause variation in non-nutrient content of foods. This has to be taken into account in the sampling protocols for food surveillance. In many cases, the maximum non-nutrient contents and the maximum exposure are of special interest. In many cases, blood levels or other biomarkers of exposure and health consequences are monitored in contaminated areas. Since health consequences of high non-nutrient intake are most likely found in certain contaminated areas, food surveillance and dietary intake studies are often directed accordingly. Examples are areas where fish is contaminated by the pulp and paper industry (Louekari, Verta, & Mukherjee, unpublished data) and areas where crops receive the fallout from

Table II. Contents of two related records in a non-nutrient database

The calculation database

Contents	Example
Name of the food item	Liver, cattle
Code of the food item	0102
Preparation status	Raw
Non-nutrient	Cadmium
Average concentration	70
Unit	µg/kg, wet weight
Number of samples	60
The range of 95 percentile of the analytical results	350
The maximum permitted concentrations	Not given
The relation code to the reference database	0502

The reference database (record 0502)

Contents	Example
Publication	Salmi A, Hirn J. The cadmium and selenium contents of muscle, liver and kidney from cattle and swine, Fleischwirtschaft 64:1984:464-465
Analytical method	AAS, graphite furnace
The analytical quality control	NBS ref.material 1577 analyzed
Description of sampling	10 slaughterhouses representing the whole country, variation caused by the age of animals was considered
Detection of limit of analysis	Not given, sensitivity was 0.005µg/20µl
Year of sampling	1981
Year of analysis	Not given

mines or refineries containing cadmium or lead.

The food nomenclature used in a non-nutrient database should be designed to cover and differentiate those foods which contain significant amounts of the non-nutrients of interest. Vegetables and fruits may contain pesticide residues; processed foods may contain food additives; mushrooms, liver and predator fish may contain high concentrations of toxic metals.

∎ Examples of Non-nutrient Databases

Non-nutrient databases are maintained for example in USA, Netherlands, Denmark and Finland (1,2,3,4,5). These databases contain data on toxic metals, selected pesticides and in some countries, also on mycotoxins, radionucleides or organochlorine compounds. Data are often generated by a governmental agency, e.g. the FDA in the United States, and the National Food Agency in Denmark as part of a food surveillance program. Studies in academic institutes can be incorporated into the database. A description of some existing non-nutrient databases and surveillance/monitoring programs has been presented elsewhere (6).

In Finland, the steering group of the recently established non-nutrient database consists of representatives from relevant authorities, research institutes and the food industry. The Finnish database includes summaries of the origin, toxicity and regulatory status of non-nutrients, in addition to concentration of non-nutrients. The first version of the database contains data on mercury, cadmium, lead, dioxins, PCBs and poly- aromatic hydrocarbons, residues of antibiotics in milk products and hormones in tissue samples of animals. Also microbial contamination by *Salmonella*, *Listeria* and *Yersinia* is covered in the database.

With this information, the maintainer of the database, the National Food Administration, can advise consumers, respond to the media about food safety questions and in future, produce certificates for food processors. It is planned that in the future the system would also enable estimation of dietary intakes using the collected analytical data.

The presentation of the data in a record of the Finnish non-nutrient database is similar to that in Table II, with a few exceptions. Preparation/processing status of the samples is not presented in the database, maximum permitted concentrations are in a separate file and basic data on sampling is given in the calculation database but not the reference database. It was found in the updating of the database that a general way of presentation could not be strictly followed but had to be adapted according to the availability and relevance of items of information for the non-nutrient in question.

■ Experiences of the Estimation of Dietary Intake and in the Analysis of Trends

Dietary Intake of Cadmium — Are the Available Data Comparable ?

It is often important to know the trend of non-nutrient concentration and/or dietary intake. However, the interpretation of the available data is difficult if changes in analytical techniques and methods of dietary intake estimation are not taken into account. For example, it has been suggested that a decreasing trend in cadmium intake in European countries could be seen (7). However, the estimates of intake used by van Assche are not comparable since studies have been made using different methods and since up to the late 1970s, analytical techniques for determination of cadmium were non-sensitive and not accurate at the level observed in foods. Furthermore the total diet method utilized earlier tends to result in overestimates (8). Using non-comparable data, no conclusions can be drawn about trends of non-nutrient concentration. A non-nutrient database with contents presented in Table II enables a decision about whether there are enough data to observe the trends of non-nutrient concentrations or dietary intake.

Trend of Total Mercury Concentration in Fish and Intake in Different Socio-economic Groups

In a recent study, we have analyzed the intake of mercury using the analytical data on these contaminants and the Finnish Household Survey for food consumption data (of Louekari, Verta, & Mukherjee, unpublished data). Some results of that and another study (9) are presented to illustrate how a non-nutrient database can be used for estimation of non-nutrient intakes in different groups of populations or in particular risk groups, and for analysis of different food groups to the total intake.

In Finland, most of the intake of mercury is caused by eating fish, which accumulate methylmercury of the food chain of the lakes. In the study on mercury intake, changes in Hg intake of people of different socio-economic groups during the period of 1967-1990 were observed in the polluted areas, which include 10-15 per cent lakes and coastal waters in Finland. In the study areas, Hg is discharged mainly by the pulp and paper industry and by chloroalkali plants. Our results show that the average pike Hg concentration decreased from 1.52 mg per kg (in 1967-68) to 0.60 mg per kg (in 1990-91).

The dietary intake of Hg among farmers and white-collar workers living in the study areas was estimated by combining the data on Hg concentrations in food with the data on food consumption during the period of 1967-1990. It was observed that total dietary Hg intake for farmers was 22 and 15 mg per day in the years 1967 and 1990, respectively. On the other hand, the total dietary Hg intake for white-collar workers was 13 and 8 mg per day in the years 1967 and 1990, respectively. The study suggests that although the fish consumption of the Finnish population (except for farmers) has increased slightly, the intake of Hg has decreased remarkably (by 39 per cent on average). This is due to the rapid decline of aquatic Hg discharge especially from the pulp and paper industry. The other reason is that consumers prefer fish species, e.g. rainbow trout, which contain much less Hg than pike and perch.

In compilation of the mercury database, the following problems were faced: First the concentration of "other fresh fish" and "processed fish" were not analyzed, and had to be estimated. We used the average concentration of those fish species, which were not covered in the food consumption study by name but had been analyzed for Hg concentration. These calculations were recorded in the

same file as other data on Hg concentration. Second, in the food consumption file some fish (e.g. herring) is presented as smoked, frozen, fresh, salted. Because the Hg concentration is not affected by processing, consumption of these different types of herring were added up and multiplied by the Hg concentration of herring to obtain the total Hg intake from herring.

The Average and Maximum Intake of PCBs

A 1993 study of the intake of polychlorinated biphenyls (PCB) from the Finnish diet was based on measurement of seven PCB indicator congeners in 99 food samples and the Household Survey data. The average PCB intake from food was 15 mg/day or 0.25 mg/kg of body weight per day, and showed no change as compared with estimates from late 1980s. Approximately half of the intake came from fish. Cheese, fats and oils contributed significantly to the intake, since their consumption is relatively high, although the concentration is not at the level observed in fish (up to 2100 mg/kg in pike) (9).

We also estimated the theoretical maximum intake of PCB of an average consumer assuming that the consumer eats food containing the maximum observed concentration of PCB. This theoretical maximum was 41 mg/day which is almost three times the average intake. This theoretical maximum is probably not too far from the actual maximum intake, since in this calculation the food consumption was at the average level. Furthermore, the maximum value in the database is dependent on the number of samples (n was between 3 and 20 in this case). The maximum observed concentration would be higher if the number of samples were greater. People having a high fish consumption and living in contaminated areas, consume the actual maximum dietary intake of PCB (9).

■ References

(1) Pennington, J. A. T. (1983) *J. Am. Diet. Assoc.* **82,** 166-173

(2) State Supervisory Public Health Service (1983) *Surveillance Program "Man and Nutrition".* Report No. 10, Hague

(3) State Supervisory Public Health Service (1987) *Surveillance Program "Man and Nutrition",* Hague

(4) Andersen, A. (1981) *Lead, Cadmium, Copper and Zinc in the Danish Diet,* Statens Levnedsmiddelinstitut, Copenhagen

(5) Southgate, D.A.T., & Walker, A.D. (1992) *Report of FLAIR Euro-foods-Enfant Project 2nd Annual Meeting,* Wageningen Agricultural University, Wageningen, pp. 40-43

(6) Louekari, K., & Salminen, S. (1991) *Trends Food Sci. Technol.* **2,** 289-292

(7) Van Assche, F., & Ciarletta, P. (1992) *Cadmium '92,* Cadmium Association, London, pp. 51-54

(8) Louekari, K., Jolkkonen. L., & Varo, P. (1988) *Food Add. Contam.* **5,** 111-117

(9) Himberg, K., Hallikainen, A., & Louekari, K. (1993) *Zeit. Lebensmitteluntersuch. -Forsch.* **196,** 1-5

Copyright, Food Industry and Food Safety Considerations

Food Composition Databases in the Food Industry

Olivier de Rham

Nestlé Research Centre,
Manufacturing, Milk and Nutrition Business Unit,
Avenue Nestlé 55, 1800 – Vevey, Switzerland

This paper covers specific aspects of the use and production of food composition data in the food industry. Two types of information are stored by manufacturers: quantitative information on an extensive list of nutrient and non-nutrient components (including contaminants, stored separately), and qualitative information about suitability for diets to reduce or eliminate components. The aim of collecting such information is usually to check product compliance with regulations or internal specifications and norms, with a special emphasis on nutritional labeling. Control of costs, processing, storage stability, taste and texture constraints are important goals along with provision of product information to consumers. The origin of the information is usually analytical, calculated or borrowed from published food composition tables, depending on availability, regulatory requirements, product type, and cost of analysis. The meaning of the information is different depending on whether natural products are processed without intentional modification of composition, or whether intentional alteration of composition occurs, thus engaging the responsibility of the processor to guarantee the declared level. However, considering the natural variability in food composition, the 20 per cent tolerance margin usually accepted tends to discourage the declaration of the actual average value when liability is engaged. A clear understanding of these constraints is important to ensure a fruitful collaboration between industry and other interested parties in the use of food composition data.

Threhe problem of an unequivocal description of a food in a table is a familiar one. The translation of food names needs not only a very good familiarity with the relevant languages, but also an intimate experience of the cultures and their local variants.

■ Foods and Food Classes

Food Names and Descriptions

The situation is also difficult with commercial product brand names, as they often have no meaning in themselves. To complicate the situation further, the same brand name can be used for different products in various parts of the world, or conversely the same food product may have different brand names. A detailed description of the food in these cases is necessary, as well as the use of the food classes and subclasses, and internally the use of codes.

Food Classification

The interest to widen the classical list of food classes (and subclasses if needed) is multiple. They help to select an ingredient for a given aim from a suitably selected screen listing of the corresponding group(s) of ingredients. They allow the origin of a nutrient in a product or in a diet to be traced. They help in checking the coherence and validity of food composition data.

Table I. List of food ingredient classes

Animal	Plant	Refined products
Meat	Cereals	Oils, fats, shortenings
Fish and seafood	Vegetables (leaves, stalks, flowers, fruits, bulbs, sprouts)	Proteins, hydrolysates, amino acids
Egg	Roots	Starches
Milk and milk products	Mushrooms	Sugars and sweeteners
	Algae	Dietary fiber concentrates
	Oilseeds	Enzymes
	Herbs and spices	Microbiological starters
	Tubers (potatoes)	Acids, alkalis, salts
	Pulses (dry beans, grain legumes)	Vitamins
	Fruits	Thickeners, emulsifiers, antioxidants, preservatives
	Berries	Processing aids
	Nuts	Colours, aromas and flavours
	Cocoa	Water
	Coffee and surrogates	
	Tea and herbal teas	
	Wine, spirits, vinegar	
	Yeast and yeast products	

Whether a food can be attributed in a table to more than one class of products is an important question. The answer is almost always negative in the printed version of food composition tables as this would mean a waste of space, but could easily be positive in computerized databases with the necessary programming precautions.

Ingredients and Ingredient Classes

Besides the traditional food ingredient classes found in published food composition tables, food manufacturers use additional raw materials for product manufacture:

- industrial "raw" materials, often already processed to some extent, e.g. peeled, cut, pureed, deboned, cooked, dehydrated, freeze-dried
- food ingredients not consumed as food in themselves and not usually accessible to consumers, constituting additional raw material classes. These include refined food components (e.g. fiber concentrates, starches, proteins, hydrolysates, amino acids, medium chain triglycerides, hydrogenated fats, trans-esterified fats), pure chemicals (acids, alkalis, salts), enzymes, microbiological starters, vitamins, additives (antioxidants, emulsifiers, thickeners, preservatives), colors, aromas and flavors (see Table I).

Out of these materials, a large number of intermediate products, subrecipes or premixes are produced, that can be either transient in processing, stored for later use, or purchased as such. These subrecipes or premixes also constitute an "ingredient" class.

Products and Product Classes

Manufactured products may be classified according to consumption characteristics that are familiar to the consumer, rather than on the basis of the major ingredient which is sometimes very difficult to define. Minimally processed foods (with only sugar, salt, fat or water added or removed) can be classified within the class of their major ingredient. However, manufactured product classes go much further than that: beverages, breakfast items, starters, snacks, main dishes, garnishes, fast foods, side dishes, sauces, desserts, infant foods and clinical nutrition products (see Table II).

Quantitative Information

Components Contents

Quantitative data on the contents of a great number of components including both nutrients and non-nutrients can be required by technologists or marketing specialists. The interest for each individual component is very variable according to the type of product concerned and the aims of the demand. Most requests do not ask for more than the proximate composition ("big 4": energy, protein, fat, carbohydrates) or slightly more ("big 8": the "big 4" plus dietary fiber, sodium, cholesterol, saturated fat), and possibly one or two vitamins and minerals, but there may be additional requests.

Dairy product specialists insist on milk fat and non-fat milk solids. Chocolate manufacturers have special requirements related to cocoa solids and fruit content. Yoghurt producers are interested in the transformation of lactose to lactic acid. Broth and stock producers ask for glutamate figures, meat and sausage manufacturers need carnitine values, coffee and cocoa beverage processors want data about methyl xanthines. In addition, there are national differences due to local legislation.

Dietetic product specialists are most demanding, including not only a list of vitamins and minerals, but also occasionally figures for fat and sugar substitutes with reduced energy value. Breast milk substitutes and clinical nutrition products

Table II. List of food product classes

Simple products[a]	Dairy	Evaporated milk, milk powder, cheese, yoghurt
	Meat	Preserved meats, sausages
	Fish	Frozen fish
	Cereals	Bread, pasta, bakery products
	Vegetables	Frozen prepared vegetables
	Tubers	Potato flakes, frozen croquettes, chips, crisps
Beverages	Alcoholic	Wine, beer, cider, drinks, punch, cocktail, spirits, liquors
	Soft	Fruit juices, vegetable juices, dairy beverages, milk modifiers
	Cereal drinks	Coffees, teas, water, mineral water, sodas
Breakfast foods		Butter, margarine, jam, spreads, cheese
		Bacon and sausages, eggs, milk, yoghurt, fruits, fruit juices
Starters		Soups, broth, stock, "hors d'oeuvres"
Snacks	Savory, salted	Appetizers, cocktail foods, chips, salted peanuts, crepes
	Sweet	Ice-creams, chocolates, cereal bars
		Pastry, confectionery, sweets, biscuits
		Yoghurts, fruits
Main dishes		With meat or fish
		Without meat or fish
Garnishes		Potatoes, cereals, pasta, bread, doughs
		Vegetables, legumes
Fast foods	Hot	Hamburgers, pizzas, quiches
	Cold	Sandwiches, savoury pies
Side dishes		Salads, cheese, bread, spreads
Sauces		Salad dressing, mayonnaise
		Meat sauces
		Seasonings, condiments, spices
Desserts		Fruits, dairy desserts, custard
		Cakes, tarts, sweet pies, fried desserts
Infant foods		Starter milks, follow-up milks
		Infant cereals, baby foods
Clinical nutrition products		Enteral
		Parenteral

[a] Simply processed, with only salt, fat, sugar or water added

require a long list of vitamins, minerals and trace elements, and some amino acids and fatty acids. The figures for fatty acid classes are being requested more and more often.

At Nestlé, the INFOODS tags (1) as such are not used, but instead a similar system of conventional abbreviations and standard units, to avoid confusion and errors arising during data transfer.

Contaminants

Data on contaminants contents is quantitative, and it is tempting to put it in the same database as the other components. But food composition data should have a predictive value, i.e. be valid in the future as well as in the past with the correct safety margins, whereas contamination levels vary greatly from batch to batch and cannot predict the values for future crops. The data should be stored with batch identification in a separate database that does not allow the usual averaging done in food composition data. This is so, for example, for aluminum levels in the ingredients for infant formulas.

∎ Qualitative Information

Elimination Diet Suitability

Elimination diets are sought for various reasons, either medical, religious or philosophical. For example, gliadin, milk protein, soy, must be eliminated from the diet of people allergic to these foods, meat from the diet of vegetarians, animal products from that of vegans, pork from kosher or halal products. This information is qualitative (present or absent) rather than quantitative (numeric).

Such qualitative criteria are delicate to handle. An error (which could have very serious consequences making somebody very ill) is easily made, whereas an occasional low figure for, say, protein on the label of the same product is harmless.

The decision whether an ingredient or a product is acceptable or not in a given elimination diet depends on a number of complex rules, especially for religious diets. In addition, in order to reach a decision on the suitability of a product *all* its ingredients must be correctly identified for the given criterion, the recipe must be strictly followed, and the processing (contamination, recycling, incompatibilities, processing equipment and conditions, processing-induced components) must be properly addressed.

Qualitative information is *not* suitable for components like sodium, cholesterol, lactose, sugar, phosphate, caffeine. In these cases, the aim is a *reduction* diet with a maximum acceptable daily intake and not an *elimination* diet. Such parameters are quantitative factors and must be handled as such.

Ingredients and Additives Usage

The recipes database gives quantitative information on the ingredients used in a product. This information is usually passed to the public in a simplified form of the qualitative list of ingredients. The additives are in this respect no different from the other ingredients. "Additives-free lists" can therefore only be obtained from the recipes database, and this information does *not* belong to the food composition database.

A frequent confusion ignores the fact that some additives are at the same time natural molecules. The absence of such an additive in the recipe does not imply the absence of that molecule in the product. Such a molecule is then a normal food component to be handled quantitatively. For example, claiming "no-phosphate added evaporated milk" or "no glutamate-added tomato ketchup" suggests that these products are, respectively, phosphate-free and glutamate- free, which is incorrect. Furthermore, at the same time such claims reinforce and perpetuate erroneous beliefs, ideas and fears about additives among consumers.

■ Quality of the Information

Aims of Information

Composition data in the food industry are usually produced to satisfy quality assurance aims: compliance with regulatory or scientific composition standards, and with internal norms and specifications. In recent years, a great deal of this activity has been geared to nutritional labeling as new regulations appeared in the US (2) and in the EEC (3) with compliance dates in 1994, and this will continue in the near future.

In addition, it is often necessary to control one or the other parameter of food composition to ensure optimal process control, taste, texture, flavor, convenience, price, shelf life. Only in a few cases does the publication of food composition information brochures and the transmission of data to dietitians or database compilers receive priority.

Origin of the Information

Food composition data are usually analytical (hopefully on multiple representative samples), calculated from the recipe, or borrowed from an external database. Whether one or the other source is to be preferred or rejected depends on the local constraints which may include, e.g. regulations, availability, facilities, costs, and needs for accuracy.

Variability

The biological nature of the materials used (e.g. ripeness, variety, soils, fertilizer use, rearing and feeding practices, post-harvest practices) introduces a large variability in the composition of ingredients. In addition, there is a variability in recipes, including intentional small variations for various technological, taste, price or regulatory reasons and non-intentional ones for practical reasons.

The cumulated variability of food composition is mastered to a certain extent by technologists, but can only increase as international comparisons are made. This raises the question of when two foods are close enough to be considered one and the same in the database. When the need for accuracy is low, such cumulations are easily accepted, whereas every batch must be recorded separately when high accuracy is needed. It is up to the user to decide the degree of precision that is needed and to handle the database accordingly.

The food industry composition data compiler enjoys some advantages over other database compilers. Purchase specifications are used for a defined list of raw materials. Fixed, precise and controlled recipes and processes are used. Manufactured products are controlled for various reasons (e.g. legal, standards of identity, cost, storage stability, taste and texture), which reduce the variability of the final composition.

In full cream milk powders we measured a relative standard deviation of 5 to 10 per cent for minerals, and 15 to 25 per cent for vitamins. It is probably greater for trace elements as well as in other less standardized products. The legislation usually allow for a 20 per cent tolerance. This is by far not large enough for minerals and vitamins, and the declared values are therefore often below the real average content, to allow a safety margin. This is unfortunate for dietitians, but largely unavoidable.

Meaning of the Information

Dietetic products are sold on the basis of medical advice, and their nutritional value is of prime importance. The technologist is required to produce a food that matches a predefined composition, and this is assured by standardization of every single batch of production. Action is taken to guarantee the required levels that are declared on the label, and the producer is responsible for ensuring that the declared figures are adhered to under normal circumstances. This is also the case when a component level is controlled (addition or reduction), but needs "overages" or safety margins in the declared values.

Normal, everyday food products on the other hand do not require such accuracy of composition data. In this case, the processor discloses what nature has produced, as influenced by processing. A yearly production average is in this case the most significant nutritional figure. One half of the production will have a content lower than the average and the other half a higher one. In order to ensure that the vast majority of packages correspond to the declaration (including possible losses during storage), the declaration might be below the actual average value for those perceived as healthy nutrients, while for those nutrients negatively perceived, such as sodium, the declaration might be higher than the actual average value.

∎ Conclusions

Food composition information that exists in the food industry is not primarily aimed at dietitians, nutritionists or database managers, and some frustrations are predictable. The cost of producing information for external use as well as the cost of its dissemination are high and may be restrictive. The risk of misunderstanding and misuse of this information is important to highlight, especially if its currency is not assured by regular updates. At the same time, the protection of that part of the information which is proprietary is a necessity.

Understanding the constraints and the reasons for producing such information will foster a common understanding of its meaning and limits, and will facilitate the dialogue and improve its use. It is in this context that a collaboration is possible and fruitful.

∎ References

(1) Klensin, J.C., Feskanich, D., Lin, V., Truswell, A.S., & Southgate, D.A.T. (1989) *Identification of Food Components for INFOODS Data Interchange*, UNU Press, Tokyo.

(2) Mermelstein, M.H. (1994) *Food Technol.* **48**, 62-71

(3) EEC (1990) *Council Directive of 24th Sept. 1990 or Nutritional Labeling of Foodstuffs 90/496/EEC.* Official Journal of the European Community L276/40-44 of 6/10/1990.

The Databases of the Australian National Food Authority

Janine Lewis, Simon Brooke-Taylor, Fay Stenhouse

National Food Authority, PO Box 7186,
Canberra, ACT 2610, Australia

The National Food Authority was established in August 1991 as a reform to the food standards setting system. Although development and variation of food standards is its primary role, the Authority is also responsible for the national references on nutrient composition and for food safety surveillance. Three databases providing the supporting information systems for these activities are described. The food composition work of the Authority (and the federal Department of Health before it), has focused on revision of the national reference on nutrient composition and the release of the data in a number of formats. Nutrient data are produced mainly from an ongoing food analytical program and managed by means of a computer system, the Australian Nutrient Data Bank. These data enable the Authority to estimate the levels of nutrients in food, and the probable nutritional impact on foods of changes to the compositional and technological aspects of food standards. The published food composition tables also provide a valuable data source for industry when formulating nutrition information for labeling of foods. The Authority also has responsibility for the Market Basket Survey which identifies whether pesticides and contaminants are at levels which pose health risks to consumers. The last completed survey in 1990 concluded that Australian intakes of pesticides and contaminants were well below international limits recommended by the World Health Organization. To facilitate a uniform interpretation, implementation and enforcement of the Food Standards Code, the Authority is developing a national food safety information database, which will link all agencies involved and provide an information network to enable effective use of resources for a rapid national response to public health emergencies related to food.

The National Food Authority (NFA) was established in August 1991 with the proclamation of the Commonwealth *National Food Authority Act 1991* (the Act), as an independent and expert body with responsibility for the development, variation and review of Australia's food standards.

■ Functions of the National Food Authority

The Act specifies a list of 13 statutory functions that the NFA is required to perform. More than half of these functions do not relate directly to the Authority's primary role of developing and revising food standards, but focus on food safety research and education, and coordination of food recalls and food safety information. In summary, the functions are:

- development and review of food standards
- co-ordination of food surveillance
- research and surveys
- food safety education
- co-ordination of food recalls
- development of assessment policies on imported food
- advice to the federal minister
- development of codes of practice for industry
- incidental functions.

Three of the functions have or will result in ongoing activities that are dependent on the databases of the Authority. They are:

- researching the nutrient composition of the Australian food supply
- monitoring the pesticide and contaminant levels in the food supply
- establishing a system of food safety surveillance.

■ Nutrient Composition Database

The responsibility for government-sponsored nutrition composition activities was transferred to the National Food Authority upon its formation. However, these activities have been conducted in Australia since the 1930s under the auspices of the federal Department of Health. Up to the 1970s, the Department issued three major revisions to the food composition tables, which were compilations of data from a number of sources mainly from overseas but including some Australian data. During the 1970s, there was a growing awareness and call for Australia to have a more comprehensive and contemporary set of food composition tables that reflected the Australian food supply (1).

The first step towards this goal was achieved in 1978 when it was decided to revise Australia's nutrient composition data completely by establishing a program to analyze the Australian food supply progressively. At that time, a Working Party of Australia's peak health advisory body, the National Health and Medical Research Council, was formed to devise a plan for the collection of food composition data including the priorities for analysis of foods and nutrients, and to review the format for publication. Their recommendations included extending the range of nutrients and foods, particularly for take-away and ethnic foods, and for publication of the tables to be in a loose-leaf format to enable easy incorporation of updates (2).

In establishing the program, it was decided that within the available funding, the data should be produced to serve nutrition and health goals before aiming to meet agricultural requirements. Thus, the overall direction of the revision program was generally to analyze one composite sample of food in preference to multiple samples, to collect data for primary pro-

Table I. Present range of constituents analyzed

Proximate constituents	Minerals	Vitamins
Moisture	Sodium	Retinol[a]
Total nitrogen	Potassium	α-carotene[a]
Total fat	Calcium	β-carotene[a]
Individual monosaccharides	Magnesium	β-cryptoxanthin[a]
Individual disaccharides	Iron	Thiamin
Starch	Zinc	Riboflavin
Ash	Phosphorus	Niacin
Dietary fiber[a]	Copper	Vitamin C[a]
Cholesterol[a]	Manganese	α-tocopherol
Fatty acids[a]	Chloride	Vitamin B6
Organic acids[a]	Fluoride	Vitamin B12[a]
	Selenium	Biotin
	Sulphur	Pantothenic acid

a Analysis of these nutrients depends on the type of food

duce prior to manufactured food products and to sample at the retail level on a regional rather than a national basis. After 13 years of the laboratory program, this approach has enabled Australian nutrient data to be produced on a broader range of foods than would otherwise have been possible given the funding constraints and the demand for comprehensive data in as short a time as possible.

The initial laboratory work was undertaken at universities in Sydney. The majority of the work during the first five years of the laboratory program was conducted by the Wills and Greenfield team at the University of New South Wales. Since 1985 however, the analyses have been conducted by the South Australian division of the Australian Government Analytical Laboratories in Adelaide.

From the commencement of the program, routine analysis of foods included:

- moisture; total fat; total nitrogen; carbohydrate components — monosaccharides, disaccharides and starch; ash;
- sodium; potassium; calcium; magnesium; iron; zinc

- retinol, α- and β-carotenes, β-cryptoxanthin; thiamin; riboflavin; niacin; vitamin C.

Other components were analyzed appropriate to the foods, such as cholesterol, fatty acids and organic acids. Special programs were also conducted for amino acids and dietary fiber analyzed by the Englyst method (3).

For the first 11 years, the program focused on obtaining a broad nutrient profile of foods commonly available in the Australian food supply. By the end of this period, over 2500 foods had been analyzed for their nutrient composition. As opportunities arose and expertise became available, the range of analyzed nutrients gradually expanded from six to ten vitamins, and from six to 13 minerals. The range of nutrients which now comprises the routinely commissioned constituents is given in Table I.

Because of the expansionary approach described above, there were some gaps in the vitamin and mineral data for foods analyzed during the early part of the program, principally for primary produce and take-away foods.

In 1992, the laboratory program began to resample foods to analyze those nutrients which were not included in the first round of analyses. The focus of the program from now on will be to build up a more comprehensive profile on all foods previously analyzed. The sampling scheme for these analyses is being maintained as close as possible to the original specifications. The "catchup" program also provides opportunities for other nutrients with previously doubtful values to be reanalyzed. In addition to the "catchup" analyses, there will be an ongoing component which will analyze new foods entering the market.

With the continuation of the food analysis program, there is now the opportunity for more detailed information to be collected. This is considered to be particularly useful for staple foods. One example of this approach is a program currently in progress to collect and analyze composite samples of three of the most commonly consumed types of bread from each of the eight Australian States and Territories. These results will further extend the information base by enabling calculation of descriptive statistics such as standard error of the mean. This project is being conducted in collaboration with the Bread Research Institute of Australia.

Over the life of the program, the food industry and other organizations have participated with government in building up the store of nutrient composition data by contributing their own data, or funding specific programs that analyze their products according to agreed specifications. Successful cooperation has occurred with industry organizations such as the Australian Meat and Livestock Corporation, the Australian Dairy Corporation and the Bread Research Institute of Australia.

An integral component of the revision process was the development of a supporting computer system for data storage, processing and reporting. The Australian Nutrient Data Bank (ANDB) was a mainframe application developed from a pilot system in 1987. A series of enhancements were made to the data bank in 1990. One of these was to provide the capability to calculate foods from recipes using factors as estimates of the weight change on cooking and nutrient retention. There is some scope now for the Authority to undertake the supporting research into weight loss factors for recipe foods. With the transfer of responsibility for the food composition program to the Authority, the databank has been relocated from a mainframe to the Authority's smaller computer system. It is anticipated that there will be future opportunities for developments to be made to this system. From a compiler's viewpoint, the opportunity to improve the system regularly is most important. It enables refinements to be made and new features to be added as well as taking advantage of improvements in software and hardware technology to enhance efficiency and functionality.

The results of the laboratory program are now published in a number of formats. Australia's national nutrition reference is a series of loose-leaf volumes entitled *Composition of Foods, Australia* (4). There are now six volumes in the series providing data on some 1430 foods. Volume 7 is presently in preparation and will add a further 100 foods, mainly restaurant dishes originating from other countries.

Additional formats are available to meet the needs of a range of data users. A summary database *NUTTAB* for use in software applications has been produced for public use since 1989, although a predecessor of this database was used to analyze the national dietary surveys conducted in the 1980s. The currently available version *NUTTAB91-92* (5) is the third publicly available update to the database and provides data on 28 nutrients and energy for some 1580 foods. A revised version is planned for release after publication of Volume 7 of the food tables series. The additional foods in this database are those from British sources which have continued to be included from the original dietary survey database. Two condensed versions of the tables also have been released. *Nutritional Values of Australian Foods* (6) was produced to meet the needs of educators and students in food, biology and health courses at upper secondary and tertiary levels while *Food for Health* (7) is a simplified guide for the general public which also includes general dietary advice. The two latter publications have proved to be among the most popular books released by the government publishing service.

The food composition tables are also used as a reference by the food industry for food labeling purposes. Part A of the *Australian Food Standards Code* (8) sets out the labeling regulations, including those for nutrition labeling, with which manufacturers must comply. When a label carries a nutrition claim, a nutrition information panel must be displayed containing, as a minimum, information on the energy, protein, fat, total carbohydrate, total sugars, sodium and potassium content of that food. Other nutrients which may be claimed and listed in the panel include amino acids, starch, cholesterol, fatty acids, and dietary fiber. The information given in the panel should represent the average quantity of the listed components allowing for seasonal variability and other known factors which could cause actual values to vary. These average quantities can be determined from three sources of information:

- the manufacturer's analysis of the food
- calculation from the actual or average quantity of nutrients in the ingredients used
- calculation from generally accepted data.

The term 'generally accepted data' is a very broad one, but now that there are Australian data on a significant range of foods and ingredients, it is being increasingly used as a reference for labeling purposes. Manufacturers need to be aware of the different modes of expression between the data tables and the Code requirements. For example, the Code specifies that total carbohydrate content should be determined by difference rather than by analysis. The Australian tables report carbohydrate data by direct analysis. A carbohydrate by difference value can be readily calculated from those data tables because a value for ash is provided routinely, together with the other proximate data that are required.

The relevant food standard which controls the claims for the vitamin and mineral content of foods is currently being revised. The term "average quantity" previously defined in the general labeling provisions is proposed to be used as the basis for determining the amount of claimed vitamin or mineral. The Australian database is and will continue to be a valuable source of information for this purpose.

Although provision of nutrient composition data is not the National Food Authority's primary role, there is a profound appreciation of the important contribution made by these data to the improved knowledge of food and its relationship to health and disease in Australia. The Authority is committed to the ongoing program of laboratory analysis of Australian foods and the publication of contemporary and comprehensive nutrient composition data for the benefit of health professionals, educators, consumers, the food industry and the development of public health policy and programs.

■ Market Basket Survey Database

The Australian Market Basket Survey (AMBS) is conducted in Australia every two years to estimate the levels of pesticides and contaminants including heavy metals and natural toxins in the Australian food supply. Responsibility for the AMBS was transferred to the Authority upon its establishment, from the federal Health Department.

The survey comprises the collection and preparation to table-ready state of a specified list of foods for analysis of particular chemical residues. These foods are selected to represent all major groups of foods in the Australian food supply. Foods are collected over one year according to one of three standard protocols and prepared according to a set of instructions. Core foods are sampled once every season and in every capital city; regional foods are sampled in every capital city but only in one season; and national foods, such as corn flakes, which are not expected to vary between regions, are sampled in only three capital cities in one season. The results are expressed on a per kilogram wet weight basis and entered into the AMBS database. The number of foods sampled has been increasing gradually over the years in which the surveys were conducted. In the 1990 survey, 53 foods were sampled, while 62 foods were sampled in the 1992 survey.

The laboratory results for each sample are identified on the database by the food name, its location and the season of the year in which it was collected. The information from each survey is maintained in separate files on the database. Currently, data from the 1985, 1986, 1987, 1990 and 1992 surveys are stored on the database. The survey was run annually until 1988 when a review was held which recommended that the survey be conducted biennially. The maximum range of the residue data for one food from the 1992 survey is given by the following example. Twenty-four samples of grilled lamb chops were analyzed for residues of 57 compounds. They were three heavy metals, 13 organochlorines plus three metabolites of organochlorines, 22 organophosphates, six synthetic pyrethroids, two fungicides and one class of fungicides, six herbicides and polychlorinated biphenyls. Analyses were conducted also on specific compounds often found in particular types of foods. For example, seafood was analyzed for mercury, peanut paste for aflatoxins and potatoes and potato crisps for solanine content. The database is sufficiently flexible so that it can store such

data when they are commissioned from time to time.

These results are used to estimate the total dietary intake of these substances by six age/sex categories covering adults and children, and thus to assess the safety of the Australian diet with respect to these substances. The intake data are derived by reference to the consumption patterns given in the most recent national dietary surveys. These values in grams/day are entered on to a spreadsheet and an estimate of the total dietary intake of each substance is then calculated for each age/sex category. Dietary intakes at the 95th percentile of energy are determined. For the 1992 survey, intakes at the mean intake of energy were also determined. These results and the summary data on the distribution of levels of pesticides and contaminants found in the sampled foods are provided in regularly published reports of each survey (9). The estimated dietary intakes are also compared to the internationally accepted safe limits which are the Provisional Tolerable Weekly Intakes (PWTIs) for contaminants and Acceptable Daily Intakes (ADIs) for pesticides.

The results of surveys over the last 23 years have indicated where additional vigilance is required in the food production chain as well as estimating the overall levels of these substances. This important monitoring function has shown to date that Australia's food supply has generally safe levels of pesticides and contaminants and these levels have been improving since monitoring began.

▮ Food Safety Information Database

The coordination of food surveillance information is a statutory function of the Authority. Currently there is no national system to collate these types of data. Most of the States and Territories however, are collecting and maintaining information on the results of food inspection and monitoring activities within their jurisdictions. Unfortunately, the data are variable in scope and are stored in a number of formats, some of which are more technologically advanced than others. The types of information currently collected include surveys of the microbiological and contaminant levels in food, food complaints, recalls and prosecutions.

Soon after the formation of the Authority, the NFA Advisory Committee (NFAAC), comprising representatives of all State and Territory Health Departments, the federal Health Department and the Australian Quarantine Inspection Service, was formed. At its first meeting, the Committee expressed general support for the concept of a national food surveillance database and agreed that a consultant should be employed to undertake a feasibility study of the project.

The feasibility report points to significant overall savings in resources at the State and Territory level, as well as the broader benefits of a shared and online system. It is proposed that a fully automated national system will include:

■ an information base to facilitate the allocation of resources efficiently and effectively by reducing unnecessary duplication in sampling activities and assisting to redirect effort to areas best serving public safety objectives

■ on-line access to current national information from a range of agencies. This will assist agencies plan activities and allocate resources, and facilitate rapid response to food safety concerns. It will also promote uniform enforcement of standards by permitting agencies immediate access to up-to-date information on investigations in other jurisdictions

■ availability of printed information on food safety issues, plans, trends, and contacts

■ potential savings in information technology development and support. These are greatest for those States supporting existing systems and for States and Territories which intend to de-

velop their own food safety related computer systems.

It is expected that the development of a national food safety information system, which by providing a unique information base of food recall, survey and sampling data, will offer significant benefits to regulatory agencies.

The Food Safety section of the Authority is currently collating information on food surveillance procedures of the States and Territories to enable the identification of relevant fields for the database and levels of security required. It is anticipated that a trial will be undertaken shortly between the Authority and a State or Territory, to gain experience in the transfer of food surveillance data, prior to any large scale implementation.

■ References

(1) Greenfield, H., & Wills, R.B.H. (1981) *Food Technol. Aust.* **33,** 101-130

(2) English, R. (1990) *Food Aust.* **42,** S5-S7

(3) Englyst, H., Wiggins, H.S., & Cummings, J.H. (1982) *Analyst* **107,** 307-318

(4) Commonwealth Department of Community Services and Health/National Food Authority (1989–) *Composition of Foods, Australia,* Australian Government Publishing Service, Canberra

(5) Commonwealth Department of Community Services and Health (1991) *NUTTAB91-92,* AGPS, Canberra, ACT

(6) Commonwealth Department of Community Services and Health (1991) *Nutritional Values of Australian Foods,* Australian Government Publishing Service, Canberra

(7) National Food Authority (1991) *Food for Health,* Australian Government Publishing Service, Canberra

(8)   *Australian Food Standards Code*, Australian Government Publishing Service, Canberra

(9)   National Health and Medical Research Council/National Food Authority (1991) *The 1990 Australian Market Basket Survey,* Australian Government Publishing Service, Canberra

Use of Databases for Nutrition Labeling in the United States

James T. Tanner

Office of Special Nutritionals, HFS-451,
Center for Food Safety and Applied Nutrition,
US Food and Drug Administration, Washington, DC 20204, USA

The Nutrition Labeling and Education Act of 1990 requires that all foods sold in the United States be nutritionally labeled. In response to the requirements of that Act, the Food and Drug Administration (FDA) published final regulations in January, 1993, on enforcement of nutrition labeling. In the regulations, provisions were made for the use of databases for labeling, and a manual was prepared to assist companies and organizations in this task. This manual gives generic information on how to develop and calculate from databases label values which will meet regulations that FDA is required to enforce. FDA does not prescribe how an individual company is to determine nutrient content for labeling purposes but does offer to review a database and to work with the manufacturer to resolve problems before taking any regulatory action. The compliance policy of FDA remains based on analysis of composite samples, performed using methods of the Association of Official Analytical Chemists (AOAC), or other validated methods if no AOAC method exists. FDA will then compare the label values with the results from laboratory analyses. The use of databases for labeling, the regulations of FDA for foods sold in the United States, the compliance policy of FDA, and the future uses of databases are discussed.

In 1973 the US Food and Drug Administration (FDA) promulgated regulations (1) that required nutrition labeling in certain circumstances. The agency took this action largely in response to recommendations of the 1969 White House Conference on Food, Nutrition, and Health (2).

▪ Overview of Database Use

The 1973 regulations required nutrition labeling only for certain foods, those with added nutrients or for which a nutrition claim was made in either labeling or advertising. Some foods such as fresh produce were specifically exempted. FDA encouraged manufacturers, however, to provide nutrition labeling voluntarily on a wider variety of food products, including the exempt foods.

Industry-wide databases were suggested as a possible means of reducing the cost of developing nutrition labeling for individual companies. In 1979 FDA, the US Department of Agriculture (USDA) and the Federal Trade Commission (FTC) encouraged this concept in a notice (3) published in the *Federal Register*, describing the agencies' policies and intentions with respect to numerous food labeling issues. In that notice, FDA, while not agreeing to approve databases, stated that it would work with industry to resolve any compliance problems that might arise for food labeled on the basis of a database that the agency had accepted. Specifically it stated, "If products bearing nutrition labeling in accordance with properly evaluated [FDA evaluated] nutrient databases and manufactured in accordance with food manufacturing practices are found not to be in compliance with applicable nutrition labeling regulations, the agency will work with the firms responsible for the product in question and with the appropriate authorities who are maintaining the applicable nutrient database to correct the problem before initiating compliance provision actions." The policy given in that 1979 notice is the same policy that is in effect today.

With the *Nutrition Labeling and Education Act* of 1990 (4) expanding mandatory nutrition labeling to nearly all foods regulated by FDA, greater interest has been expressed in using industry-wide databases for some food products. Some manufacturers of food products not currently labeled have expressed interest in using data available from other sources, for example, the open scientific literature, as the basis for labeling their products.

The policy of the Food and Drug Administration is that the choice of a data source is the prerogative and the responsibility of the firm or organization that provides a nutritionally labeled product. The firm or organization needs to be judicious in this selection, however, to ensure that the product labeling is in compliance with the regulations for that product. FDA has developed a manual (5) which will be of assistance in identifying data that are of sufficient quality to provide an adequate basis for nutrition labeling. In addition, guidance has been given on when average values may be used and when calculated values using the equations given in the manual should be used. The agency understands that most companies will not have sufficient information to meet the suggested criteria listed in the manual; however, we view this as the "gold standard" and hope that by making a diligent effort there will be sufficient analytical data available in five to ten years' time to comply fully with the different criteria given in the manual.

Historically, label values based on calculation of nutrient content from ingredients were considered unacceptable for a mixed product for the following reasons: 1) There are no quality indicators of the data for the components; 2) there are no indicators of the methods of analysis and sampling used to obtain the data for the components; 3) there are no indicators of the design and execution of quality control procedures used to monitor the sampling and analysis of the com-

Table I. Formulas for calculating label values

(1)	Class I nutrients (fortified): Computed value = mean - $t_{(0.95;df)}(1/k + 1/n)^{1/2}(s)$
(2)	Class II nutrients (naturally occurring) $\geq 80\%$ label value: Computed value = $[mean - t_{(0.95;df)}(1/k + 1/n)^{1/2}(s)](5/4)$
(3)	Class II nutrients (naturally occurring): calories, sugars, total fat, saturated fat, cholesterol, and sodium, $\leq 120\%$ label value: Computed value = $[mean + t_{(0.95;df)}(1/k + 1/n)^{1/2}(s)](5/6)$
where	mean = sample mean $t_{(0.95;df)}$ = 95th percentile of the t-distribution df = n-1 degrees of freedom n = sample size used to calculate the mean k = number of future units making up the future mean.

ponents; and 4) there are no indicators of nutrient loss during the processing and handling of the mixed product. In addition, inclusion of sugars as mandatory in nutrition labeling and a change in the definition of fat limit the use of most ingredient databases.

Use of data from the open literature and use of ingredient databases present similar problems because the values given are generally averages based on an undetermined number of analyses. Average values based on numerous analytical values representing the different variables associated with a nutrient may be sufficient if they are within the range (per cent CV) represented by the coefficient of variation given in the manual. If the coefficient of variation is large, then the equation given in the manual should be used to ensure that the regulatory requirements can be met. This applies to indigenous nutrients only; for fortification nutrients the value must be at least 100 per cent of the label value. If average values are used, then the value will be correct only 50 per cent of the time. The manual gives equations for calculating label values for indigenous and fortification nutrients that would have the highest probability of meeting the regulatory requirements which the agency must enforce.

■ Equations for Use in Calculating Label Values

For label values computed to reflect the variability of individual units, the one-sided 95 per cent prediction interval is constructed to contain the result of a single (k = 1) future retail unit or to contain the mean of k = 12 future retail units. Suppose there are n individual values of a nutrient in the database, from which the sample mean and SD are computed. The calculation of a lower or upper limit of the one-sided 95 per cent prediction interval also depends on the nutrient classes (i.e., Class I or II). The computed limit for Class II nutrients is adjusted for the 20 per cent margin of allowance in the FDA compliance evaluation.

The computing formulas are given in Table I. Label values computed using these equations have the highest assurance of meeting FDA requirements.

■ Class I and Class II Nutrients and Compliance Policy

Compliance with nutrition labeling is determined in the following manner: A collection of primary containers or units of the same size, type, and style produced under conditions as nearly uniform as possible, designated by a common container code or marking, or in the absence of any common container code or marking, a day's production, constitutes a "lot."

The sample for nutrient analysis shall consist of a composite of 12 subsamples (consumer units), one from each of 12 different randomly chosen shipping cases, taken to be representative of a lot. Unless a particular method of analysis is specified, composites shall be analyzed by appropriate methods as given in the *Official Methods of Analysis of the Association of Official Analytical Chemists*, 15th Edition (1990) (6), or in the supplements issued annually. If no AOAC method is available or appropriate, other reliable and appropriate analytical procedures should be used.

Two classes of nutrients are defined for purposes of compliance: Class I nutrients: added nutrients in fortified or fabricated foods; and, Class II nutrients: naturally occurring (indigenous) nutrients. If any ingredient which contains a naturally occurring nutrient is added to a food, the total amount of such nutrient in the final food product is subject to Class II requirements unless the same nutrient is also an added ingredient.

A food with a label declaration of a vitamin, mineral, protein, total carbohydrate, dietary fiber, other carbohydrate, poly- or monounsaturated fat, or potassium shall be deemed to be misbranded under Section 403(a) of the *Federal Food, Drug, and Cosmetic Act* (the Act) (7) unless it meets the following requirements:

- Class I vitamin, mineral, protein, dietary fiber, or potassium: The nutrient content of the composite is at least equal to the value for that nutrient declared on the label
- Class II vitamin, mineral, protein, total carbohydrate, dietary fiber, other carbohydrate, poly- or monounsaturated fat, or potassium: The nutrient content of the composite is at least equal to 80

per cent of the value for that nutrient declared on the label

- Provided: That no regulatory action will be based on a determination of a nutrient value that falls below this level by a factor less than the variability generally recognized for the analytical method used for that food at the level involved (8).

A food with a label declaration of calories, sugars, total fat, saturated fat, cholesterol, or sodium shall be deemed to be misbranded under section 403(a) of the Act if the nutrient content of the composite is greater than 120 per cent of the value for that nutrient declared on the label. Again, the same statement on analytical variability applies.

Reasonable excesses over labeled amounts of a vitamin, mineral, protein, total carbohydrate, dietary fiber, other carbohydrate, poly- or monounsaturated fat, or potassium are acceptable within current good manufacturing practice. Reasonable deficiencies under labeled amounts of calories, sugars, total fat, saturated fat, cholesterol, or sodium are acceptable within current good manufacturing practice.

Compliance with these provisions may be provided by use of a database that has been compiled by following FDA guideline procedures and submitted to FDA for approval and with foods that have been handled in accordance with current good manufacturing practice to prevent nutrient loss. Guidance in the use of databases may be found in the *FDA Nutrition Labeling Manual — A Guide for Developing and Using Databases* (5).

∎ Nutrient Database Development and Use

The development of a database (a collection of related information) is a complex task that consists of several general steps such as development of a sampling plan, collection of the samples, analysis of the laboratory samples, and statistical analysis and interpretation of the results. Each of the steps can be performed in several different ways, and decisions made regarding the alternatives may directly affect the available resources, the quality of the data, and the risk of making incorrect decisions.

The process of developing a sampling plan involves the resolution of a series of interrelated tasks that may be broadly classified as follows:

- defining the sampling objective
- defining the target product population
- developing the sampling frame
- selecting the sampling methods (i.e., stratified multistage plan)
- selecting the analytical methods.

To increase the chance that the data will be of the desired quality, it is essential that these tasks, as a minimum, be given careful consideration, and that specific questions be addressed and resolved in the planning stage of the data collection effort.

In using a database for the purpose of labeling, consideration has to be given to:

- the variability of the factors that influence nutrient content
- the distribution that the nutrient values follow
- the statistical methodology that is applied in deriving label values.

To resolve these tasks effectively, information on the variability of the nutrient levels in the product is needed. Variables such as variety or geographic growing area for fruits and vegetables need to be determined. For mixed products and/or products requiring processing, the nutrient content may change during processing or during storage before sale. Information on the variability of the analytical method for the nutrients of interest is also needed.

If sufficient information is not available, it will be necessary to perform a pilot study or perform a literature search to obtain the necessary information before developing the sampling plan.

A database that would be adequate for the purpose of nutrient labeling will reflect a satisfactory degree of data quality, and hence database accuracy. Data quality (determined by the amount of error that is contained in data) depends primarily on the effectiveness of the activities stated earlier for database development. The accuracy of a database depends on its data quality, which is expressed in terms of four characteristics:

- precision (magnitude of the error of the estimate)
- representativeness (how accurately samples reflect the population)
- comparability (similarity of data from different sources)
- completeness (amount of information collected).

It is necessary that satisfactory degrees of these characteristics be reflected in the data.

▮ Calculation of Label Values

Once an acceptable amount of analytical data of satisfactory quality has been accumulated, a value must be determined for the label, which will reflect the nutrient content of the product. This number may be calculated in several ways.

The first and perhaps the most straightforward way is to use the mean of the analytical data. If the analytical data are within certain limits indicated by the coefficient of variation (usually 11 per cent or less), then the mean value may be used. This applies only to Class II nutrients. The coefficient of variation is the standard deviation times 100 divided by the mean. The reason for using the coefficient of variation is that numbers which are applicable to all concentrations can be given in the guidelines.

For nutrients that are highly variable, i.e., that have coefficients of variation higher than the maximum limits given in the guidelines, there is an equation for Class I nutrients (which must be at least 100 per cent of the label claim) and two for Class II nutrients, one for those nutrients that must be 80 per cent of the label claim, or greater, and one for those nutrients that may not exceed 120 cent of the label claim.

Once the nutrient content has been calculated, various rounding rules must be used, such as rounding to the nearest gram or half-gram, etc.

■ "Recipe Databases"

Although FDA has stated that it would not accept label values generated by computer from ingredient or component composition values or "recipe databases," it was stated that FDA would work with various trade organizations and companies to develop a model which could be used to calculate label values based on ingredient composition and determination of nutrient loss (if any) during processing. To date we have worked with several organizations but have not yet accepted any models. In the comments received after the manual was announced in the *Federal Register*, a large number stressed the need for recipe databases. FDA still believes that most ingredient composition databases are not useful for calculating the final composition of a mixed product for the following reasons:

■ such databases are usually not accompanied by indicators of the quality of the data for the components

■ such databases have no indicators of the methods of analysis and sampling used to obtain the data for the components

■ such databases have no indicators of the design and execution of quality control procedures used to monitor the sampling and analysis of the components

■ such databases have no indicators of nutrient loss during the processing and handling of the mixed product.

To successfully validate a model to calculate final composition based on ingredient composition, extensive analyses of ingredients and final product composition would be required. The application of this model would be limited by the products for which it was developed.

FDA believes that in the future ingredient composition databases may have the necessary validation to be used in calculating the final composition of mixed products for an acceptable range of food products. At this time, however, the agency believes that the data making up ingredient databases are of mixed quality and, therefore, of limited value. Companies that wish to use ingredient databases must evaluate the individual analytical values for each ingredient to assure themselves that the data are representative, valid from an analytical perspective, and sufficient to account for any variation in the ingredient.

During the comment period several principles were given by companies and trade associations that would be useful and instructive for developing recipe databases. Keeping in mind the general requirements for databases, these proposed principles are given as general guides:

■ Confidence in the quality of data, supported by documentation of data sources. Companies maintaining or using ingredient composition databases must be able to demonstrate the data source used for each type of product and each nutrient for which ingredient composition databases are utilized.

■ Proper maintenance of the database. Companies developing or using ingredient composition databases must have procedures in place to ensure that the values in the ingredient composition databases are reviewed and updated as needed and on a regular basis.

■ Specificity with respect to ingredients, product formulations, and processes. Companies using ingredient composition databases must have procedures in place to ensure that the nutrient values are used only for specific applications. For example, a company should have a procedure to ensure that nutrient data specific for one product formulation or process are not used to prepare nutrient declarations for similar product formulations or processes, when there is no assurance that the data are applicable to those products or processes.

- Validation of the database. Companies developing or using ingredient composition databases must have procedures in place to ensure that nutrient values receive reviews, audits, and confirmation through nutrient analyses as often as necessary.

Several other companies offered equivalent guidelines and one other guide that is important:

- Companies making nutrient content or health claims should substantiate the claim by analysis of the final product. This applies to products labeled with a health message or those making claims such as low or reduced in certain nutrients.

■ Confidentiality of Databases

During the comment period many companies/trade associations objected to the lack of confidentiality of submitted databases. They did not want the information gained through analyses of products and ingredients to be released through freedom of information requests or used in unacceptable ways or for inappropriate products. In addition, in developing databases, costs are shared among the participating companies; these companies sought assurance that the data would not be available without cost to companies that did not participate in development. Formulations that are used to produce mixed products are also regarded as confidential company information, and there should be some assurance that this information will not be available to anyone who requests it. The agency is aware that the development of a database is costly, and that it may contain confidential information. FDA agrees that release of a database could reveal substantial proprietary interests in documents that

have been submitted to the agency. Furthermore, it has never been the agency's intent, nor does it have the resources, to maintain and manage databases that are developed by manufacturers or associations. The agency believes that the availability of a database is, therefore, the primary responsibility of the developer.

FDA will continue with the policy of assisting the developers of databases, providing guidance to those who ask for it, and evaluating databases for the products submitted for review. Confidentiality of such data will be determined and maintained in accordance with regulations.

Those database developers who choose to do so are encouraged to make their information available through such compilations as the *USDA Handbook No. 8* (9), so that all may benefit from the additional analytical information. In the long run, recipe databases will be useful after extensive information is gathered and placed in these compilations of public information.

The information and procedures given in the manual are generic, and only the parts that pertain to the food or product under study should be used. Because preparation of a different manual for each food type was not practical, all the information is contained in one manual. FDA is always available to help companies with problems or those needing assistance in determining how to proceed in attaining the best label possible while continuing to satisfy the regulations that the agency must enforce.

■ References

(1) Anon. (1993) *Federal Register* **38**, 20702

(2) *White House Conference on Food, Nutrition, and Health* (1969) U.S. Government Printing Office, Washington, DC

(3) Anon. (1979) *Federal Register* **44**, 75990

(4) *Nutrition Labeling and Education Act* (1990), P.L. 101-535

(5) FDA (1993) *Nutrition Labeling Manual — A Guide for Developing and Using Databases*; available by sending a self-addressed mailing label to: James T. Tanner, HFS-451, Center for Food Safety and Applied Nutrition, U.S. Food and Drug Administration, Washington, DC 20204

(6) *Official Methods of Analysis* (1990) 15th Ed., AOAC, Arlington, VA

(7) *Federal Food, Drug, and Cosmetic Act* (1938), P.L. 75-717

(8) Horwitz, W., Kamps, L.R., & Boyer, K.W. (1980) *J. Assoc. Off. Anal. Chem.* **63**, 1344-1358

(9) US Department of Agriculture (1976–) *Composition of Foods: Raw, Processed, Prepared*, Agric. Handbook No. 8 series, USDA, Washington, DC

Functional Foods for Specific Health Use — The Needs for Compositional Data

Kazuki Shinohara

National Food Research Institute, MAFF, Tsukuba, Ibaraki, Japan

National projects on the physiological functions of foods, which have been carried out by university groups and the Ministry of Agriculture, Forestry and Fisheries in Japan, revealed that foods have functions controlling homeostasis in the body, as well as nutritional and sensory functions, leading to the introduction of the terminology of functional foods, and in 1991, a system for licensing "Foods for Specified Health Use". To obtain a license for a "Food for Specified Health Use", the following evidence is required: a) potential to contribute to the improvement of dietary habits and the maintenance and enhancement of health; b) medical and nutritional data on specific health aspects; c) data on intakes determined medically and nutritionally; d) safety data; e) physicochemical data; f) data on nutritional composition, and others. As such foods proliferate there will be a need to collect comprehensive data on them and to make these data systematically available to doctors, dietitians and others.

A t present, one can obtain nutritious and appetizing foods whenever necessary in industrialized countries and the daily diet is becoming satisfactory in terms of quantity. Longevity has increased considerably due to improved nutrition and medical treatment. However, with a change in food habits, food-related diseases such as allergy, obesity and geriatric diseases are increasing in Japan. Because of the costs of treatment of geriatric diseases, total medical expenditure is expected to increase. Furthermore, the aged population is expected to reach a maximum in the next century. From these points of view, new health aspects of foods are a public concern. In order to respond to the need for improved foods, it is important to elucidate the physiological functions of food components.

■ Research on the Physiological Functions of Food Components

National projects on the physiological functions of food components have been carried out by university groups in Japan under the following headings:

- systematic evaluation of the physiological functions of foods (1984–1986)
- evaluation of bioregulatory functions of foods (1988–1990)
- analysis of functional foods and molecular design (1992–1994).

These projects have revealed that foods have biomodulating functions (tertiary) which control homeostasis in the body, as well as nutritional (primary) and sensory (secondary) functions. The biomodulating functions include regulation of immunological functions, regulation of biorhythms, prevention of ageing, prevention of food-related disease, and facilitation of recovery from food-related disease. In the Ministry of Agriculture, Forestry and Fisheries, the following projects have been carried out:

- the Japanese R&D Association for a new separation system in the food industry (1989–1991)
- the Japanese R&D Association for new food materials (1990–1993)
- elucidation of the functions and molecular structures of food components (1989–1992)
- integrated research program for effective use of biological activities to create new demand (1991–2000)

- development of technology for evaluation and utilization of functional properties of agricultural products in relation to health (1993–1999).

From these projects, the physiological functions of components of vegetables, soybeans, milk and other foods or their metabolites have been discovered, such as antimutagenicity, anticarcinogenicity, antioxidant activity, immunostimulation, modifying endocrine function, hypotensive effect, cholesterol control, intestinal control, and others.

■ Functional Foods

These projects exerted a great influence on the Japanese food industry and the Ministry of Welfare and Health (MWH) leading to the introduction of the terminology of "functional foods". A functional food was defined as a food containing compounds which satisfy the following criteria: clear effectiveness for a specific health purpose, defined chemical structure, clear mode of action at cellular level, proven effectiveness by oral administration, safety, stability in foods, acceptability as food, and potential for use in a range of diverse food products. In comparison with most conventional nutritious foods, functional foods have more potential efficacy for health. Functional foods claim to control homeostasis, resulting in the prevention of geriatric diseases. In contrast to conventional healthy foods, these foods have direct scientific evidence about their functionality. The member companies of the Japan Health and Nutritional Food Association collaborate in working groups which are responsible for collecting scientific evidence about 11 identified categories of functional components: dietary fibers; oligosaccharides; sugar alcohols; polyunsaturated fatty acids; peptides and proteins; glycosides, isoprenoids and vitamins; alcohols and phenol; choline; lactobacteria; minerals; and others.

■ Physiological Functionality of Food Components

The physiological functions of food components are as follows:

Dietary Fibers

Dietary fibers such as polydextrose, wheat, bran, corn, apple, soybean, and beet fibers have been recognized to have beneficial effects. Fibers are considered to be promising candidates for functional components of foods. The physiological functions of dietary fibers are claimed to be: a) regulation or control of intestinal functions, including prevention of constipation, improvement of bacterial flora in the intestine, inhibition of absorption of harmful substances and promotion of their excretion, prevention of colon cancers, and immuno-stimulation, b) regulation or control of blood sugar content, including inhibition of insulin secretion, inhibition of glucagon secretion, and prevention of diabetes mellitus, and c) regulation or control of cholesterol levels, prevention of gallstone formation, decrease in fat deposition, prevention of obesity, and hypotensive effects. Dietary fibers can be used in foods (insoluble fibers) and beverages (soluble fibers). Polydextrose has been used in beverages as a substitute for sugar.

Oligosaccharides

Oligosaccharides such as lactulose, fructo-, galacto-, isomalto-, and xylo-oligosaccharides, and cyclodextrins are considered to have potential for use as functional ingredients in foods. They can be used as food modifiers that do not affect the texture and physicochemical properties of foods and can be replacements for sugar. The physiological functions are claimed to be: low energy, prevention of tooth decay, intestinal control, and bifidobacterium activation. Products containing oligosaccharides are believed to have great sales potential in Japan.

Sugar Alcohols

Sugar alcohols such as malcitol, erythritol, and reduced palatinose are promising materials which have low energy content and preventative effects against obesity and tooth decay.

Polyunsaturated Fatty Acids

Polyunsaturated fatty acids, especially eicosapentaenoic acid (EPA), docosahexaenoic acid (DHA), and linolenic acid, have great potential for sales and development into functional foods. EPA and DHA are derived from fish body oils. Their functionalities are claimed to be: decrease in fat deposition, decrease in plasma cholesterol, hypotensive effect, decrease in viscosity of blood, and prevention of cancers of the breast, colon and prostate gland.

Peptides and Proteins

These include casein phosphopeptide (CPP), lactoferrin, and peptides from casein, fish, and soybean. CPP prepared from milk is a promising functional ingredient which enhances the absorption of calcium and iron. Recently, hypotensive peptides have been recovered from milk casein, fish proteins and soybean. Their functional properties are claimed to be: hypotensive effect, control of cholesterol level, detoxification of harmful substances, antiviral effects, and promotion of bone and tooth growth.

Glycosides, Isoprenoids and Vitamins

The functions of this class which includes saponins, carotenoids, flavonoids, and tocopherols are claimed to be: antioxidant activity, intestinal control, improvement of stomach, liver, and kidney metabolism, decrease in blood sugar and cholesterol levels, and hypotensive effects.

Alcohols and Phenols

The functions of this class which includes tea polyphenols, oryzanol, and octacosanol are claimed to be: prevention of tooth decay, deodorant effect, hypotensive effect, and decrease in plasma cholesterol. Among tea polyphenols, catechin, epicatechin, epicatechin gallate, and epigallocatechin gallate have received considerable attention.

Cholines

This class of compounds, including soybean and egg yolk lecithins, is claimed to have functions such as improvement of plasma lipid metabolism, prevention of arteriosclerosis, and prevention and improvement of fatty liver.

Lactobacteria

Fermented foods with lactobacteria and bifidobacteria are popular in Japan, because they have the function of intestinal control, decrease in cholesterol, and immuno-stimulation.

Minerals

The claimed benefits of minerals (e.g., calcium salts, heme-iron, magnesium include: promotion of bone and teeth growth, prevention of osteoporosis, and prevention of anemia.

Others

The last category are classified as health-enhancing foods which cannot be as-signed to any of the categories above. It includes fermented vinegar, and Chlorella. The claimed benefits are: improvement of plasma lipid metabolism, immuno-stimulation, and anticarcinogenic effects.

■ Foods for Specified Health Use

In 1991, a system for licensing "Foods for Specified Health Use" was established by MWH. According to this system a food for specified health use is "a food which, based on knowledge concerning the relationship between foods or food components and health, is expected to have certain health benefits, and has been licensed to bear a label claiming that a person who uses it for specified health use may expect to obtain the health use through the consumption thereof" (1).

"Foods for Specified Health Use" are defined as a category of food for special dietary uses within the establishment frame of the Special Nutritive Foods under article 12 of the *Nutrition Improvement Act* (Figure 1).

To obtain a license for a "Food for Specified Health Use", evidence that the food meets the following requirements must be produced :

- potential to contribute to the improvement of dietary habits and the maintenance and enhancement of health

- medical and nutritional data on specific health aspects

- appropriate serve size of the food or relevant compound, based on medical and nutritional information

- safety data of the food or relevant compounds

- physicochemical properties, test methods and methods of qualitative and quantitative determination

- data on nutritional composition, since the nutritional composition of the product should not be defective when compared with the composition of the

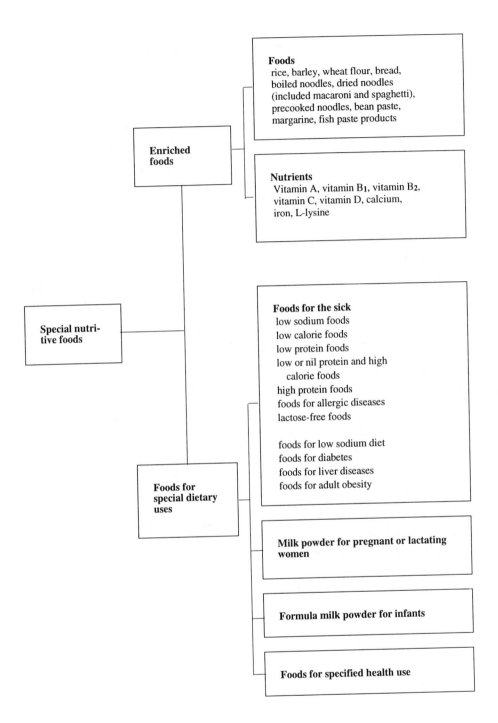

Figure 1. Types of special nutritive foods

regular food product that it may replace.

In addition to these requirements, the product should preferably be a food that is consumed regularly in the general diet, rather than a food consumed only occasionally. The product should be in the form of ordinary food, rather than pills or capsules. Only functional foods which satisfy these requirements will be approved by MHW as a Food for Specified Health Use.

Official permission for licensing a Food for Specified Health Use is under the control of the MHW. In the system for licensing, overseas applicants need to apply directly to the MHW (Office of Health Policy on Newly Developed Foods, Environmental Health Bureau). The application for licensing by the MHW must be in writing and must be accompanied by a product sample. The MHWs minimum requirements for an application are: brand name of food, list of ingredients by percentage, details of manufacturing procedure, analysis of ingredients, matters for which permission or approval is sought, name, address, and date of birth of applicant, name and address of main office, reason for seeking permission or approval, statement of energy value, list of nutritive elements by amount, instructions for storage, preparation, and administration, and any precautions to be observed in use of such foods.

Future Prospects

Recently, allergen-free rice (fine rice) and low phosphate (LPK) were approved by the HMW as the first Foods for Specified Health Use. Allergen-free rice in which 99 per cent of allergic globulin protein is removed is effective for patients with atopic disease. Low phosphate content milk is effective for patients with chronic renal diseases who are instructed to reduce the intake of phosphate. The phosphate content of the product is 20 per cent of that of regular milk while the protein content remains the same. In addition to these, foods such as beverages containing soybean-, fructo-, xylo-oligosaccharides, or calcium salts, table sugars containing soybean- or fructo-oligosaccharides, and gums containing malcitol and palatinose have also been approved as Foods for Specified Health Use. Foods for Specified Health Use containing dietary fibers, oligosaccharides, lactobacteria and others will be licensed. As such foods proliferate there will be a need to collect data on them and to make this available to doctors, dietitians and others, particularly those concerned with nutritional epidemiology and controlled dietary intervention trials.

▮ Reference

(1) *Nutrition Improvement Act* (1991) Article 12, Ministry of Health and Welfare, Tokyo

**The Second International Food Data Base
Conference**

Food Composition Research:
The Broader Context

August 28–30, 1995
Lahti, Finland

Eurofoods–Enfant Meeting as a satellite
August 31

For further information:

The Second International Food Data Base
Conference:

Prof. Lea Hyvönen
Dept. Food Technology
P.O. Box 27 (Viikki, Building B)
FIN-00014 University of Helsinki
Finland
Tel: +358 0 7085215
Fax: +358 0 7085212
E-Mail: Lea.Hyvonen@Helsinki.Fi

The Eurofoods-Enfant Meeting:

Prof. Clive West
Dept. Human Nutrition
Wageningen Agricultural University
P.O. Box 8129 Wageningen 6700 EV
The Netherlands
Tel: +31 8370 8 25 89
Fax: +31 8370 8 33 42